# Sports Injuries

### diagnosis and management
### for physiotherapists

# Sports Injuries

## diagnosis and management
## for physiotherapists

**Christopher M Norris** MSc, CBA, MCSP, SRP

*Director of Norris Associates, Chartered Physiotherapists, Altrincham, Cheshire, UK*

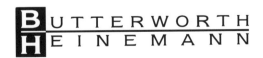

Butterworth–Heinemann Ltd
Linacre House, Jordan Hill, Oxford OX2 8DP

A member of the Reed Elsevier group

OXFORD LONDON BOSTON
MUNICH NEW DELHI SINGAPORE SYDNEY
TOKYO TORONTO WELLINGTON

First published 1993

**British Library Cataloguing in Publication data**
Norris, Christopher M.
    Sports Injuries: Diagnosis and Management
    for Physiotherapists
    I. Title
    617.1

ISBN 0 7506 0156 6

**Library of Congress Cataloguing in Publication Data**
Norris, Christopher M.
    Sports injuries: diagnosis and management for physiotherapists/
    Christopher M. Norris.
        p.    cm.
    Includes bibliographical references and index.
    ISBN 0 7506 0156 6
    1. Sports–Accidents and injuries.    2. Sports physical therapy.
    I. Title.
    [DNLM: 1. Athletic Injuries – diagnosis.    2. Athletic Injuries –
    rehibilitation.    3. Physical Therapy. QT 260 N854a]
    RD97.N67
    617.1'027–dc20                                    92–22841
                                                      CIP

Typeset by TecSet Ltd, Wallington, Surrey

Printed and bound in Great Britain by Thomson Litho Ltd
East Kilbride.

# Contents

# Preface

Injuries relating to sport and exercise are by no means restricted to the elite athlete. The Sunday footballer, the twice-a-week aerobics devotee, and the pensioner playing badminton all deserve the same high quality of care that the professional sportsperson receives. Increases in life expectancy and changes in employment have led to an increased number of retired individuals in our society. These people are quite rightly encouraged to remain active, and exercise classes and sports centres are now being filled with older people. This trend has inevitably led to a change in the nature of those we see with sports injuries. It is now commonplace to see a fifty-year-old badminton player with an injury, and the individual with a frozen shoulder is as likely to complain that it affects their tennis serve or golf swing as much as it does the activities of everyday living. For this reason a number of complaints are included in this book which at first appear to be out of the realm of sports injuries. Conditions such as frozen shoulder, carpal tunnel syndrome and thoracic outlet syndrome are more commonly noticed when an elderly person starts exercising.

The subject area of the book is very diverse and draws on many aspects of sports science as well as sports physiotherapy. Part One deals with general aspects of injury and management, while Part Two looks at specific injuries. Part Two is arranged in individual body areas purely for convenience. Considerable overlap exists, and treatment will be far more effective when an holistic approach is taken. The book is selective in its approach, placing greater emphasis on the more commonly seen complaints. It draws on the diverse body of knowledge of sports injuries and combines this with practical experience, in an attempt to produce an academic but freely readable format. Some attention is paid to functional anatomy of the injured area, as to continue to treat well and to fully understand dysfunction we must regularly revise and update our knowledge of the normal human body. Chapter 2, which deals with the tissue response to injury, is equally important from this standpoint.

Over the years, the athletes I have treated have come from all competition levels, and the variation of sports practised by them have been countless. One central theme throughout the management of all these individuals however, has been the emphasis on active healthcare, especially by the use of therapeutic exercise in all its forms. It has always been my practice when treating injured athletes to ask the simple question, 'how can I teach this patient to help him or herself?' It is my firm belief that active therapy, by encouraging an individual to take part in his or her own treatment, places an emphasis on the patient to take a greater responsibility for their own wellbeing. I have seen countless numbers of athletes regain self-esteem and take charge of their injury, through exercise therapy. The facial expression of depression and defeat gradually gives way to confidence and the athlete becomes a 'winner' once more. In Chapter 3 we deal with the psychological consequences of injury, and the importance of changing an individual from a 'pain sufferer' to a 'pain manager'. Exercise therapy can produce this change.

It is no coincidence that Chapter 6 on physical training and injury is one of the longest in the book, and that many of the chapters include autotherapy techniques for athletes to apply themselves. Successful management of sports injuries requires an in depth knowledge of exercise therapy, and the sports physiotherapist must ensure that their standard of treatment in this area is as good as that of manual therapy or electrotherapy. Much of the material in this chapter is taught by the author on the Advanced Certificate in Sports Physiotherapy, at Alsager College, and on other postgraduate physiotherapy courses in the UK and abroad.

It is not intended that the book be read from cover to cover, but rather that it is 'dipped into', and so cross-referencing is used where appropriate. The text is written for a variety of practitioners, reflecting the multidisciplinary approach to the care of the injured athlete. It will be of particular interest to physiotherapists, at both student and postgraduate levels, and should be useful to doctors, sports scientists, coaches and athletes.

Some may say that the use of the word 'diagnosis' in the title of this book is inappropriate for physiotherapists. However, the physiotherapist dealing with the injured athlete is usually the first, and sometimes only, practitioner to see a patient.

He or she must therefore take a greater responsibility for determining the nature of an injury, and be able to distinguish those conditions which are suitable for physiotherapy management from those which require referral. In this context both the therapist and medical practitioner must realize the limitations of their particular skills and recognize when a condition would be more suitably treated by each other. In Chapter 4 we look briefly at assessment techniques, and pay particular attention to the evaluation of function. This is an ongoing process, and as treatment progresses more information becomes available to the practitioner and so the exact diagnosis may change.

C.M.N.

# Acknowledgements

I am thankful to the following individuals for their assistance during the preparation of this text. Jacquelyn Bradford for secretarial services. The staff at the London Sports Medicine Institute for library services, and the staff at Crewe and Alsager College of Higher Education for use of their CD ROM facility. The staff at Butterworth–Heinemann. Finally, I am indebted to HC for unceasing tolerance and encouragement.

# Part One

# 1 Biomechanics of injury

Human tissue is governed by the laws of mechanics in the same way as other materials. While mechanics is concerned with forces, the effect of these forces on living organisms is the realm of biomechanics. The association between biological and mechanical aspects of movement has been said to give human motion its sophistication (Williams and Sperryn, 1976). For this reason, the study of biomechanics has a direct application to injury and recovery, and knowledge of this subject is essential for an understanding of the prevention, diagnosis and treatment of sports injuries.

## Biomechanical principles

### Forces

Force may be defined as the physical action which tends to change the position of a body in space (Stallard, 1984), consequently it is an entity which will produce motion. The unit of measurement of a force is the newton (N), one newton being the force which would produce an acceleration of $1 \text{ m/s}^2$ when acting on an object with a mass of 1 kg.

The most common forces affecting the human body are those produced by muscles, and those occurring as a result of gravity, inertia and contact. There are four important considerations when dealing with forces, the magnitude and direction of the force, and its line and point of application.

Forces can be represented graphically by an arrow, the direction of which gives the direction of the force. The arrowhead represents the force's point of application, and the magnitude is given as a value in newtons. Forces may be added and subtracted from each other. For forces acting in parallel, this is a simple task (Fig. 1.1), but when forces act at angles to each other a parallelogram of forces must be constructed. Here, the two forces form the adjacent sides of the parallelogram, and the force which represents the two combined (the resultant) is the diagonal of the parallelogram (Fig. 1.2).

Another method is the triangle or polygon of forces (Bowker, 1987). In this case, the two forces are drawn so that one starts where the other ends, the resultant being the line joining the free ends of the force lines. Provided all the forces have the same point of application (that is they are concurrent), a polygon may be used to determine the magnitude and direction (the vector) of the resultant (Fig. 1.3).

The principles of resolution of forces work equally well in reverse. If the resultant force is known, its two components, acting at 90° to each other, may be determined. Thus, when the foot strikes the ground (Fig. 1.4) two component forces exist causing both shear and compression.

### Newton's laws of motion

Newton's first law of motion is the law of inertia. It states that an object remains in its existing state of motion unless acted on by an external force. A stationary object will not begin to move unless acted on by an external unbalanced force, and a body which is moving will continue to move in the same direction and at the same velocity unless it is similarly affected by an external force. Consequently, objects have a resistance to change in motion, and this property is called *inertia*.

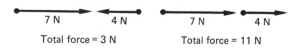

Figure 1.1 Calculation of forces acting in parallel.

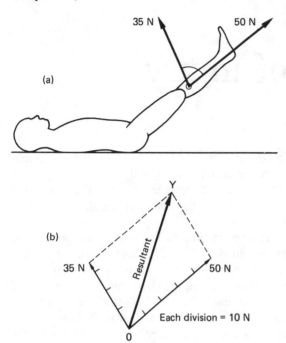

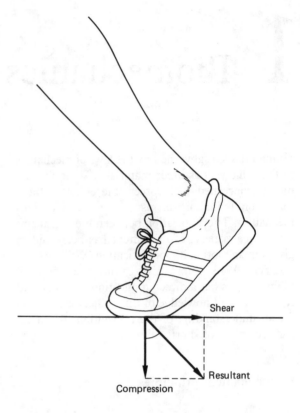

**Figure 1.2**   Parallelogram of forces. The two forces acting parallel to (50 N) and at right angles to (35 N) the lower leg (a) may be resolved into a single force represented by the resultant (b). From Bowker (1987), with permission.

**Figure 1.4**   Components of ground reaction force in a runner.

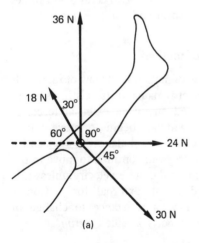

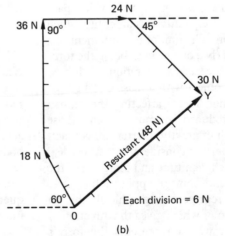

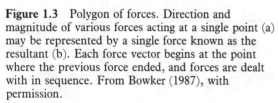

**Figure 1.3**   Polygon of forces. Direction and magnitude of various forces acting at a single point (a) may be represented by a single force known as the resultant (b). Each force vector begins at the point where the previous force ended, and forces are dealt with in sequence. From Bowker (1987), with permission.

When a ball is rolling along the ground, it requires more energy to start or stop the ball rolling than it does simply to keep it rolling at the same speed. Similarly, in a vigorous kicking action, inertia will have to be overcome to start the limb moving. If the force required to do this is large enough and rapid enough, muscle damage may occur.

A joint has a certain inertia as a result of its osteological format and the properties of the joint structures. Following immobilization, the inertia is likely to be greater because the joint tissues will have stiffened and the joint fluid will have become more viscous. Gentle, rhythmic swinging exercises are often used to mobilize stiff joints. The continuous motion is more effective than stopping, pausing, and then starting again. In cases of severe weakness after injury, a muscle may be unable to overcome joint inertia to initiate movement. Once the movement has been started by the therapist, the patient's muscles may be strong enough to continue the action. This technique is applied in sling suspension.

Heavier objects will be more difficult to start or stop than light objects travelling at the same speed, because heavier things possess more *momentum*. Momentum is the product of an object's mass and its velocity, and is an important consideration during exercise. Rapid, full range weight training exercises, for example, can be dangerous when muscle fatigue sets in. The combined momentum of the limb and the weight may continue movement beyond the full physiological joint range, thus causing tissue damage. Gleim (1984) showed momentum to be a significant factor in injuries to American football players. Taunton, McKenzie and Clement (1988) claimed that the most serious injuries in adolescent football and hockey players occur in the largest athletes, who create larger momentum forces.

Newton's second law is that of acceleration. This law states that the rate of change of momentum of a body occurs in the direction of the force and is proportional to the size of the force and the duration for which it acts.

When a hockey player hits a ball, the force (F) with which he or she hits acts for the specific time (t) that the stick is in contact with the ball. The ball

has a certain mass (m), and changes its velocity from that at the start (u) to that at the finish of the action (v). We know that momentum is the product of mass and velocity, and we know the velocity at the start and at the finish, so the rate of change of this momentum can be obtained by dividing the difference in velocities by time, thus:

$$\text{Rate of change of momentum (F)} = \frac{mv - mu}{t}$$

Factorizing this we are left with

$$F = \frac{m(v - u)}{t}$$

since $(v - u)/t$ is the same as change in velocity/t and this is acceleration (a), we are left with the equation $F = ma$.

The amount by which the velocity of an object is increased is dependent both on the magnitude of the force imposed on the object, and the time for which this force acts. This is an important consideration in throwing sports. A greater range of movement will allow a force to be applied on an object for a longer time, and as a consequence the velocity obtained will be greater. These principles are used in events such as the shot-put and discus throw, in which the athlete 'winds up' and spins to apply the greatest force over the greatest time.

Newton's third law is the law of reaction, which states that action and reaction are equal in magnitude but opposite in direction. When a ball is hit with a cricket bat, the player applies a force (action force), and the ball pushes back (reaction force). From Newton's second law we know that:

$$F = \frac{m(v - u)}{t}$$

Suppose the mass of the ball (m) is 0.1 kg, the velocity at the start (u) and finish (v) are 15 m/s and 40 m/s, respectively, and the ball strikes the bat for only 0.05 s (t). Because the initial velocity and the final velocity act in opposite directions, the difference in velocity is now obtained by summing the two values.

$$F = \frac{0.1(15 - (-40))}{0.05}$$

$$= 110 \text{ N}$$

To avoid injury when a ball travelling with this force is caught, it is necessary to reduce its momentum. Similarly, when landing from a vertical jump, body momentum must be reduced if injury (such as a fractured calcaneus) is not to result. The aim in each of these cases is to extend the time taken to dissipate the reaction force (Watkins, 1983). If the cricket ball is stopped with the arms and wrists locked, injury may result from the sudden impact of the force. However, if the arms are extended to meet the ball, and flexed as the ball is brought into the body, the time taken to dissipate the ball's force (deceleration period) is extended, and the injury risk reduced. In the case of landing from a jump, the knees should be bent to dissipate the reaction force, rather than falling directly onto the heels with straight legs.

## Stress and strain

When a force acts on an object, the force, expressed per unit area, is called mechanical stress. Pushing, pulling or twisting are all examples of such forces, but three major categories of stress are important in the context of sports injury. These are tension, compression and shear (Fig. 1.5).

Tension stress is a pulling force. When the ankle is twisted by an inversion injury, the lateral ligament stretches and tension stress is applied. Simi-larly, when the spine is flexed, the posterior spinal ligaments are tightened and subjected to a tension stress.

Compression stress is the opposite of tension. It is a pushing force, applied along the length of a tissue. In the upright posture, the menisci of the knee take weight and are subjected to compression stress. Another example occurs when the quadriceps contract in a bent knee, the patella is pulled against the femur and compression stress is applied to the patello-femoral joint.

Shear stress occurs when opposite forces are applied to a tissue, causing one part of the tissue to slide over another. For example, shearing stresses may be applied to the sacro-iliac joint during a fall, or to a finger which is subluxed when hit by a hard ball.

Both compression and tension stresses occur in line with the tissue fibres, the direction in which the tissues are strongest. Shearing stresses are imposed at an angle to the fibres, making this type of stress potentially the most dangerous in terms of injury. A fall onto the straight leg, for example, will cause compression stress on the joint structures, especially the cartilage and menisci of the knee. These forces will largely be absorbed, but, if severe, compression fracture may occur. Tension stress will be imposed on the muscles if the joints bend during the fall. The elastic capacities of the muscles will now take some of the stress away from the joint. Falling at an angle will also cause some compression and tension, but, in addition, shearing will occur between the body tissues, and the foot and ground. This type of stress could cause valgus or varus strain at the joint, with associated ligament damage or joint subluxation if the force is great.

When a stress is applied to a tissue, the tissue will deform, and the deformation is called strain. The relationship between stress and strain is shown graphically by the stress–strain curve (Fig. 1.6). Different materials will each have specific curves, but the general shape of the curves will be the same.

Initially, the tissue obeys Hooke's law and its deformation is proportional to the force applied to it, so the relationship between stress and strain at the start of the curve is linear. This part of the curve represents the elastic range of a material. At any point along this line, the material which is put

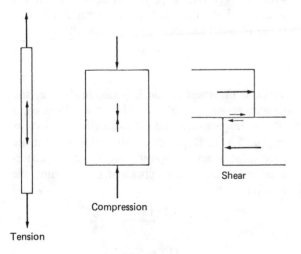

Tension

Compression

Shear

**Figure 1.5** Tension, compression and shear stresses.

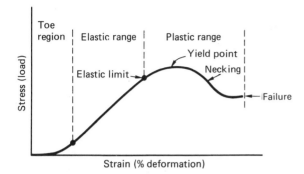

**Figure 1.6** The stress–strain curve. From Kisner and Colby (1990), with permission.

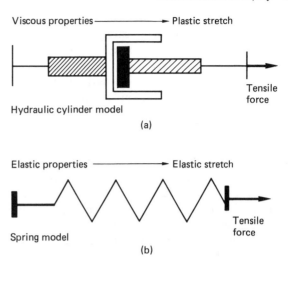

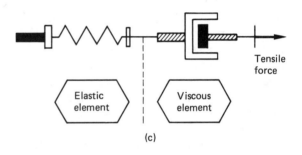

**Figure 1.7** Viscoelastic tissues. (a) Schematic representation of a viscous element in material capable of permanent (plastic) deformation. (b) An elastic element in material capable of recoverable (elastic) deformation. (c) A simplified model of collagenous tissue. Connective tissue is a viscoelastic material: when stretched, it behaves as if it has both viscous and elastic elements connected in series. From Sapega et al. (1981), with permission.

under stress will return to its original size and shape when the stressing force is released.

When the material is stressed beyond the elastic range, it will reach a point at which deformation becomes permanent. At this point, known as the elastic limit, the object will not return to its original form when the force is released. Going past this point, further along the stress–strain curve, the material moves into the plastic range. Here, the object will permanently deform, but not rupture. The greater the force, the greater the permanent deformation. As the stress imposed on the material increases still further, the yield point (Y) is reached. Now the material continues to deform even though the stress applied to it remains constant. The stress–strain curve reaches its peak at this point.

Some materials (including connective tissue) demonstrate both plastic (viscous) and elastic properties, and so are termed viscoelastic. A simple mechanical model of a spring (elastic) and hydraulic cylinder (plastic) linked in series may be used to illustrate this property (Fig. 1.7). As greater stress is applied to the material, and we move still further along the curve, the material fails rapidly. Only a little extra force is required to increase the rate of deformation that is already occurring. This is known as the necking region. The final load required to produce complete material failure (rupture) is the breaking strength.

### Factors influencing the stress–strain curve

The stress–strain curve may be influenced by a number of mechanical features of tissue. Of these,

we will look at stiffness, creep, fatigue, resilience and toughness.

Structural stiffness occurs when a tissue is less elastic. In this case the initial slope of the stress–strain curve is steeper as less deformation occurs when stress increases. Scar tissue would fall into this category. Scar tissue within a ligament for example may be as strong or stronger than the ligament itself, but will not be as elastic and will not therefore respond to stress in the same manner.

Creep occurs when a load (usually a small load) is imposed on a material over a long time period, causing the material to deform very gradually. Viscoelastic materials demonstrate this property. They deform at a constant rate regardless of the speed with which a force is applied to them. The degree of deformation in this case is determined not just by the amount of force applied to a tissue, but also by the duration for which the force is applied. Creep is therefore time dependent. A lesser load applied over a greater time period will produce a larger amount of creep. Creep is related to the viscosity of a tissue, and elevation of temperature will cause corresponding increases in creep. This fact can be used to good effect when stretching tight connective tissue. A warmed tissue that is stretched and held is more pliable than a cold tissue that is stretched rapidly.

Fatigue is the characteristic of materials to fail before the yield point is reached, when a load is applied repeatedly (cyclically). The larger the load, the fewer repetitions are required to produce failure, although a certain minimum load (the endurance limit) must be applied. An example of fatigue through cumulative loading is that of continually bending a wire until it breaks. Fatigue (stress) fractures occur in some athletes who place too much stress on a bone through training. Other things being equal, a heavier athlete is likely to produce fatigue more quickly than a lighter one because the heavier athlete is placing his or her tissues under greater load.

Both resilience and toughness are related to the ability of a material to absorb and release energy. Resilient materials absorb energy well in the elastic range while tough materials absorb energy well in the plastic range. A resilient material will absorb energy and deform, returning to its original shape when the load is released. A tough material will also deform, but will not return to its original shape. Highly resilient materials tend to be bouncy. For example, a rubber ball will deform and absorb energy when dropped. It will quickly release this stored energy and return to its original shape as it bounces back.

Tough materials will absorb a lot of energy without breaking, but when their failure point is reached, they rupture quickly. Putty is an example here. If something is dropped onto it, it will absorb energy by deforming but will not return to its original shape when released. If subjected to slow tension stress it will stretch, but if stretched quickly it will snap.

## Leverage

### Types of lever

A typical lever is a rigid bar with one point (the fulcrum or pivot) about which the lever revolves. Two forces are applied to a lever, the effort which tries to move the lever, and the resistance which tries to stop movement. The product of the force, and the horizontal distance between the point of application of the force and the fulcrum, is known as the 'moment' of the force, or torque, and is measured in newton-metres (Nm).

The distance from the effort to the fulcrum is called the effort arm, and that from the resistance to the fulcrum, the resistance arm. The ratio of the effort arm to the resistance arm gives a value for the mechanical advantage. If the effort arm is greater than the resistance arm the mechanical advantage is greater than one. The mechanical advantage is less than one if the resistance arm is the greater of the two.

The relationship between the fulcrum, resistance and effort within a lever system determines the type or 'order' of lever.

The first type, or 'first order lever', is one of balance. A typical example is a child's see-saw, in which the fulcrum lies between the force and effort. For the lever to balance, the leverage created by the effort must equal that created by the resistance. Figure 1.8 shows a simple first order lever. A resistance of 6 kg is placed 3 m away from the fulcrum. Multiplying these together gives a torque of 18 Nm. To balance this out, the effort has to be of the same magnitude. So, a 9 kg weight has to be placed only 2 m from the fulcrum on the other side for the lever to balance. An example of a first order lever in the body is the skull pivoted on the atlas. The line of gravity of the skull passes anterior to the vertebral column, and to stop the head falling forwards under its own weight, the neck extensors must exert an equivalent balancing force.

In the second order lever, the resistance lies between the fulcrum and the effort. With this type,

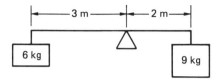

**Figure 1.8** A first order lever.

which is commonly illustrated by a wheelbarrow, the torque produced by the effort is always greater than that produced by the resistance, so the mechanical advantage is also greater than one. The second order lever is consequently used to produce power, but is rarely found in the human body.

The third order lever is the one found most commonly in the body, for example the deltoid muscle abducting the arm. The shoulder joint is the fulcrum, the weight of the arm acts around elbow level, and the deltoid applies a force to the top of the humerus. Here, the resistance arm is the full length of the lever, and the mechanical advantage is always less than one. The effort is applied between the fulcrum and resistance. Unlike the second order lever, this does not favour power, but rather distance and speed. With this type of lever, a contraction of a muscle (the effort) will cause a large movement of the resistance (the limb).

*Leverage and injury*

Increased leverage will multiply the effect of a force on body tissue, often making injury more likely. For example lifting a 10 kg weight is not, in itself, dangerous. However, lifting it at arm's length in a bent over position with the legs straight will place excessive leverage on the spine, increasing the effect of the weight on the lumbar spine and making injury more likely. As another example, performing a bilateral straight leg raising movement will place excessive strain on the spine, while simply bending the legs will reduce the leverage effect of the legs and so reduce the likelihood of injury.

Some types of athletic equipment may increase the risk of injury by their leverage effects. Running shoes (see Fig. 14.8, page 221) with flared heels increase the leverage effect on the ankle joints and

may, under certain circumstances, predispose the athlete to injury. The face-guard on an American football helmet will increase the leverage of neck extension, and a ski will increase leverage forces acting on the tibia.

**Centre of gravity**

The centre of gravity of an object is the point at which all the weight of the object can be considered to act. This is also the point at which the object would balance. In a symmetrical object, such as a ball, the centre of gravity will be at the centre of the object. But, with asymmetrical objects, such as the human body, the centre of gravity will be nearer to the larger and heavier end.

In the human body standing in the anatomical position, the centre of gravity is at the S1/2 spinal level, but this point will vary as the body position changes. As the centre of gravity is partially determined by an object's weight, it will shift when something is carried. The centre of gravity of a hiker carrying a heavy rucksack for example, is shifted up and back and would probably lie behind the lower thoracic spine.

By extending the centre of gravity in a line towards the floor, we can calculate the line of gravity, and, importantly, the point at which it passes through an object's base of support.

In order for any object to remain upright, its line of gravity must always pass through its base of support. When the line of gravity moves outside this area, the object will fall over. It follows that an object will be more stable when its line of gravity lies well within its base of support, because it will take a large movement to push the line of gravity to the edge of the supporting base. Take as an example an athlete performing an arm curl exercise with a heavy barbell. In the normal standing position without the barbell his line of gravity will fall between his feet. However, when he holds the weight in front of him, his centre of gravity moves forwards, and the line of gravity will now fall nearer to his toes. As the line of gravity is now closer to the edge of his base of support, it will take only a small movement to push it outside his supporting base, and cause him to lose balance.

## Stability

During most sports and exercises, an unstable position is a dangerous one, particularly when the body becomes fatigued. An object is more stable when its centre of gravity is lower. Moreover, we say that an object is in stable equilibrium if moving it would cause its centre of gravity to rise. In Fig. 1.9c, the pyramid can either slide sideways, or it would have to be moved onto its side to raise its centre of gravity.

Unstable equilibrium exists when an object's centre of gravity would fall if it were moved (Fig. 1.9b). If the centre of gravity remains the same in all positions, as with a ball, then an object is said to be in neutral equilibrium (Fig. 1.9a).

In addition to the position of the centre of gravity, the size of an object's base of support will also affect its stability. A wide base of support is more stable than a narrow one. Take as an example an ice skater skating a line. With only the thin blade of the skate on the ice and her feet close together, her base of support is very small. In addition, she is standing tall, lifting her centre of gravity. The combination of these two features makes her quite unstable. However, a judo exponent with her feet wide apart has a wide base of support, her knees are bent lowering her centre of gravity and making her much more stable.

When moving, the base of support should be widened in the direction of movement. A pulling action such as in a tug-o-war is therefore safer when a wide stance is taken, with one foot in front of the other, thus increasing the base of support. Sideways actions, such as lateral flexion of the spine, become more stable and much safer with the feet astride in the frontal plane.

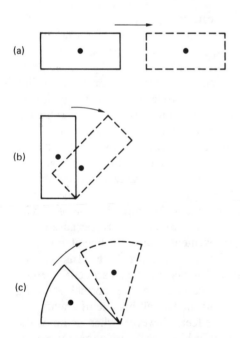

**Figure 1.9** Equilibrium and stability (a) Neutral equilibrium. The centre of gravity remains level as the object is moved. (b) Unstable equilibrium. The centre of gravity moves down as the object is moved. (c) Stable equilibrium. The centre of gravity moves up as the object is moved.

## Biomechanics and kinesiology of muscle

### Form of muscle

A great number of muscle types exist, but, generally speaking, muscles may be grouped according to the orientation of their fibres. The fibres may be arranged either in parallel, obliquely, or in a spiral fashion, and the arrangement will dictate the power and range of motion that the muscle can produce.

When the fibres are arranged in parallel, the muscle may be strap-like, with individual fibres running the whole length of the muscle (e.g. sartorius). The fibres may run between adjacent tendinous intersections which divide the muscle as a whole into sections (e.g. rectus abdominis). Alternatively, the fibres may be grouped into discrete bundles, producing a fusiform muscle belly which attaches to a tendon (e.g. biceps). Another fibre arrangement is the sheet attaching to a broad flat tendon or aponeurosis (e.g. external abdominal oblique).

In the oblique or 'pennate' grouping the muscle fibres are attached to a central tendon. Fibres which join to only one side of a tendon are termed unipennate. When the fibres bind to both sides of a central septum the muscle is termed bipennate, and when the muscle has several septa it is termed multipennate.

In each case, the muscle fibres can only shorten to half their original length, so the shorter fibres of a pennate muscle will produce a smaller range of motion than the long fibres of a parallel muscle (Fig. 1.10). However, the power of a muscle is determined by the total cross-sectional area of the fibres. With a pennate muscle the total cross-sectional area is much larger than that of a parallel muscle and so the power produced is significantly greater (Fig. 1.11).

The third type of fibre arrangement is spiralized (Fig. 1.12). Here, the muscle fibres twist as they travel between the two ends of the muscle (e.g. pectoralis major). As the muscle contracts, the fibres tend to de-rotate and straighten out, imparting a rotation force to the bone on which they attach. In this way, a spiralized muscle not only approximates the bones of the joint over which it acts, but pulls the bones into the same plane.

## Muscle attachment

The position of the muscle attachment to the bone, and the direction of the muscle will largely determine its action. As a muscle contracts, the force exerted onto its tendon may be resolved into three distinct components (Fig. 1.13a). The first component acts at 90° to the bony lever and tends to move

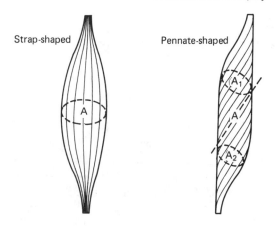

**Figure 1.11** Muscle power is proportional to fibre cross-sectional area (A). The total area ($A_1 + A_2$), and so the power, is greater for a pennate-shaped muscle than for a strap-shaped one.

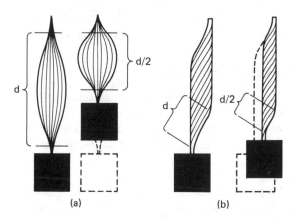

**Figure 1.10** Muscle shortening. A muscle fibre can only shorten by half its original length (d/2), so the range of motion is greater for a parallel arrangement of muscle fibres (a), than for a pennate arrangement (b).

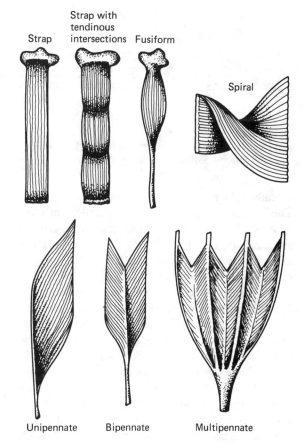

**Figure 1.12** Various muscle fibre arrangements. From *Grays Anatomy* (35th edn), with permission.

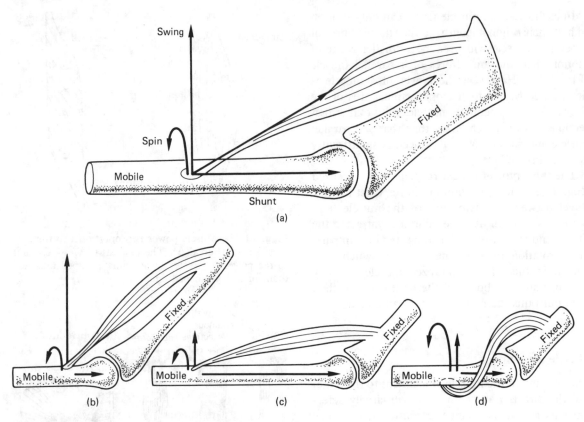

**Figure 1.13**  The components of the force exerted by a muscle on its tendon (see text for details). From *Gray's Anatomy* (35th edn), with permission.

it, causing a rotatory (swing) action at the joint. The second component acts in parallel with the bony lever and pulls it into the joint causing approximation (shunt). Finally, the offset arrangement of the muscle insertions causes the bone to rotate about its longitudinal axis (spin).

The three movements will vary tremendously between muscles and are altered by the restriction of bony configuration and soft tissue tightness. However, each of the three components is emphasized differently in various muscles. Where the muscle attachment is wrapped around the bone (Fig. 1.13d), the spin component is emphasized (e.g. pronator quadratus). The positions of the distal and proximal muscle attachments will dictate the relative amount of swing and shunt. When the distal attachment is close to the joint (e.g. brachialis) the swing component dominates (Fig. 1.13b),

but when the distal attachment is placed some distance from the joint (e.g. brachioradialis) the shunt component is greater (Fig. 1.13c).

## Group action of muscles

The properties of muscle contraction are often described for isolated muscle fibres in the laboratory. Functionally, however, muscles do not contract singly, but in a group. The group action of muscles is an important consideration, both in injury and the process of rehabilitation.

When stimulated, a muscle fibre will develop tension tending to shorten the muscle as a whole. Whether the tension developed is sufficient to cause shortening, or indeed joint movement, will depend on a number of factors. The amount of tension developed, the resistance opposing the muscle, the mechanical leverage system, and contraction of neighbouring muscles will all have an effect.

The most effective muscle at producing a particular movement is called the prime mover (agonist). Any muscle which helps to create this same movement but is less effective at doing so is called an assistant mover. In different situations a muscle may take on both actions. Take as an example a bench-press movement in weight training. If a wide grip is taken, the prime mover will be the pectoral muscles, and an assistant mover will be the triceps. If a narrow grip is taken, pulling the arms in close to the side, the pectorals are shortened and become less effective (length–tension relationship). Now, the triceps becomes the prime mover and the pectorals act as assistant movers.

The muscle which, if it contracted, would tend to oppose the action of the prime mover is called the antagonist. Normally, through reciprocal inhibition, the contraction of the antagonist is reduced. With a co-contraction, however, both prime mover and antagonist may contract. This type of contraction can represent a lack of skill (Wells, 1966), and its reduction has been cited as one way in which strength increases are produced early on in training (Sale, 1988). In actions such as gripping, two joint muscles (see below) are acting, and there may also be a rapid alternation between opposing muscle groups or isometric action to stabilize the joint. The interaction of muscles in co-contraction is complex, and the interested reader is referred to Basmajian and Deluca (1985) for a full review.

A muscle acts as a fixator or stabilizer when it anchors or supports a body part to supply a firm base for another muscle (usually the prime mover) to pull on. When a muscle contracts, it will tend to pull both of its ends towards each other. To produce movement at one end only, the bony attachment of one end of the muscle must be stabilized. An example is the contraction of the medial rotators of the scapula as the teres major adducts the humerus. Another situation in which a fixator can act is to resist the pull of gravity to stabilize a body segment. An example of this is a press-up action, in which the abdominal muscles contract to prevent the spine sagging into extension.

A neutralizer is a muscle which contracts to prevent an unwanted action of the prime or assistant mover. Most muscles are capable of several actions, and those not required must be counteracted by activity of a neutralizer. For example, biceps will both flex the elbow and supinate the forearm. If we wish to flex the elbow without forearm rotation, the pronators must neutralize the unwanted supinatory action of the biceps.

### Ballistic and reciprocal actions

In rapid actions, such as throwing or kicking, the prime mover will contract powerfully, but briefly, to move the limb, allowing momentum of the moving limb to maintain the action. At the end of the desired range of motion, the antagonist contracts eccentrically to decelerate the limb, finally the prime mover works again to control the final position of the limb. This triphasic muscle action (Fig. 1.14) is known as a ballistic contraction. An overlap may be present between the initial contraction of the prime mover and that of the antagonist, in which case a co-contraction occurs. The ballistic action is obviously a highly skilled co-ordination, and when, with fatigue, the action becomes uncontrolled, injury frequently results.

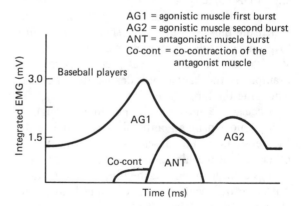

**Figure 1.14**  Triphasic muscle action. Initially the arm is propelled forwards by the agonist muscles (AG1). As the arm reaches its target, the antagonists contract to eccentrically slow the limb (ANT). Some overlap of muscle contraction occurs (CO-CONT). Finally, the agonist contracts again to finely position the limb (AG2). From McArdle *et al.* (1986), with permission.

When an eccentric action immediately precedes a concentric one, a reciprocal contraction occurs, giving a more powerful contraction. LaGasse (1983) demonstrated an 11.4% greater force output from the quadriceps when knee flexion was performed prior to knee extension. Reciprocal contractions occur in most functional movements, such as walking and running, and form the basis of power training using plyometrics (p. 101). The stretch incurred by the elastic components of the muscle when working eccentrically is released with the concentric contraction, increasing the force output. In addition the stretch reflex is stimulated in the stretched muscle, facilitating a more powerful contraction through increased recruitment and activation of motor units.

## Two joint muscles

Most joint complexes contain two joint or 'biarticular' muscles, and these are frequently the muscles which are torn in sport. Examples in the lower limb are the rectus femoris, hamstrings, and gastrocnemius. The important characteristic of these muscles is that they are unable to permit full movement at both joints simultaneously.

When full movement is limited by passive stretch of the muscle, passive insufficiency is present. An example is passive hip extension combined with knee flexion being limited by rectus femoris. When the muscle is unable to shorten sufficiently to produce a full range movement at both joints simultaneously, active insufficiency exists. An example is the hamstrings flexing the knee and extending the hip.

Because the muscles are not long enough to permit movement at both joints simultaneously, the tension in one muscle is transferred to the other. Using the hip as an example, as the hamstrings contract to extend the hip, tension is transmitted to the rectus femoris enabling it to extend the knee (Wells, 1966). This type of action, involving either extension or flexion at both joints at the same time, is called concurrent movement. The muscle shortens at one end but lengthens at the other, and so maintains its length and conserves tension. When the hip is flexed but the knee extended, the rectus femoris is shortened and

rapidly loses tension, while the hamstrings are lengthened and rapidly gain tension, an example of countercurrent movement (Rasch, 1989).

## Force–velocity relationship

When a muscle is contracting, a relationship exists between the speed of the movement it creates and the force which the muscle can develop. The torque generated by the muscle decreases as the velocity of movement increases (Pipes and Wilmore, 1975; Coyle 1981; Burnie and Brodie, 1986). The greatest force is produced at the slowest speeds. One theory for the force–velocity relationship is that the myosin cross-bridges within the muscle continually move through thermal agitation. The probability of union between the actin and myosin filaments is therefore reduced at higher speeds (Bray et al., 1986).

## Length–tension relationship

A further biomechanical relationship exists between the initial length of the muscle and its force production, the so-called length–tension relationship. In the laboratory, an isolated muscle can exert its maximal force or tension while in a resting stretched state. If the muscle is shortened or overstretched, less tension can be exerted

Physiologically, this can be explained in terms of the sliding filament mechanism. In the shortened position, an overlap of the muscle filaments occurs, interfering with cross-bridge coupling. If the muscle is overstretched, the filaments are pulled completely apart, the cross-bridges will not come into contact, and no tension can be developed (Fig. 1.15).

As the relaxed muscle is stretched, however, a passive force due to muscle elasticity is created. This varies between muscles, for example the spinal extensors in humans resist a stretching force by purely passive means. The total force developed by the muscle will be the sum of the active and passive forces, as shown in Fig. 1.16.

The length–tension relationship can be used to advantage where two muscles work together to produce a movement as primary and secondary movers. We can emphasize the prime mover by

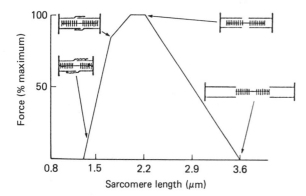

**Figure 1.15** Relationship between sarcomere length and contractile force.

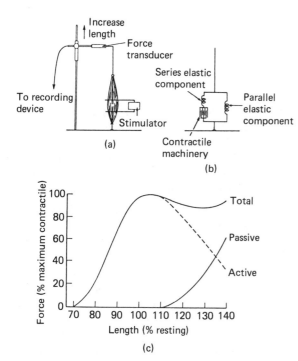

**Figure 1.16** Contractile and elastic properties of a muscle. (a) Experimental set-up. (b) Diagrammatic model. (c) Force generation. From Bray et al. (1986), with permission.

shortening (and therefore 'weakening') the secondary mover. For example, in a sit up movement with the legs straight both the hip flexors and abdominal muscles are working. However, the hip flexors are generally strong anyway through use in everyday living, so the training effect on these muscles has to be reduced. This is accomplished by bending the knees and hips. The length–tension relationship dictates that the hip flexors will now be able to produce less force.

## Joint mechanics

### Accessory movements

The movements of a joint are of two types, physiological and accessory. Physiological movements are those which the athlete can perform actively, for example flexion and extension of the knee. Accessory movements cannot be produced actively as individual movements, but occur automatically between articulating surfaces of a joint as it moves. Three accessory movements are of particular importance when treating sports injuries, these are roll, slide and spin (Fig. 1.17).

Roll occurs when points at certain intervals on a moving surface contact points at the same intervals on the opposing surface. This is similar to a car tyre rolling over the road. If one point on the moving surface stays in contact with a variety of points on the opposing surface, slide is occurring. Spin is a pure rotation around a mechanical axis (Barak, Rosen and Sofer, 1990). Usually when a joint moves, both slide and roll must take place. If roll alone were the only movement, the joint would sublux before any appreciable range had been achieved. If only slide occurred, the edges of the concave aspect of the joint would impinge on the opposing convex lip.

### Concave-convex motion

Synovial joints in general consist of both concave and convex surfaces created by the shapes of the bone ends within the joint and their covering cartilage. When a concave surface moves on a convex surface, roll and slide occur in the same direction, the bone sliding towards the direction of movement. When a convex surface moves on a concave surface roll and slide occur in opposite directions, the bone sliding away from the direction

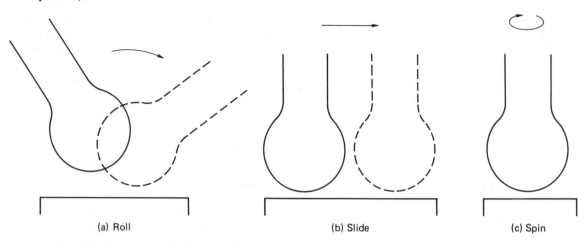

(a) Roll      (b) Slide      (c) Spin

**Figure 1.17** Accessory joint movements. (a) Roll, (b) slide, and (c) spin.

of movement. Take as an example knee movement. If the tibia extends on a fixed femur in a leg extension exercise (concave on convex) the joint surface of the tibia rolls and slides forwards in the direction of extension. Conversely, if the femur extends on a stationary tibia, as with standing up from a chair (convex on concave), the femoral condyles will roll forwards but slide backwards in the opposite direction to the movement. Knowledge of the direction of accessory movements is important when using joint mobilization techniques. For example, if shoulder flexion is limited, although the movement of the humerus is upward, because a convex surface is moving on a concave one, gliding of the joint should be directed downwards (caudally).

When gliding a joint, the direction of movement is altered with the angle of the joint. The glide direction chosen is called the treatment plane, and is the one in which most translatory motion is possible. In peripheral joints the joint line can be established fairly easily by palpation, and so the treatment plane is determined directly. In the spine, however, the treatment plane is determined by the joint angles of the facets, and is horizontal for C0–C1, angled at 45° between C2 and T12, and almost horizontal for the lumbar area.

**Close and loose pack**

The two opposing surfaces of a joint do not fit together exactly; they are said to be non-congruent. But, with the joint in one particular position its surfaces will come as close together as they are able, and this is known as 'close pack'. In this position the joint capsule and ligaments twist and pull the joint surfaces together into approximation. The joint space is at a minimum and the concave surface of one bone fits tightly into the convex shape of the other. No further movement is possible in a joint which is close packed, and so this position is avoided when trying to mobilize the joint.

The loose pack position is exactly the opposite. As the joint surfaces are released from their close pack position, elastic recoil of the soft tissues surrounding the joint enables its surfaces to move apart, maximizing the joint space. The loose pack position is the resting position often taken up after injury because more joint fluid can accumulate. In loose pack positions joint play is possible. This consists of small accessory movements which give the joint its 'spring'. These are essential to the normal functioning of the joint and play a part in joint nutrition and combined movements.

Many fractures of the upper limb occur with a fall onto the outstretched arm, which is a close packed position, and many ligament sprains occur in a loose packed position (Kessler, 1990). Examples of close and loose pack positions are given in Table 1.1.

## Axes and planes

The human body may for descriptive purposes be divided into three planes. The sagittal plane passes through the body from front to back, dividing it into right and left halves. The frontal plane divides the body into anterior and posterior sections, and lies at right angles to the sagittal plane. The transverse plane divides the body into upper and lower portions, and lies at right angles to the other two planes.

Each of the three body planes has an associated axis which passes perpendicularly through it (Fig. 1.18). Movement occurs *in* a plane but *about* an axis. Abduction and adduction occur in the frontal plane about a sagittal axis, flexion and extension occur in a sagittal plane about a frontal axis, and rotations occur in a transverse plane about a vertical axis.

**Table 1.1  Close packed and loose packed positions of selected joints**

| Joint(s) | Close packed position | Loose packed (resting) position |
|---|---|---|
| Facet (spine) | Extension | Midway between flexion and extension |
| Temporomandibular | Clenched teeth | Mouth slightly open |
| Glenohumeral | Abduction and external rotation | 55° abduction, 30° horizontal abduction, rotated so that the forearm is in the transverse plane |
| Acromioclavicular | Arm abducted to 30° | Arm resting by side, shoulder girdle in the physiological position |
| Sternoclavicular | Maximum shoulder elevation | Arm resting by side, shoulder girdle in the physiological position |
| Ulnohumeral (elbow) | Extension | 70° elbow flexion, 10° forearm supination |
| Radiohumeral | Elbow flexed 90°, forearm supinated 5° | Full extension, full supination |
| Proximal radioulnar | 5° supination | 70° elbow flexion, 35° forearm supination |
| Distal radioulnar | 5° supination | 10° forearm supination |
| Radiocarpal (wrist) | Extension with ulnar deviation | Midway between flexion–extension (so that a straight line passes through the radius and third metacarpal) with slight ulnar deviation |
| First carpometacarpal | Full opposition | Midway between abduction-adduction and flexion-extension |
| Metacarpophalangeal (fingers) | Full flexion | Slight flexion |
| Metacarpophalangeal (thumb) | Full opposition | |
| Interphalangeal | Full extension | Slight flexion |
| Hip | Full extension, internal rotation and abduction | 30° flexion, 30° abduction, and slight external rotation |
| Knee | Full extension and external rotation of the tibia | 25° flexion |
| Talocrural (ankle) | Maximum dorsiflexion | 10° plantarflexion, midway between maximum inversion and eversion |
| Subtalar | Full supination | Midway between extremes of inversion and eversion |
| Midtarsal | Full supination | Midway between extremes of range of movement |
| Tarsometatarsal | Full supination | Midway between extremes of range of movement |
| Metatarsophalangeal | Full extension | Neutral |
| Interphalangeal | Full extension | Slight flexion |

From Clarkson and Gilewich (1989), with permission.

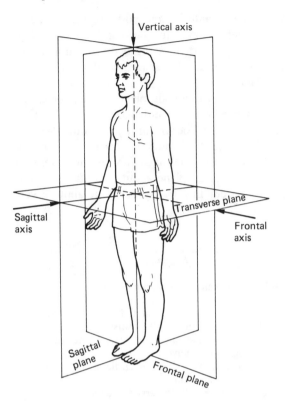

**Figure 1.18**  Axes and planes of the body. From Clarkson and Gilewich (1989), with permission.

In reality, movements do not occur in one plane, but in several. For example we talk of 'tri-plane motion' of the sub-taloid joint in a runner (see page 151). This is because a complex series of movements link together to give a motion which occurs in all three planes about an oblique axis.

## Biomechanical analysis

### Video movement analysis

Analysis of human movement is vital for the prevention and rehabilitation of sports injuries. The most basic analysis may be performed by the clinician simply observing the subject. This type of analysis may be useful, but is limited by the visual memory of the observer. The clinician is unable to follow and retain much of the important detail in even the slowest movement. Although the trained observer may extract considerably more data than the layperson, even when an action is repeated a number of times, precise analysis is not possible.

The situation is improved considerably when an action is recorded on videotape or cine film to be played back later for accurate analysis. This procedure has previously been complex and expensive, but with the steadily reducing cost and increasing standard of video equipment the task is much easier.

### Observing and recording movement

In order to accurately record an action, the subject and environment in which he or she performs must be prepared. Subjects should be suitably dressed in shorts or bathing costume to enable accurate location of body segments and joints. Bony reference points or centres of motion are marked on the skin with adhesive tape. The background is cleared, where possible, to allow unobscured vision of the whole movement. The video camera is set up on a stand at a set distance from the subject. The camera should be capable of recording in poor lighting conditions, and have a timing/counting facility. If two or more analyses are to be made, the distance from the camera to the subject must remain the same to reduce parallax error. Complex motions are better recorded with two synchronized cameras placed at 90° to each other.

Lighting must be adequate to illuminate the subject in all positions, and where this cannot be controlled (on the field) a low-light camera should be used. Reference points, such as a measuring stick placed in the field of view, can be useful to give a comparison of distance. Ideally, the whole action should be filmed without moving the camera. To do this the observer must be far enough away from the subject to get a wide field of view.

### Analysing movement

The simplest way to analyse a movement is to slow the action down and use an experienced clinical eye. Where the video image is sufficiently clear and reference markers are visible this is an inexpensive and extremely useful method. The analysis may be taken further, by digitizing the image. Essentially this involves establishing X-Y coordinates of the various marked reference points. The video film is played back on a large flat-screen monitor, using a freeze-frame facility to stop the action at a predetermined point. The relative positions of the various reference points are then recorded. A number of commercially available computer software programs allow the clinician to do this using a 'digitizing pen'. Alternatively, a 'mouse' is used to move the computer cursor to the selected reference point. The software package then records the position of the point in two dimensions. Gradually an image is built up, which may be used to create a stick figure (Fig. 1.19).

By progressing frame to frame, the limb and centres of rotation for the subject are recorded

throughout the movement. Various parameters such as linear and angular displacements and accelerations of the body segments are then calculated. The overall action is reviewed by analysing the stick figure display, and the path described by individual reference points (loci) (Fig. 1.20) are studied. In addition, if sufficient joint locations are used, the body's centre of gravity may be determined.

Video analysis still has limitations, particularly with respect to joint rotation and three dimensional images, although the use of two synchronized cameras reduces this problem. However, with the increasing availability of these systems, they are useful clinical tools for the sports physiotherapist.

### Force plates

The force that an athlete exerts on a sports surface may be measured using a force plate. This is essentially a rigid plate set flush into the floor. Beneath the plate, at each corner, sit four transducers capable of recording various components of the ground reaction force (Fig. 1.21). The vertical component ($F_z$) is a compression force, while the horizontal components ($F_y$ and $F_x$) are shearing forces. $F_y$ is in line with the long edge of the force plate and is parallel to the direction of travel, whereas $F_x$ is at right angles to the line of travel and parallel to the short edge of the force plate.

In addition to these three fundamental measurements, the force plate will show the moment (turning force) about a vertical axis through the contact point of the foot on the force plate. The

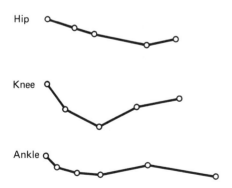

**Figure 1.19** Stick figure compiled by digitizing a video image.

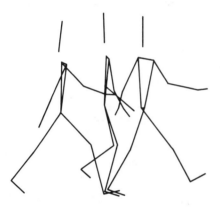

**Figure 1.20** Paths desribed by the hip, knee and ankle reference points. From Williams and Davies (1990), with permission.

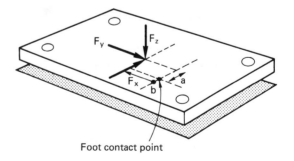

Foot contact point

**Figure 1.21** Three force components of a force plate. a and b represent 'offset' position from centre of force plate.

position of the line of action of a force is shown by measuring the distance from the force to the centre of the plate, represented by the values a and b.

# References

Barak, T., Rosen, E.R. and Sofer, R. (1990) Basic concepts of orthopaedic manual therapy. In *Orthopaedic and Sports Physical Therapy* (ed. J.A. Gould), C.V. Mosby, St Louis, pp.195—211.

Basmajian, J.V. and Deluca, C.J. (1985) *Muscles Alive*, Williams and Wilkins, Baltimore.

Bowker, P. (1987) Forces and their effects. *Physiotherapy*, **73**, (6) 264–70

Bray, J.J., Cragg, P.A., Macknight, A.D.C., Mills, R.G. and Taylor, D.W. (1986) *Lecture Notes on Human Physiology*, Blackwell Scientific, Oxford.

Burnie, J. and Brodie, D.A. (1986) Isokinetics in the assessment of rehabilitation: a case report. *Clinical Biomechanics* **1**, 140–146

Clarkson, H.M. and Gilewich, G.B. (1989) *Musculoskeletal Assessment*, Williams and Wilkins, Baltimore

Coyle, E.F., Feiring, D.C., Rotkis, T.C., Cote, R.U. and Roby, F.B. (1981) Specificity of power improvements through slow and fast isokinetic training. *Journal of Applied Physiology*, **51**, 1437–1442

Gleim, G.W. (1984) The profiling of professional football players. *Clinics in Sports Medicine*, **3**, (1) 185–197

Hertling, D. and Kessler, R.M. (1990) *Management of Common Musculoskeletal Disorders*, J.B. Lippincott, Philadelphia

Kisner, C. and Colby, L.A (1990) *Therapeutic Exercise: Foundations and Techniques*, F.A. Davis, Philadelphia, p.117.

LaGasse, P. (1983) Neuromuscular facilitation of muscle tension output by reciprocal muscle work. *Ann. French-Canadian Association for the Advancement of Sciences*, **50**, 222

LeVeau, B.F (1990) Basic biomechanics in sports and orthopaedic therapy. In *Orthopaedic and Sports Physical Therapy* (ed. J.A.Gould), C.V. Mosby, St. Louis, pp.65–83

Macdonald, F.A. (1978) *Mechanics for Movement*, Bell and Hyman, London

McArdle, W.D., Katch, F.I. and Katch, V.L. (1986) *Exercise Physiology. Energy, Nutrition and Human Performance*, Lea and Febiger, Philadelphia, p. 383

Pipes, T.V. and Wilmore, J.H. (1975). Isokinetic vs isotonic strength training in adult men. *Medicine in Science and Sports*, **7**, 262–274

Rasch, P.J. (1989) *Kinesiology and Applied Anatomy*, Lea and Febiger, Philadelphia

Sale, D.G. (1988) Neural adaptation to resistance training. *Medicine and Science in Sports and Exercise*, **20**,(5) 135–145

Sapega, A.A., Quedenfeld, T.C., Moyer, R.A. and Butler, R.A. (1981) Biophysical factors in range of motion exercise. *Physician and Sports Medicine*, **9**, 57–65

Stallard, J (1984) The mechanics of lower limb orthoses. In *Cash's Textbook of Orthopaedics and Rheumatology for Physiotherapists*, (ed. P.A. Downie), Faber and Faber, London pp.21–42

Taunton, J.E. McKenzie, D.C. and Clement, D.B. (1988) The role of biomechanics in the epidemiology of injuries. *Sports Medicine*, **6**, 107–120

Warwick, R. and Williams, P.L. (Eds)(1973) Gray's Anatomy (35th edn), Longman, p.494

Watkins, J. (1983) *An Introduction to Mechanics of Human Movement*, MTP Press, Lancaster

Wells, K.F. (1966) *Kinesiology*, W.B. Saunders, Philadelphia

Williams, J.G. and Davis, M. (1990) KINEMAN: a microcomputer-based video digitising system for movement analysis. *Physiotherapy*, **76**, (6)

Williams, J.G.P. and Sperryn, P.N. (1976) *Sports Medicine*, Edward Arnold, London

# 2 Healing

The basic processes of soft tissue healing underlie all treatment techniques for sports injuries. We need to know what occurs in the body tissues at each stage of healing to be able to select the most appropriate treatment technique.

A technique aimed at reducing the formation of swelling, for example, would be inappropriate when swelling had stopped forming and adhesions were the problem. Similarly, a manual treatment designed to break up adhesions and mobilize soft tissue would not be helpful if inflammation was still forming and further injury might be caused.

The stages of healing are, to a large extent, purely a convenience of description, since each stage runs into another. Traditionally, the initial tissue response has been described as inflammation, but some authors consider inflammation to be a response separate from the processes that occur at the time of injury. Van der Meulen (1982) described both in terms of the 'reaction phase', arguing that the classical inflammatory period is preceded by a short (10 min) period before the inflammatory mechanism is activated. The second stage of healing has been variously called repair, proliferation and regeneration. The tertiary stage has been termed remodelling (Van der Meulen, 1982; Kellett, 1986; Dyson, 1987). The terms injury, inflammation, repair and remodelling will be used in this book.

When describing the stage of healing, the terms acute, sub-acute and chronic are helpful. The acute stage (up to 48 hours following injury) is the stage of inflammation. The sub-acute stage, occurring between 14 and 21 days after injury, is the stage of repair. The chronic stage (after 21 days) is the stage of remodelling.

## Injury

This stage represents the tissue effects at the time of injury, before the inflammatory process is activated. With tissue damage, chemical and mechanical changes are seen. Local blood vessels are disrupted causing a cessation in the supply of oxygen to the cells they perfused. These cells die, and their lysosome membranes disintegrate, releasing the hydrolysing enzymes the lysosomes contained. The release of these enzymes has a two-fold effect. First they begin to break down the dead cells themselves, and secondly, they release histamines and kinins which have an effect on both the live cells nearby, and the local blood capillary network.

The disruption of the blood vessels which caused cell death also causes local bleeding (extravasated blood). The red blood cells break down, leaving cellular debris and free haemoglobin. The blood platelets release the enzyme thrombin which changes fibrinogen into fibrin. The fibrin in turn is deposited as a meshwork around the area (a process known as walling off). The dead cells intertwine in the meshwork forming a blood clot. This network contains the damaged area.

The changes occurring at injury are affected by age (Lachman, 1988). Intramuscular bleeding, and therefore haemorrhage formation, are more profuse in individuals over 30 years of age. The amount of bleeding which occurs will be partially dependent on the vascularity of the injured tissues. A fitter individual is likely to have muscle tissue which is more highly vascularized, and therefore greater bleeding will occur with muscle injury. In addition, exercise itself will affect gross tissue responses.

Muscle blood flow is greatly increased through dilatation of the capillary bed, and bleeding subsequent to injury will be greater.

## Inflammation

The next stage in the healing sequence is that of inflammation. This may last from 10 min to several hours, depending on the amount of tissue damage that has occurred. The inflammatory response to injury is the same regardless of the nature of the injuring agent or the location of the injury (Hettinga, 1990).

Inflammation is not simply a feature of soft tissue injuries. It occurs when the body is infected, in immune reactions and when infarction stops blood flowing to an area. Some of the characteristics of the inflammatory response have even been described as excessive (Cyriax, 1982) and better suited to dealing with infection, by preventing bacterial spread, than to healing injury (Evans, 1990).

The cardinal signs of inflammation are heat (calor), redness (rubor), swelling (tumor) and pain (dolor). These in turn give rise to the so called fifth sign of inflammation—disturbance of function of the affected tissues (functio laesa).

### Heat and redness

Heat and redness take a number of hours to develop, and are due to the opening of local blood capillaries and the resultant increased blood flow. Chemical and mechanical changes, initiated by injury, are responsible for the changes in blood flow.

A number of substances act as chemical mediators in the inflammatory process. The amines, including histamine and 5–hydroxytryptamine (5–HT or serotonin) are released from mast cells, red blood cells and platelets in the damaged capillaries and cause vessel dilatation and increased permeability lasting 10–15 min (Lachman, 1988).

Kinins (physiologically active polypeptides) cause an increase in vascular permeability and stimulate the contraction of smooth muscle. They are found normally in an inactive state as kininogens. These in turn are activated by the enzyme plasmin, and degraded by kininases.

The initial vasodilatation is maintained by prostaglandins. These are one of the arachidonic acid derivatives, formed from cell membrane phospholipids when cell damage occurs, and released when the kinin system is activated. The drug aspirin acts to inhibit this change—hence its anti-inflammatory action. The prostaglandins E1 and E2 are two of the substances responsible for pain production.

The complement system, which consists of a number of serum proteins circulating in an inactive form, is switched on and has a direct effect on the cell membrane as well as helping to maintain vasodilatation. Various complement products are involved, and these are activated in sequence.

Finally, polymorphs produce leucotrienes, which are themselves derived from arachidonic acid. These help the kinins maintain the vessel permeability.

Changes in blood flow also occur through mechanical alterations initiated by injury. Normally, the blood flow in the venules in particular, is axial. The large blood proteins stay in the centre of the vessel, and the plasmatic stream, which has a lower viscosity, is on the outside in contact with the vessel walls. This configuration reduces peripheral resistance and assists blood flow.

In a damaged capillary, however, fluid is lost, and so the axial flow slows. Marginization occurs as the slower flow rate allows white blood cells to move into the plasmatic zone and adhere to the vessel walls. This, in turn, reduces the lubricating effect of this layer and slows blood flow. The walls themselves become covered with a gelatinous layer (Wilkinson and Lackie, 1979), as endothelium changes occur (Walter and Israel, 1987).

Some four hours after injury (Evans, 1980) diapedesis occurs as the white cells pass through the vessel walls into the damaged tissue. The endothelial cells of the vessel contract (Hettinga, 1990), pulling away from each other and leaving gaps through which fluids and blood cells can escape (Fig. 2.1). Various substances, including

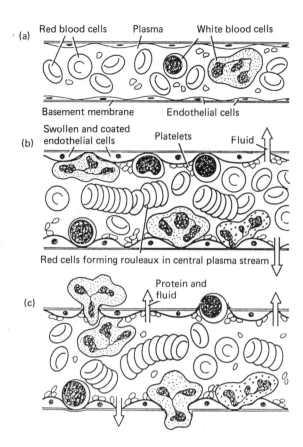

(a) Red blood cells    Plasma    White blood cells

Basement membrane    Endothelial cells

(b) Swollen and coated endothelial cells    Platelets    Fluid

Red cells forming rouleaux in central plasma stream

(c)    Protein and fluid

**Figure 2.1** Vascular changes which occur in inflammation. (a) Blood vessel starts to dilate. (b) Dilated vessel showing marginization. (c) White blood cells and fluid pass into tissue. From Evans (1990), with permission.

histamine, kinins and complement factors, have been shown to produce this effect (Fox, Gayley and Wayland, 1980; Walter and Israel, 1987).

## Swelling

The normal pressure gradients inside and outside the capillary, balance the flow of fluid leaving and entering the vessel (Fig. 2.2). The capillary membrane is permeable to water, and so water will be driven out into the interstitial fluid. However, because the tissue fluids usually contain a small amount of protein, and the blood contains a large amount, an osmotic pressure is created which tends to cause water to move back from the tissue fluid and into the capillary once more. The magnitude of

this osmotic pressure is roughly 25 mmHg. At the arteriole end of the capillary the blood pressure (32 mmHg) exceeds the osmotic pressure and so tissue fluid is formed. At the venous end of the capillary the blood pressure has reduced (12 mmHg) and so, because the osmotic pressure now exceeds this value, tissue fluid is reabsorbed into the capillary.

During inflammation the capillary bed opens and blood flow increases (heat and redness). The larger blood volume causes a parallel increase in blood pressure. Coupled with this, the tissue fluid now contains a large amount of protein, which has poured out from the more permeable blood vessels. This increased protein concentration causes a substantial rise in osmotic pressure, and this, together with the larger blood pressure in the capillary, forces fluid out into the interstitium, causing swelling.

Protein exudation in mild inflammation occurs from the venules only and is probably mediated by histamine (Evans, 1990). More severe inflammation, as a result of trauma, results in protein exudation from damaged capillaries as well.

During inflammation, lymphatic vessels open up and assist in the removal of excess fluid and protein. The lymph vessels are blind-ending capillaries which have gaps in their endothelial walls which enable protein molecules to move through easily. The lymph vessels lie within the tissue spaces, and have valves preventing the backward movement of fluid. Muscular contraction causes a pumping action on the lymph vessels and the excess tissue fluid is removed to the subclavian veins in the neck.

## Pain

Pain is the result of both sensory and emotional experiences, and is associated with tissue damage or the probability that damage will occur. It serves as a warning which may cause us to withdraw from a painful stimulus and so protect an injured body part. Unfortunately, pain often continues long after it has ceased to be a useful form of protection. Associated muscle spasm, atrophy, habitual postures, guarding, and psychological factors all combine to make chronic pain almost a disease entity in itself.

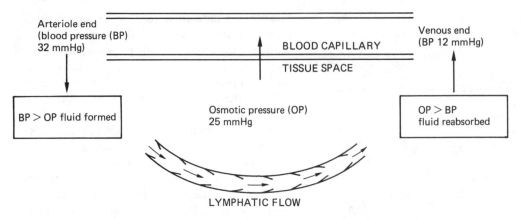

**Figure 2.2**   Formation and reabsorption of tissue fluid.

### Types of pain

Pain may be classified as somatogenic (acute or chronic), neurogenic or psychogenic. Chronic pain may be considered generally as that which lasts for more than six weeks, while acute pain is that of sudden onset which lasts for less than six weeks (Donley and Denegar, 1990).

Musculoskeletal pain is not in general well localized, the surface site where the pain is felt rarely correlates directly with injured subcutaneous tissue. In general, the closer an injured tissue is to the skin surface, the more accurate the athlete can be at localizing it.

Deep pain is normally an aching ill-defined sensation. It usually radiates in a characteristic fashion, and may be associated with autonomic responses such as sweating, nausea, pallor, and lowered blood pressure (Lynch and Kessler 1990). Pain referral corresponds to segmental pathways, most often dermatomes. The extent of radiation of the pain depends largely on the intensity of the stimulus. The pain normally radiates distally, and does not usually cross the midline of the body.

Neurogenic pain is different again. Compression of a nerve root gives rise to ill-defined tingling, especially in the distal part of the dermatome supplied by the nerve. This is a pressure reaction, which quickly disappears when the nerve root is released. Greater pressure causes the tingling to give way to numbness. Compression or tension to the dural sleeve covering the nerve root causes severe pain generally over the whole dermatome. In contrast, pressure on a nerve trunk usually causes little or no pain, but results in a shower of 'pins and needles' as the nerve compression is released. Pressure applied to a superficial nerve, distally, gives numbness and some tingling, with the edge of the affected region being well defined (Cyriax, 1982).

### Irritability

Irritability may be defined as 'the vigour of activity which causes pain' (Maitland, 1991). It is determined by the degree of pain which the patient experiences, and the time this takes to subside, in relation to the intensity of activity that brought the pain on in the first place. The purpose of assessing irritability is to determine how much activity (joint mobilization, exercise, etc.) may be prescribed without exacerbating the patient's symptoms.

An assessment of irritability may be made at the second treatment session. The amount of movement which the patient was subjected to in the previous session is known, as is the discomfort that he or she feels now. These subjective feelings are then used to determine the intensity of the second treatment session. Similarly, at the beginning of each subsequent treatment session the irritability is again assessed.

## Pain production

Free or 'bare' nerve endings (type IV) respond to painful stimuli and are termed nociceptors (from the Latin *nocere*, to damage). They are largely unresponsive to normal stimuli, but have a low threshold to mechanical and thermal injury, anoxia, and irritation from inflammatory products. Tissues vary in the intensity of pain they will produce when stimulated. The joint capsule and periosteum are the most sensitive to noxious stimuli. Subchondral bone, tendons and ligaments are the next in line in terms of sensitivity, followed by muscle and cortical bone. The synovium and cartilage are largely insensitive.

The pain receptors are supplied by a variety of different nerve fibres. Skin receptors are supplied by thinly myelinated (A delta) fibres which carry 'fast' pain and respond to strong mechanical stimuli and heat above 45°C (Low and Reed, 1990). They give the initial sharp well-localized pain feeling. The function of fast pain is to help the body to avoid tissue damage, and it often provokes a flexor withdrawal reflex.

Impulses from free nerve endings found in deeper body tissues are carried by non-myelinated C fibres. This is 'slow' pain, which tends to be aching and throbbing in nature, and poorly defined. Its onset is not immediate, and the sensation it produces persists after the pain stimulus has gone. The function of slow pain seems to be to enforce inactivity and allow healing to occur and it is therefore often associated with muscle spasm. The C fibres respond to many different types of stimuli and, as such, are said to be 'polymodal'. However, they are most sensitive to chemicals released as a result of tissue damage. Histamine, kinins, prostaglandins E1 and E2, and 5–HT have all been implicated in this type of pain production during inflammation (Lachman, 1988; Walter and Israel, 1987).

It can be seen that the pain experienced as a result of sporting injury will usually be either mechanical or chemical in nature. Mechanical pain is the result of forces which deform, or damage the nociceptive nerve endings, and so may be caused by stretching contracted tissue or by fluid pressure. This type of pain is influenced by movement.

Chemical pain on the other hand, results from irritation of the nerve endings, and is less affected by movement or joint position, but will respond to rest.

## Articular neurology

In addition to pain receptors (type IV), three other joint receptors are important. Type I receptors are located in the superficial layers of the joint capsule. They are slow adapting, low threshold mechanoreceptors, which respond to both static and dynamic stimulation. These receptors provide information about the static position of a joint, and contribute to the regulation of muscle tone and movement (kinaesthetic) sense. The type I receptors sense both the speed and direction of movement.

Type II receptors are found mainly in the deeper capsular layers, and within fat pads. These are dynamic receptors with a high threshold, and they adapt quickly. They respond to rapid changes in direction of joint movement.

The type III receptors are found in the joint ligaments, and are also high-threshold dynamic mechanoreceptors, but are slow adapting. These receptors monitor the direction of movement, and have a 'braking' effect on muscle tone if the joint is moving too quickly or through too great a range of motion.

The type IV receptors are the nociceptors described above. Table 2.1 provides a synopsis of the various movement categories to which the receptors respond.

Alteration in the feedback provided by joint receptors is of great importance following sports injury. The importance of balance exercises follow-

**Table 2.1 Function of joint receptors**

| Function | Receptor |
| --- | --- |
| Static position | Type I |
| Speed of movement | Type I |
| Change in speed | Type II |
| Direction of movement | Types I and II |
| Postural muscle tone | Type I |
| Tone at initiation of movement | Type II |
| Tone during movement | Type II |
| Tone during harmful movements | Type III |

Adapted from Hertling and Kessler (1990).

ing ankle injury has been emphasized by a number of authors (Freeman, Dean and Hanham, 1965; Glencross and Thornton, 1981; Gauffin, Tropp and Olenrick, 1988; Lentell, Katzman and Walters, 1990), and reflex quadriceps weakness following joint distension has been described (De Andrade, Grant and Dixon, 1965; Stokes and Young, 1984) .

### Pain pathways

Three categories or 'orders' of neurone make up the pain pathways. First order neurones travel from the pain receptors to the spinal cord, second order neurones travel within the spinal cord to the brainstem and third order neurones travel from the brainstem to the higher centres of the cerebral cortex.

Seventy percent of the C fibres (slow pain) enter the spine via the dorsal root, while 30% enter via the ventral root. The C fibres synapse with second order neurones in the substantia gelatinosa of the spinal cord and these neurones ascend in the anterolateral funiculus on the opposite side of the spinal cord (Fig. 2.3). From here they travel via the reticular formation to the intralaminar nuclei of the thalamus. The neurones synapse here once more and travel to the prefrontal region of the cerebral cortex.

The A delta fibres (fast pain), on the other hand, synapse in the outer part of the posterior horn of the cord and cross to ascend in the spinothalamic tract to the ventrobasal nuclei in the thalamus, and then to the postcentral gyrus of the cortex.

Fast pain is registered in the parietal lobe and visceral pain in the insula cortex. Emotional res-

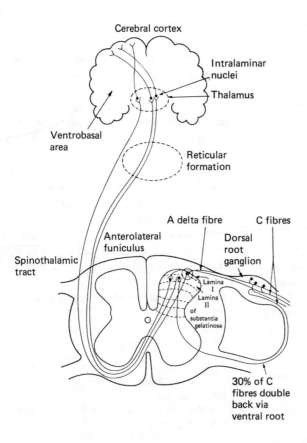

**Figure 2.3**  Pain pathways. From Low and Reed (1990) with permission.

ponses to pain (see p.52) are generated in the limbic system and states of anxiety, fear and dread of pain are generated by the frontal lobes.

### Pain relief mechanisms

Three concepts of pain control are generally used in physiotherapy. First, stimulation of ascending fibres to block pain messages (pain gate theory), secondly, endogenous opioid formation, and thirdly, descending fibre stimulation within the dorsal horn of the spinal cord (descending inhibition).

### The pain gate

The pain gate theory (Melzack and Wall, 1965) proposed that pain perception was regulated by a 'gate' which could be opened or closed. When stimulated, mechanoreceptors in the skin send impulses via A beta fibres to the posterior horn of the spinal cord. Here, collateral branches are given off. These collaterals affect A delta and C pain fibres in the substantia gelatinosa (SG), reducing their excitability by presynaptic inhibition. Stimulation of A delta fibres by low intensity, high frequency transcutaneous electrical nerve stimulation (TENS) (100–200 Hz) will therefore reduce pain through this gating mechanism (Fig. 2.4).

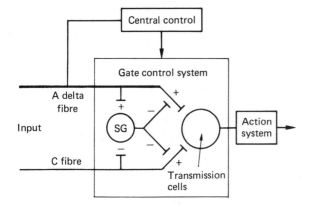

**Figure 2.4**  The pain gate mechanism. Central control — effects caused by higher centre (brain); action system — pain response. SG, substantia gelatinosa. From Melzack and Wall (1965), with permission.

### Endogenous opioids

Interneurones within the substantia gelatinosa are able to produce endogenous (made in the body) opioid peptides, with similar effects to opioids such as morphine, heroin, and codeine, which are some of the most powerful analgesics known. These opioids inhibit C fibre cells. Collateral branches of A delta fibres in the posterior horn connect to the interneurones and stimulate them to produce opioids.

The opioids, including enkephalins and endorphins are produced in various areas of the central nervous system, including the limbic system and thalamus, the pituitary gland, the substantia gelatinosa, and nerve terminals. These substances inhibit transmission in the A delta and C fibre pathways and so block pain before it reaches sensory levels. Stimulation of the A delta fibres with high intensity low frequency TENS (2–10 Hz) will damp down C fibre activity and reduce pain through this method.

### Descending inhibition

In addition, activity of the A delta fibres may provoke impulses from the periaqueductal grey matter of the midbrain. These impulses travel back down the spinal cord to inhibit nociceptor neurones. Inhibition is by the release of serotonin and possibly noradrenaline. Stimulation at frequencies above 50 Hz may affect this system (De Domenico, 1982).

## Management of inflammation

The effects of acute inflammation can be reduced by slowing the body's response represented by the cardinal signs. Redness and heat are therefore treated by trying to reduce localized bleeding by the use of cold or ice and compression. Swelling is similarly managed by the use of compression to contain local oedema, and gentle movement to assess lymphatic drainage. By reducing the chemical and mechanical effects of the three inflammatory signs above, pain is also reduced.

Various anti-inflammatory drugs are used to reduce acute inflammation, and especially pain. Their effects are usually by modification of prostaglandins. The effects of various types of electrotherapy and cryotherapy are discussed in Chapter 7. The amount of rest prescribed during inflammation will depend on the stage of inflammation and the amount of tissue damage.

## Repair

Inflammation may continue for up to five days, but with minor trauma it is usually finished by the third day after injury (Evans, 1980). Tissue repair can then take place. Repair is by resolution, organization or regeneration, depending on the severity of the injury and the nature of the injured tissues.

A minor injury will result in acute inflammation as described above, and the phagocytic cells will clear the area. If there is little tissue damage, the stage of resolution will result in a return to near normal (Lachman, 1988). True resolution rarely occurs with soft tissue injuries, but is more common with inflammatory tissue reactions, such as pneumonia.

On the periphery of the injured area, macrophages and polymorphs are active because they can tolerate the low oxygen levels present in the damaged tissue. Cellular division by mitosis is seen in the surrounding capillaries about 12 hours after injury. During the next three days capillary buds form and grow towards the lower oxygen concentration of the injured area. These capillaries form loops and blood begins to flow through them. This new capillary-rich material is known as granulation tissue. Plasma proteins, cells and fluid pour out of these highly permeable vessels. The gradually increasing oxygen supply to the previously deoxygenated area means phagocytosis can now begin.

New lymphatic vessels bud out from the existing lymphatics, linking to form a renewed lymphatic drainage system. As this process is occurring, fibroblast cells multiply and move towards the injured tissue. By the fifth day after injury they begin to lay down fibrils of collagen, a process requiring adequate amounts of vitamin C.

The individual fibrils form into parallel bundles lying in the direction of stress imposed on the tissue. If no movement occurs to stress the collagen bundles, they are laid down in a haphazard and weaker pattern (Cyriax, 1982). Controlled movement causes the fibrils to align lengthways along the line of stress of the injured structure (Burri, Helbing and Spier, 1973). External mechanical factors then, and not the previous organization of the tissue, dictate the eventual pattern of fibril arrangement (Stearns, 1940). Total rest during this stage of healing is therefore contraindicated in most cases.

In some tissue, regeneration occurs, damaged cells are replaced by functioning normal tissue. Fractured bone exhibits this property, as do torn ligaments and peripheral nerves, providing conditions are suitable (Evans, 1990).

## Remodelling

The remodelling stage overlaps with repair, and may last from three weeks to 12 months (Kellett, 1986). During this stage, collagen is modified to increase its functional capacity. Remodelling is characterized by a reduction in the wound size, an increase in scar strength and an alteration in the direction of the collagen fibres (Van der Meulen, 1982).

Contraction of granulation tissue will occur for as long as the elasticity of the fibres will allow (Van der Meulen, 1982). Fibroblast cells transform into myofibroblasts which then form intercellular bonds. These contain contractile proteins (actomyosin) and behave much like smooth muscle fibres.

Three weeks after injury, the quantity of collagen has stabilized (Van der Meulen, 1982) but the strength of the fibres continues to increase. Strength increases are a result of an expansion in the number of cross-bonds between the cells, and the replacement collagen cells themselves. There is a continuous turnover of collagen, a process influenced by a number of factors, including the age of the patient, the type of tissue injured, the quantity of scar tissue present, the site and direction of the scar and external forces (Van der Meulen, 1982; Frank et al., 1983).

# Tissue response to injury

In this section the responses of the individual tissues to injury, and the effects these have upon subsequent rehabilitation are examined. Aspects of tissue structure relevant to sports injury are discussed.

## Synovial membrane

The synovium consists of two layers, the intima, or synovial lining, and the subsynovial (subintimal) tissue. The intimal layer is made up of specialized cells, known as synoviocytes, arranged in multiple layers. Two types of synoviocytes are present, type A cells, which are phagocytic, and type B cells, which synthesize the hyaluronoprotein of the synovial fluid. The two types are not distinct however, and appear to be functional stages of the same basic cells (Hettinga, 1990).

The subsynovial tissue lies beneath the intima as a loose network of highly vascular connective tissue. Cells are interspaced with collagen fibres and fatty tissue. The subsynovial tissue itself merges with the periosteum of bone lying within the synovial membrane of the joint. Similar merging occurs with the joint cartilage through a transitional layer of fibrocartilage.

The blood vessels of the joint divide into three branches, one travelling to the epiphysis, the second to the joint capsule and the third to the synovial membrane (Paget and Bullough, 1981). From here the vessels of the subsynovium are of two types. The first is thin walled and adapted for fluid exchange, and the second thick walled and capable of gapping to allow particles, especially nutrients, to pass through.

Once free of the vessels, any material must pass through the synovial interstitium before entering the synovial fluid itself. The passage of this material is by diffusion on the whole, but by active transport for glucose molecules.

The synovium must adapt to movement with normal function of the joint. Rather than stretching, the synovium unfolds to facilitate flexion. The synovium is well lubricated by the same hyaluronate molecules found within the synovial fluid itself, and so the various layers slide over each other. Since the synovium must alter shape within the confines of the joint capsule, the process of synovial adaptation is at its best when the fluid volume of the joint is at a minimum.

Synovial fluid plays a significant role in joint stability. The negative atmospheric pressure within the joint creates a suction effect, which, aided by the surface tension of the synovial fluid, draws the bony surfaces of the joint together.

### Response to injury

With minor trauma the synovium is not microscopically disturbed, but will instead suffer a vasomotor reaction (Hettinga, 1990). The capillaries of the synovium will dilate and fluid filtration increase. Protein will leak into the interstitium, changing the osmotic pressure and causing local oedema and joint exudation. This process constitutes a post-traumatic synovitis.

The slight hyperaemia gives way later to alterations of the intimal layer, the total number of layers increasing three-fold. If the trauma does not continue, the protein molecules which were released are cleared by the lymphatics and the osmotic pressures return to normal. If mechanical irritation persists, the intimal layer will continue to thicken. The deep synovial cells now show increased activity and protein synthesis escalates.

Alterations occur in the number of type A and type B synoviocyte cells. The number of type A cells reduces as some of these move into the synovial fluid to become macrophages. The synovial lining becomes filled with fibroblasts, which in turn change into type B cells. Neutrophil cells die, releasing proteolytic enzymes which attack the near joint structures. This process can self-perpetuate the synovitis even in the absence of further trauma, giving rise to a reactive synovitis.

Onset of symptoms following post-traumatic synovitis usually occurs between 12–24 hours after injury and can last for between one and two weeks. Patients complain mainly of joint tightness, with warmth, erythema and pain being encountered less often. The tightness is due to joint effusion, the increased fluid volume causing the normally negative intra-articular pressure to become positive.

The stability of the joint, no longer created by a negative intra-articular pressure, comes from joint distension instead. This places a traction force on the joint capsule and surrounding ligaments. Pressures are greatest in the effused joint in extremes of flexion and extension, and are reduced at about 30° flexion, this being the resting position (loose pack) taken up by the patient (Table 1.1, p. 17). Haemarthrosis is usually present if swelling occurs within two hours of injury, and pain is intense.

### Synovial fluid

Synovial fluid is similar in many ways to blood plasma. The main difference being that synovia does not contain fibrinogen or prothrombin and so is unable to clot. The mucopolysaccharide hyaluronate (hyaluronic acid), secreted by the synoviocytes, is contained within the fluid.

The amount of synovial fluid present in a joint is very little, about 0.5–4 ml in large joints such as the knee, and this is spread throughout the joint by structures such as the cartilage, menisci and fat pads.

Synovial fluid is highly viscous and becomes more elastic as the rate of joint movement increases. As weight is taken by the joint, synovial fluid is squeezed out from between the opposing joint surfaces. This is resisted by the tenacity of the fluid itself.

As the joint moves, the synovial fluid is pulled in the direction of movement and so a layer of fluid is maintained between the joint surfaces. Any friction produced by movement will therefore occur within the synovial fluid rather than between the joint surfaces. When the joint is statically loaded, however, fluid flows away from the point of maximal load and the joint relies on the articular cartilage to provide lubrication (see below). The synovial fluid provides nutrition for about two thirds of the articular cartilage bordering the joint space.

Following injury, the fluid volume may increase as much as ten or 20 times, with a decrease in hyaluronate and, with it, fluid viscosity. Pain due to the accumulation of synovial fluid is dependent

not on the amount of fluid present, but on the speed with which it forms. Blau (1979) claimed that as much as 100 ml may be extracted from an injured joint which caused little pain because the fluid took a long time to form, while 15 ml may be exquisitely painful if formed rapidly following trauma.

With injury in which bleeding is not present, the constituents of the synovial fluid remain basically the same. In reactive synovitis, the protein concentration is slightly elevated, and the number of white blood cells increases somewhat from normal values of 100/ml to as much as 300/ml. With post-traumatic synovitis however, the white cell count is further increased, to as much as 2000/ml.

Haemarthrosis (blood within the joint) causes rapidly developing fluid, which contains fibrinogen. If the synovial membrane is torn, fat may enter the joint from the extrasynovial adipose tissue and will be seen in the synovial fluid. The blood from haemarthrosis will mostly remain fluid, and is quickly absorbed by the phagocytic cells, to disappear after several days.

### Bone

*Types*

Bone is essentially a fibrous matrix impregnated by mineral salts (mainly calcium phosphate), and it therefore combines the properties of both elasticity and rigidity. It is a living tissue, which is continually remodelled, and subject to hormonal control.

Two sorts of bone are generally described, cancellous or spongy bone and compact bone, and important differences exist in both their mechanical properties and methods of healing. Cancellous bone is found at a number of sites, including the bone ends and block like bones of the foot and wrist. It is arranged in a system of trabeculae aligned to resist imposed stresses. The shaft of a long bone consists of a ring of compact bone surrounding a hollow cavity. This structure is surrounded in turn by a further layer of compact bone. The bone cavity contains bone marrow. In infants the bone marrow is red, but this is gradually replaced by yellow bone marrow until, by puberty, only the cancellous bone cavities at the ends of the long bones contain red bone marrow. With age, the bone marrow in these cavities too is replaced, but red bone marrow may still be found in the vertebrae, sternum, and ribs, as well as the proximal ends of the femur and humerus.

The bone is enclosed in a dense membrane called the periosteum, which is absent in the region of the articular cartilage. The periosteum is highly vascular and responsible for the nutrition of the bone cortex which underlies it. The deep layers of periosteum contain bone-forming cells (osteoblasts). These lay down successive layers of bone during growth, and so the periosteum is responsible for alterations in the bone width, in addition these cells play an important part in bone healing. A direct blow to the bone which produces bleeding beneath the periosteum will lift it, causing bone deposition by the osteoblasts. This is a common problem over the anterior tibia in footballers and hockey players.

The bone cavity is lined by bone destroying cells (osteoclasts) which erode the inner surface of the bone. The balance between bone deposition by osteoblasts and bone reabsorption by osteoclasts keeps the bone width constant.

Bone may be further classified into four major types according to shape. The long bones are found within the limbs, and consist of a shaft and two enlarged ends. Short bones have a block-like appearance, such as those of the carpals, and are mainly cancellous bone. Flat bones are thinner, and consist of two layers of compact bone sandwiching a thin layer of cancellous bone, examples are the skull vaults and the ribs. Finally, irregular bones consist of a thin layer of compact bone surrounded by cancellous bone, for example the vertebrae.

## Development

Skeletal development begins with loosely arranged mesodermal cells which are mostly converted to hyaline cartilage. Between the seventh and twelfth intrauterine week a primary ossification centre appears within the shaft of the long bone, and spreads towards the bone ends. The centre of the shaft is hollowed out and filled with red bone marrow, and the whole shaft is called a diaphysis.

At the end of the bone, secondary centres of ossification appear, usually after birth. The main part of the cartilage is gradually replaced, leaving only the articular cartilage, and a cartilage plate (epiphyseal growth plate) between the shaft and end of the bone.

The growth plate is of great importance in paediatric sports medicine. This cartilage layer is responsible for the increase in bone length. As the cartilage grows it becomes thicker, and its upper and lower surfaces are converted to bone. Eventually, the cartilage stops growing, but its ossification continues, so that the cartilage becomes thinner, until it eventually disappears. At this point, the diaphysis and epiphysis are united, and growth in length of the bone is no longer possible. The point at which this occurs may be influenced by a number of factors, including impact stresses (see below).

Intramembranous ossification occurs in the mandible, clavicle and certain bones of the skull (Palastanga, Field and Soames, 1989). Here, the intermediate stage of cartilage formation is omitted and the bone ossifies directly from connective tissue.

## Epiphyseal injury

There are two types of epiphysis. Pressure epiphyses are found at the end of long bones, and are interarticular. They are subjected to compression stress with weightbearing, and are responsible for changes in bone length. Traction epiphyses (apophyses) occur at the insertion of major muscles. They experience tension stress as the muscles contract, and alter bone shape.

The growth plate itself forms a weak link in the immature skeleton, and shearing or avulsion stresses can cause it to be dislodged. Because the epiphyses are weaker than the major joint structures, injuries which in the adult would cause dislocation or tendon rupture, may cause epiphyseal injury in the child.

Five types of injury have been described (Salter and Harris, 1963) as shown in Fig. 2.5. Gentle manipulation under anaesthetic is normally used to realign the epiphysis in the first three types. Crush injuries and those through the growth plate may

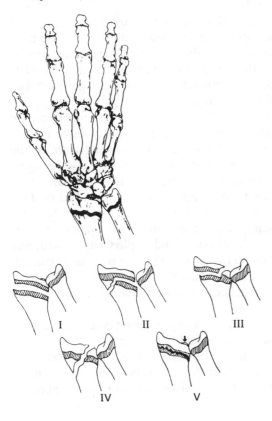

Figure 2.5   Epiphyseal injuries. After Salter and Harris (1963).

cause more severe problems of growth disturbance. When a fracture crosses the growth plate, bone may fill the gap formed, causing unequal growth. Crush injuries may lead to premature closure of the plate with associated deformities of shortening and altered bony angulation.

## Osteochondrosis

Osteochondrosis (osteochondritis) affects the pressure epiphyses during their growth period. There is interference with the epiphyseal blood supply, causing avascular necrosis to the secondary ossification centre. The bone within the epiphysis softens, dies, and is absorbed (Fig. 2.6). Because the cap of articular cartilage surrounding the epiphysis receives nutrition from the synovial fluid, it remains largely unaffected. The combination of softening bone contained within an intact articular cap leads to flattening of the epiphysis. Gradually the dead

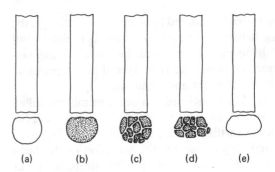

Figure 2.6   Stages of osteochondritis. (a) Normal epiphysis. (b) The bony nucleus undergoes necrosis, loses its normal texture and becomes granular. (c) The bony nucleus becomes fragmented during the process of removal of dead bone. (d) If subjected to pressure the softened epiphysis becomes flattened. (e) Re-ossification with restoration of normal bone texture, but deformity may persist. The whole process takes two to three years. From Gartland (1987), with permission.

bone is replaced by new bone by a process of 'creeping substitution'. Trauma may be one factor which initiates the ischaemic process, either through direct injury or vascular occlusion as a result of traumatic synovitis (Gartland, 1987).

Any pressure epiphysis may be affected, the condition taking the name of the person who first described it in that region. Perthes' disease affects the hip, Freibergs's disease the second metatarsal, Kohler's disease the navicular bone. In addition, three other epiphyseal disorders are important in sport, Scheuermanns' disease affecting the thoracic spine, Sever's disease affecting the calcaneal insertion of the Achilles tendon, and Osgood–Schlatter's disease affecting the tibial tubercle. These have traditionally been described as osteochondrosis, but they do not show avascular necrosis and so are different histologically.

## Healing

Bone healing is governed by a number of factors, including the type of tissue which is damaged, the extent of the damage and the position of the bony fragments, the amount of movement present at the fracture site as healing progresses, and the blood supply. In a long bone, healing may be divided into five stages, as shown in Fig. 2.7 (Crawford-Adams,

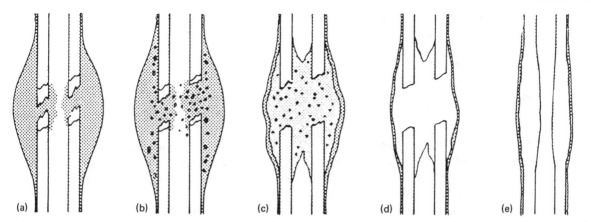

**Figure 2.7** Stages in fracture healing. (a) Haematoma: tissue damage and bleeding occur at the fracture site, the bone ends die back a few millimetres. (b) Inflammation: inflammatory cells appear in the haematoma. (c) Callus: The cell population changes to osteoblasts and osteoclasts, dead bone is mopped up and woven bone appears in the fracture callus. (d) Consolidation: woven bone is replaced by lamellar bone and the fracture is solidly united. (e) Remodelling: the newly-formed bone is remodelled to resemble the normal structure. From Apley and Solomon (1988), with permission.

1978; Apley and Solomon, 1988). The first stage is that of tissue destruction and haematoma formation. As local blood vessels are torn at the time of injury, blood is released, forming a haematoma within and surrounding the fracture site. The bone periosteum and surrounding soft tissues contain the blood, and the periosteum itself is lifted from the bone surface. The deprivation of blood to the bone surfaces immediately adjacent to the fracture line causes these surfaces to die back for up to two millimetres. Some eight hours after fracture, inflammation and proliferation may be detected as stage two of healing. The deep periosteal cells, and those of the damaged medullary canal, proliferate, and cellular tissue begins to grow forward to meet similar material from the other side of the fracture site and bridge the area. Capillary growth into the region allows the haematoma to be slowly reabsorbed. The congealed blood itself takes little part in the repair process.

The appearance of osteogenic and chondrogenic cells marks the beginning of the third stage of healing. New bone and, in some cases, cartilage is laid down, while osteoclastic cells remove remaining dead bone. The cellular mass which forms is called a callus, and becomes increasingly mineralized into woven bone, uniting the fracture. The callus is larger where there has been much periosteal stripping, when bone displacement is marked, and if the haematoma has been large. The woven bone is transformed into lamellar bone by osteoblasts in the fourth stage of healing.

As the fracture site is bridged by solid bone, the fifth and final stage of healing commences, that of remodelling. A combination of bone reabsorption and formation reshapes the callus, laying down thicker lamellae in areas of high stress and removing excessive bone. The medullary cavity is reformed.

The rate of healing is dependent on a number of factors. The type of bone is important, cancellous bone healing far more quickly than cortical bone. Also, the fracture type will dictate the speed of healing, with a spiral fracture healing more quickly than a transverse type. If the blood supply has been compromised at the time of injury, or if the fracture has occurred in an area with a poor blood supply, the healing rate will be slower. The age and health of the patient are other determining factors, with fractures in children healing almost twice as fast as those in adults. In general terms, callus may be visible radiographically within two to three weeks of injury, with firm fracture union taking about four to six weeks for upper limb fractures and eight to 12 weeks for those in the lower limb. Full consolidation may take as much as eight and

16 weeks for upper and lower limb fractures, respectively.

In contrast to long bone, cancellous bone remains fairly immobile when fractured, and heals by 'direct repair' with a minimum of callus formation. The difference mainly occurs because there is no medullary canal in cancellous bone, and the area of contact between the two injured bone fragments is much greater. Following haematoma formation, new blood vessels and osteogenic cells penetrate the area and meet similar tissue from the opposite bone fragment. The intercellular matrix which is laid down by osteoblasts is calcified into woven bone. This type of healing also occurs when internal fixation is used.

### Mechanical properties

Bone responds to mechanical stress in similar ways to other connective tissue, but at a considerably slower rate. Its ability to adapt its structure, size and shape depends on the mechanical stresses placed upon it. When stress is reduced, by prolonged bed rest for example, mineral reabsorption occurs and the bone reduces in strength. Raising stress to an optimal level, by exercise, leads to an increase in bone strength. In addition to changes in total mineral content, bone varies its strength according to the direction of the imposed stress. At bony attachment sites, such as tubercles, the alignment of collagen fibres is parallel to the direction of the imposed force. In the shaft of a long bone, fibre orientation is along the bone axis, indicating that this part of the bone is designed to resist tension and compression forces. In cancellous bone at the epiphysis, shear stresses are maximal and so fibre alignment is in the direction of the shearing forces.

A number of mechanisms have been proposed to explain how the bone remodels to imposed stress. Bassett (1965) argued that, in theory, mechanical stresses on bone create electrical charges (piezoelectric effect). Areas of compression were said to develop negative charges, while those subjected to tensile stress are more positive. The suggestion is that bone deposition by osteoblasts occurs in negatively charged areas, while reabsorption by osteoclasts takes place in regions of positive excitation. Experiments with dogs (Bassett and Pawlick,

1964) have shown that new bone is laid down at an implanted cathode site, although other authors have described bone deposition at both negative and positive sites (Hert and Zalud, 1971) so the effects of polarity are still uncertain.

Electrical fields formed in bone as a result of imposed stresses have been shown to stimulate protein synthesis in frog osteogenic cells (Becker and Murray, 1970), and increased rate of bone formation has been shown as a result of direct current (d.c.) administered through implanted electrodes (Becker, Spadaro and Mariho, 1977).

Bone trabeculae subjected to maximum stress will be strengthened by bone deposition, in the direction of the imposed force. Regions of high stress have denser trabeculae, aligned to minimize the bending effect on a bone. When a bone is subjected to an unbalanced force which would tend to bend it, remodelling occurs as a result of changes in surface strain (Riegger, 1990). On the convex surface of the bone, osteoclastic activity leads to bone reabsorption, while on the concave surface the reverse occurs and bone deposition is seen. Bone therefore moves towards the concavity which has been induced through loading of the shaft, to minimize the bending effect, a process known as flexural-drift. The stress imposed on the bone causes an increase in the calcium concentration in the interstitial fluid, as a result of changes in bone crystal solubility.

### Stress fractures

Stress fractures are usually the end point in a sequence of overuse. A number of causal factors usually co-exist to begin the development of the condition. Training errors may account for 60–75% of such injuries in runners (McBryde, 1985). Common faults include high intensity work carried out for too long with an inadequate recovery. A distance runner who suddenly increases mileage, or a throwing athlete whose training is too intense are typical examples. Faulty footwear, which fails to attenuate shock, and exercising on unforgiving surfaces will also contribute to lower limb pathology. These factors, coupled with an underlying malalignment problem of the lower limb, or biomechanical faults in technique of upper limb actions will exacerbate the problem. With novice runners, an additional factor is muscular weakness in the lower extremity, leading to a reduction in shock-absorbing capacity of the soft tissues. In each case the overload on the tissues exceeds their elastic limit, causing a plastic deformation of the bone (p.7).

Far from being inert, bone is a dynamic tissue which is continually remodelling in response to mechanical stress. A balance usually exists between bone proliferation and reabsorption, which maintains the bone integrity. The result of athletic activity is normally that the bone strengthens, but if unbalanced stresses cause bone reabsorption to exceed proliferation, the bone weakens. Examining excessive running and jumping in rabbits, Li et al. (1985) demonstrated that osteoblastic activity occurred from seven to nine days later than osteoclastic activity. Remodelling began on day two, with the haversian blood vessels dilating and by day seven osteoclastic activity was noted in the bone cortex. New bone formation began in the periosteum by the fourteenth day of excessive stress. The adaptation to this excessive stress was reabsorption, which occurred for some time before the formation of new cortical bone, thus weakening the bone structure. Abnormal X-rays were not found until day 21 after the stress was imposed.

Angular stresses in particular may cause failure of the bone with a resultant stress fracture. Two theories are generally accepted for the mechanisms by which stress affects bone. The first (fatigue), proposes that training which is too intense causes the muscles to fatigue so that they are no longer able to support the skeleton and absorb shock. The strain passes to the bone causing the fracture. The second theory (overload) suggests that when certain muscles contract, they cause the bones to bend slightly. Training which is too intense will exceed the capacity of the bone to recover from this stress.

Symptoms include warmth and tenderness over the injured area, made worse with sporting activity and better with rest. Initially, radiographs are usually negative, it taking at least two weeks for X-ray changes to be apparent (Li et al., 1985; Rzonca and Baylis, 1988). A bone scan, however, is normally revealing at the onset of symptoms and is generally more reliable. Taunton and Clement (1981) found radiographs to be positive in only 47.2% of cases, while bone scan was accurate in 95.8%. However, bone scan is expensive and not widely available in some countries so clinical examination must be relied on. Pain may be produced over the superficial fracture site by vibration. This may be produced from a tuning fork or ultrasound unit (Moss and Mowat, 1983; Lowden, 1986), and is generally of more use in low risk areas such as the foot and shin. Where there is a risk of complication through displacement, such as in the neck of the femur, bone scan with possible surgical intervention may be more appropriate. The most common areas for stress fracture in runners are the tibia (34%), fibula (24%), and metatarsals (20%)(McBryde, 1985).

Treatment of a stress fracture is primarily that of rest. Ice may be used to reduce pain, and electrical stimulation used to increase the rate of bone healing (see p.132). Removal of the causal stress is important for the prevention of recurrence. This may mean adaptation of training or modification of malalignment in the lower limb.

### Osteoporosis

Osteoporosis involves a progressive decrease in bone density, due to an imbalance between bone formation and bone reabsorption. Bone loss occurs normally in both sexes with ageing, but the rate is increased markedly with osteoporosis. Normal bone loss of 3% per decade may increase to as much as 10% per decade for trabecular bone.

Osteoporosis may be either primary, governed by age and sex, or secondary, as a result of disease. The most common primary types are postmenopausal osteoporosis and senile osteoporosis. The loss of mass makes the bone suspectible to fracture, particularly as a result of microtrauma. Common fracture sites include the distal radius and vertebrae for post-menopausal osteoporosis, and the proximal femur for senile osteoporosis. Fracture of the distal radius presents as a Colles' fracture, while vertebral wedging gives rise to an increased thoracic kyphosis or 'dowagers hump'. Three main factors are important in the development of this condition, diet, oestrogen level, and physical activity.

## Diet

Modern diet can fail to provide an adequate daily intake of calcium. Recommended requirements as high as 1500 mg of calcium and 400 IU of vitamin D have been made for post-menopausal women (MacKinnon, 1988), but many women may consume as little as 300 mg of calcium (McArdle, Katch and Katch, 1986), thus placing themselves in negative calcium balance.

Calcium deficiency in animals has been shown to lead to osteoporosis (Martin and Houston, 1987), but effects in humans are less clear. Studying early post-menopausal women, Nilas, Christiansen and Rodbro (1984) gave a 500 mg calcium supplement over a two year period and assessed bone density in the distal radius, while Ettinger Genant and Cann (1987) gave a 1000 mg supplement and assessed the lumbar vertebrae. Both of these studies failed to show any significant differences between the treatment and non-treatment groups. However, in late post-menopausal women calcium supplementation may be beneficial (MacKinnon, 1988).

Adequate calcium is clearly necessary for health, and those individuals who show a deficiency in their calcium intake may need dietary supplementation. Others should receive advice on good diet to enable them to maintain an adequate intake of calcium and vitamin D, remembering that excessive vitamin D intake can be toxic.

## Exercise

Weight-bearing exercise creates bone stress and acts as a stimulus for maintaining bone mass. Loss of bone mass has been reported both as a result of prolonged bed rest (Donaldson, Hulley and Vogel, 1970) and following weightlessness (Mazess and Whedon, 1983). Similarly, athletes have been shown to have greater bone density than non-athletes (Nilsson and Westlin, 1977), and tennis players have been shown to have a greater bone density in their dominant arm (Huddleston, Rockwell and Kuland, 1980).

A number of authors have demonstrated the beneficial effects of weight-bearing exercise in slowing bone loss. Smith, Smith and Ensign (1984) assessed the effects of exercise (45min, three days per week) on bone loss in post-menopausal women and showed a 1.4% increase in bone mass during the second and third years of their study. Krolner, Toft and Nielsen (1983) studied the effects of exercise (one hour, twice per week) on post-menopausal women. They showed a 3.5% increase in bone mineral content of the lumber spine for the exercising group compared with 2.7% for their control.

Clearly, regular weight-bearing exercise is important in the prevention and management of osteoporosis. However, the increased risk of fracture in this group means that care must be taken. Repeated spinal rotation or flexion should be avoided, as should high impact activities, especially if osteoporosis already exists.

## Hormone replacement therapy

The use of low dosage oestrogen in hormone replacement therapy (HRT) to slow or even halt bone loss in post-menopausal women is widely recommended. HRT is used to compensate for the decline in oestrogen levels that occurs during the menopause. Oestrogen plays an important part in calcium absorption by the body. Secreted by the ovaries and corpus luteum, oestrogen (a steroid hormone) stimulates regeneration of the endometrium, increases mucus output from the cervical glands, and promotes epiphyseal closure and growth of the bones and skeletal muscle.

HRT has been linked with an increased risk of endometrial carcinoma, although the risk is reduced when oestrogen is combined with progesterone (Hedlund and Gallagher, 1988).

## Articular cartilage

Cartilage is essentially a connective tissue consisting of cells embedded in a matrix permeated by fibres. Two major types are recognized, hyaline cartilage and fibrocartilage. Hyaline cartilage is found over bone ends and is described in more detail below. Fibrocartilage may be either white or yellow. White fibrocartilage is found in areas such as the intervertebral discs and glenoid labrum. Yellow fibrocartilage is found in structures such as the ears and larynx.

Articular (hyaline) cartilage is made up of collagen fibres, a protein–polysaccharide complex, and water. Fibres of collagen are embedded in a ground substance of gel-like material. The water content of cartilage is high, between 70 and 80% of its total weight (Bullough, 1981).

Cartilage has no blood vessels, lymphatics or nerve fibres. Nutrition is supplied directly from the synovial fluid, and by diffusion of blood products from the sub-chondral bone. The tangled structure of cartilage causes it to behave in some ways like a microscopic sieve, filtering out large molecules such as plasma proteins. Fluid movement through the cartilage is by osmosis and diffusion. Movement of the joint increases the rate of diffusion, but in the mature joint there is no transfer across the bone–cartilage interface (Hettinga, 1990).

Intermittent loading creates a pumping effect, squeezing fluid from the cartilage and allowing fresh fluid to be taken up as the load is released. Prolonged loading will gradually press fluid out of the cartilage, without allowing new fluid to be taken up. As much as a 40% reduction in cartilage depth can occur by compression (Hettinga, 1990).

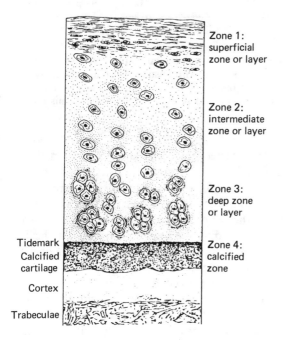

**Figure 2.8** Zones in articular cartilage. From Gould (1990), with permission.

The cartilage is arranged in four layers (Fig. 2.8). The collagen fibres of the calcified zone bind the cartilage to the sub-chondral bone, resisting shear stresses. Within the mid-zone the fibres are randomly oriented. With joint compression, these fibres stretch and will resist the tension forces created within them (Fig. 2.9). This property of elastic deformation (spring) occurs instantly. However, the fluid within the matrix of the cartilage will be compressed. As it does so, proteoglycans within the cartilage will tend to retain water and control its movement through the cartilage matrix. The cartilage will slowly flow away from the compression force, demonstrating the property of creep. When the load is removed, the fluid lost at the time of compression is reabsorbed. These two properties of instant spring and slower creep make cartilage a viscoelastic material (see p.7).

Cartilage assists joint lubrication by two processes, called boundary and weeping lubrication. Boundary lubrication occurs when hyaluronic acid molecules found in the joints' synovial fluid adhere momentarily to the cartilage surfaces of the joint. As the joint moves, the two molecular layers slide, a system which occurs mostly under light loads.

Weeping or fluid lubrication occurs when the cartilage is loaded and releases fluid which lies between the opposing surfaces—so-called squeeze film lubrication. The layer of fluid (the squeeze film) is under pressure and so keeps the cartilage surfaces apart. The fluid molecules act almost as tiny ball-bearings rolling between the opposing joint surfaces (Pascale and Grana, 1989).

### Injury

Articular cartilage is to a great extent protected from injury by the elasticity of other joint structures, and the neuromuscular reflexes. Reflex muscular contraction and soft tissue 'give' will largely dampen shock before it reaches the cartilage. However, unexpected loading (such as trauma) which occurs too rapidly to invoke reflex protection, will cause injury, but this is more frequently bony fracture than damage to the cartilage itself.

If cartilage injury does occur, it is most likely to be due to slip or shear. Three injury stages have

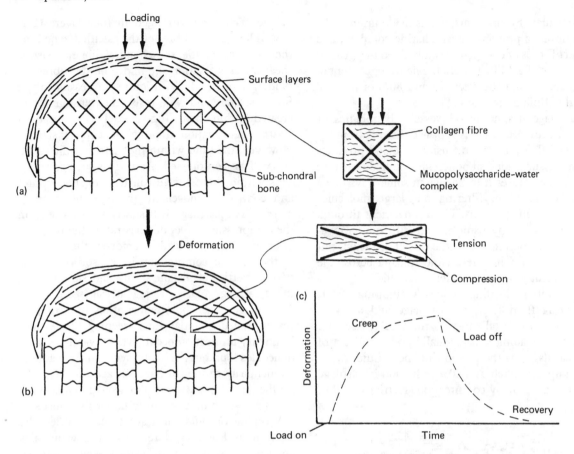

**Figure 2.9** Effects of joint compression on articular cartilage. (a) Compressive loading of the cartilage results in (b) tension stress to the collagenous elements and compression stress to the mucopolysaccharide – water complex. (c) The total response is viscoelastic. The viscous creep with sustained loading is largely the result of a time-dependent squeezing out of fluid. From Hertling and Kessler (1990), with permission.

been described (Hettinga, 1990). First, splitting of the cartilage layer at the tide mark between the calcified and uncalcified tissue. Secondly, cartilage depression into the sub-chondral bone, and, thirdly, fissuring of the cartilage and underlying bone.

Partial thickness injuries, limited to the articular cartilage alone, heal poorly. The healing which does occur is by proliferation and invasion from soft tissue, and the further away from this tissue the injured area is, the poorer the healing. Full thickness defects, extending through the sub-chondral bone, heal by superficial tissue bridging the break. Blood vessels grow into the uncalcified cartilage. Osteogenic cells and granulation tissue from the base of the break invade the area, resulting in the formation of fibrous tissue, bony trabeculae and fibrocartilage. There is obvious demarcation of the region into zones, with a chondrin-free ring surrounding the uninjured tissue. The healed defect appears as a slightly discoloured roughened area of fibrous tissue.

Intra-articular injection of hydrocortisone has resulted in a temporary reduction in cartilage matrix synthesis (Mankin and Conger, 1966) and destructive changes to the cartilage itself (Salter, Gross and Hall, 1967).

## Arthritis

The term arthritis tends to be used to describe any chronic inflammatory reaction affecting a joint. However, the term simply means 'joint inflammation', and as such must be qualified by a description of the cause of inflammation. Acute joint injury which causes intracapsular swelling may be termed 'traumatic arthritis'. True osteoarthritis involves cartilage degeneration, initially with little inflammation, so the term osteoarthrosis would seem more appropriate. This condition must be differentiated from inflammatory states affecting multiple joints such as rheumatoid arthritis. The following description is concerned with osteoarthritis and its connection with sport and exercise.

The initial changes that occur in osteoarthritis are usually painless and show no swelling. Mild fraying or flaking of superficial collagen fibres within the hyaline cartilage occurs. This happens firstly at the periphery of the joint in the non-weight-bearing region. Later damage (fibrillation) is to the deeper cartilage layers in the weight-bearing areas of the joint, extending down to one third of the cartilage thickness. Small cavities form (blistering) between the cartilage fibres which gradually extend to become vertical clefts. If cartilage fragments break off, they may float free in the joint fluid as loose bodies, giving rise to joint locking and sudden twinges of pain. The presence of a loose body and the byproducts of cartilage destruction causes the synovium to inflame, and it is only at this point that many patients become aware that a problem exists.

Turnover of proteoglycan and collagen within the cartilage ground substance is increased, and the proteoglycan molecules near the fibrillated cartilage are smaller than normal. Mechanically, this altered cartilage is weaker to both compression and tension stresses, but it is still resistant to gliding, and its coefficient of friction remains low (Threlkeld and Currier, 1988). As the cartilage thins the joint space is reduced.

The sub-chondral bone beneath the fibrillated cartilage becomes shiny and smooth (eburnated). Below the eburnated region the area becomes osteoporotic and local avascular necrosis causes cyst formation where there is complete bone loss. Osteophytes covered with fibrocartilage form at the periphery of the joint, and may protrude into the joint space or, more frequently, into surrounding soft tissue.

The synovial membrane becomes thickened and its vascularity increases in line with an inflammatory response (see above). The joint capsule demonstrates small tears filled with fibrous tissue causing thickening. Contracture usually alters both physiological and accessory movements (see p.15). For example when osteoarthritis affects the knee joint, flexion is often limited and mediolateral stability reduced.

### Arthritis secondary to sports injury

The changes which occur in osteoarthritis, if detected early enough may be reversible (Hertling and Kessler, 1990). Altered biomechanics of a joint, if corrected, can result in regrowth of fibrocartilage. However, subtle alterations in normal joint mechanics which may remain long after an injury has 'resolved' may be largely undetectable to a patient or physician. It is not until these changes are well developed and limit physiological joint movement or cause deformity that they become readily apparent. Accessory movements when limited, are, however, detectable to a manipulative physiotherapist at a much earlier stage. It would seem logical therefore to assess and restore accessory movements after joint injury rather than simply full range physiological movement and muscle strength. In this way the onset of osteoarthritis may be slowed or even avoided.

The use of biomechanical analyses after injury, using apparatus such as video playback, isokinetic dynamometry and force plates is helpful to ensure that joint function has been restored.

### Arthritis and exercise

Arthitis is often considered a normal ageing process. However Panush and Brown (1987) cite a study of a population in the age range 70–79 years in which 85% had osteoarthritis. Importantly, the result indicated that 15% of this age group did not suffer osteoarthritis, so it seems likely that although ageing is an important factor other considerations must exist.

Animal studies have failed to show a direct link between exercise and arthritis. Radin, Eyre and Schiller, (1979) found no evidence of cartilage deterioration in sheep forced to walk for four hours daily on concrete for 12 and 30 months. Videman (1982) found that running did not affect the development of osteoarthritis in rabbits. Experimentally induced osteoarthritis was not increased when the animals were forced to run over 2000 m per week for 14 consecutive weeks.

Studies of runners have also failed to show any significant difference from non-runners. Puranen et al. (1975) found less hip osteoarthritis in Finnish distance runners than in non-runners of a similar age. Panush et al (1986) found no greater clinical or radiological evidence of osteoarthritis in male runners of average age 55 years.

Studies have linked osteoarthritis of particular joints with specific sports. In a review on the subject, Panush and Brown (1987) cited studies describing osteoarthritis in the cervical spine and lower extremities of ballet dancers, the upper limbs of baseball pitchers, the hands of boxers, cricketers, and downhill skiers and the ankles and feet of soccer players. Whether these results reflect overuse of the joints involved, or altered mechanics following injury to these more frequently used body parts remains uncertain.

It would seem logical that maintaining the normal mobility and strength of a joint throughout life could help maintain the health of the joint structures and perhaps delay the onset of osteoarthritis. Conversely, high impact loading of an already degenerating joint, such as may occur with running or aerobics on hard unforgiving surfaces may exacerbate symptoms.

The advice to a patient with osteoarthritis must be to reduce impact but maintain mobility and strength in a controlled fashion. Athletes must also be made aware of the danger of 'running through the pain' and training with an injury which alters the forces across a joint. Similarly, athletes must be conscious that the cessation of pain following injury does not indicate that full function has returned.

Total rehabilitation has only occurred when normal joint mechanics have been restored.

## The joint capsule

The joint capsule is in two parts. The outer part (stratum fibrosum) is fibrous and thickened in areas to form ligaments. The inner layer (stratum synoviale) is loose and highly vascular and blends with the synovial membrane. The capsule consists of parallel fascicles of collagen and some fibrocytes. Blood vessels enter the subchondral bone at the line of capsular attachment and small vessels are found between the individual cartilage fascicles. The nerve supply is very rich, with large fibres giving proprioceptive feedback and small fibres terminating in pain endings.

The capsular response to trauma is an increase in vascularity and eventually the development of fibrous tissue. Cross-linking of collagen fibres occurs, causing a palpable thickening of the capsule. Capsular shrinkage combined with fibrous adhesions will cause loss of movement and occurs particularly after immobilization.

Accumulation of joint fluid through swelling will stretch the capsule and capsular ligaments. The nerve endings situated between the collagen fascicles of the capsule will be stretched, giving rise to mechanical pain. Should the fluid accumulation exceed the elastic limit of the joint capsule, rupture may result.

Joint effusion will stretch portions of the capsule which are normally lax to facilitate movement. The patient will tend to rest the joint in a position in which the joint cavity is of maximum volume (loose pack, see p.17); in addition, passive movements will be limited in characteristic 'capsular patterns' (Table 2.2).

## Ligaments

When a ligament is put under stress, it responds by becoming progressively stiffer before later deforming in a regular manner (Amis, 1985). There are two reasons for this. First the collagen fibres within the ligament are not in line, and so the initial tensile stress is used to pull the fibres straight. Secondly,

**Table 2.2  The capsular patterns**

*Shoulder* — so much limitation of abduction, more than that of lateral rotation, less than that of medial rotation

*Elbow* — flexion usually more limited than extension, rotations full and painless except in advanced cases

*Wrist* — equal limitation of flexion and extension, little limitation of deviations

*Trapezio-first metacarpal joint* — only abduction limited

*Sign of the buttock* — passive hip flexion more limited and more painful than straight-leg raise

*Hip* — marked limitation of flexion and medial rotation, some limitation of abduction, little or no limitation of adduction and lateral rotation

*Knee* — gross limitation of flexion, slight limitation of extension

*Ankle* — more limitation of plantiflexion than of dorsiflexion

*Talocalcanean joint* – increasing limitation of varus until fixation in valgus

*Mid-tarsal joint* — limitations of adduction and internal rotation, other movements full

*Big toe* — gross limitation of extension, slight limitation of flexion

*Cervical spine* — equal limitation in all directions except for flexion which is usually full

*Thoracic spine* — limitation of extension, side flexion and rotations, less limitation of flexion

*Lumbar spine* — marked and equal limitation of side flexions, limitation of flexion and of extension

From Cyriax and Cyriax (1983), with permission.

the fibres are not attached to a single point, but to an area of bone, and so are of slightly different lengths. When the fibres are stretched, there will be a progressive tightening of the ligament, with some fibres becoming taut sooner than others.

Ligaments demonstrate viscoelastic properties. Rapid stretch has been shown to increase stiffness by as much as 20% (Woo, Gomez and Akeson, 1981), and sustained stretch to cause ligament tension to reduce significantly after two minutes (Viidik, 1966). The mode of failure also changes with speed, avulsion occurring at slower speeds, and ligamentous rupture at higher speeds (Noyes et al., 1974).

Clinically, three grades of ligament injuries are recognized (Fowler, 1984). Grade I sprains involve minimal tissue damage with some local tenderness. Swelling is only slight, and function is almost normal. With the grade II sprain, more ligament

fibres are injured or the ligament may become partially detached from its bony attachment. Local pain is more intense and movement more limited. Grade III injuries constitute a complete rupture. There is a rapid onset of effusion with considerable pain. The joint is unstable and loss of function is complete. Noyes, Kelly and Grood (1984) argued that this traditional classification, although useful, could be misleading. The grade II injury could refer equally to an injury in which only a few ligament fibres are torn, or to a lesion in which virtually the total ligament was affected. The grade III injury, they claimed, represented not total rupture, but total loss of function of the ligament, actual continuity of the ligament often being maintained.

With grades I and II ligament injury, pain is increased by placing the ligament on stretch. With a grade II injury, some instability may be present, but with a complete rupture instability is always present. However, this may be difficult to assess clinically in instances of severe pain and muscle spasm.

Ligamentous viscosity changes with age. The collagen fibres within the ligament enlarge, reducing the water content in the ground substance. Noyes and Grood (1976) showed marked reductions in tensile strength of ligament in the 48–83 year age group compared with the 16–26 year age group.

Noyes et al. (1984) showed three-fold decreases in maximum stress, elastic modulus and strain energy between the ligaments from donors aged 50 years and those aged 20 years. The older ligaments failed by bony avulsion rather than ligamentous failure as occurred in the younger tissues. They claimed that ageing produced changes in the ligament/bone systems similar to those found due to disuse.

Immobility also has marked effects on ligaments. Laros, Tipton and Cooper (1971) showed strength reductions of 39% after 9 weeks' immobilization. Full strength was not regained for 30 weeks. Exercise has been shown to have a beneficial effect on ligament tensile strength (Adams, 1966; Heikkinen and Vuori, 1972; Cabaud et al. 1980). Exercise seems to act as a 'mechanical stimulant', causing increased collagen turnover within the ligament (Weisman, Pope and Johnson, 1980). This has important implications for rehabilitation following ligament injury. Wherever possible, complete immobilization should be avoided. While an injured ligament should be protected against excessive external forces which could cause further damage, gentle exercise within the pain-free range should still be encouraged.

The effect of corticosteroids on ligament failure is important, since corticosteroid usage in sport is still popular. Decreases in maximum load of 21% and 39% have been shown six and 15 weeks after large dosage cortisone injection (methyl prednisolone acetate), with a load reduction remaining for one year. In addition, fibrocyte death was seen within the ligament, with delay in reappearance of new fibrocytes for 15 weeks (Noyes et al., 1984).

## Muscle

The term 'strain' is generally used to imply a minor injury to any soft tissue structure. However, in this book strain will be confined to injury of muscle while the term 'sprain' will be used for injured joint structures. Strains may be subdivided into acute and chronic types. Acute strains are usually the result of a single violent stretch to a contracting muscle (Fowler, 1984; Keene, 1990), while chronic strains develop over a period of time as a result of repetitive loading.

Fowler (1984) classified strains into four grades, to include complete rupture as a grade four injury, while Keene (1990) used three grades and described complete rupture as a separate entity. The diversity of opinion makes it essential when describing an injury not to use a number alone.

The grade one (mild) strain is a contusion in which there is tearing of a small number of muscle fibres with the fascia remaining intact. Bleeding is minimal, and pain and spasm are localized. Muscle function is normal, but endurance may be reduced.

Grade two (moderate) strains result from more severe trauma. A larger number of muscle fibres are injured, and injury occurs over a greater area. The fascia still remains intact so bleeding is contained within the muscle, forming an intramuscular haematoma. The contained bleeding will cause an increase in intramuscular pressure, which in turn will compress the bleeding points and stop further haemorrhage (Williams and Sperryn, 1976). A definite palpable mass is evident with this injury, and pain to palpation is considerable. The function of the muscle is impaired, and contractility and extensibility are greatly reduced.

With grade three (severe) strains, a larger area of muscle is affected. The muscle fascia is partially torn, and more than one muscle may be involved. Bleeding is more profuse, and spread over a larger area, as the haemorrhage is no longer contained by the muscle sheath. The torn fascia releases the blood to form an intermuscular haematoma (Fig 2.10). The grade four injury is a complete rupture. The muscle ends contract and a definite gap is apparent. In some cases a snapping sound may be heard at the time of injury. Bleeding and swelling

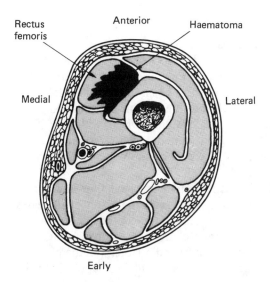

Rectus femoris — Anterior — Haematoma

Medial — Lateral

Early

**Figure 2.10** An intermuscular haematoma affecting the rectus femoris. From Fowler (1984), with permission.

are considerable, and active contraction of the muscle is not possible.

The site of the injury is especially important with regard to the treatment regime chosen. Muscle-tendon injuries can be to the muscle belly itself, the musculotendinous (MT) junction or the teno-osseous (TO) junction. Garrett (1990) showed that both passive stretching, and stretching a pre-contracted isolated rabbit muscle consistently caused failure at the MT junction. A small (0.1–1 mm) amount of muscle tissue remains attached to the tendon.

Garrett (1990) also showed that pre-contracted muscles absorbed 100% more energy than passively stretched muscle fibre, and used these results to emphasize the importance of muscles as energy absorbers. He argued that conditions which interfere with the contractile ability of a muscle, such as fatigue or muscle weakness, might diminish the energy absorbing ability of the muscle and possibly predispose to injury.

Cyriax (1982) claimed that muscle belly injuries would respond to therapeutic exercise. Muscle contraction causes broadening of the fibres and, he claimed, would reduce intramuscular scarring. Injury at the MT or TO junctions would not respond

to exercise as no muscle broadening occurs at these points. Cyriax argued that passive therapy, such as transverse frictional massage or injection, were more appropriate to these sites.

### Myositis ossificans traumatica

Myositis ossificans traumatica (MOT) is soft tissue ossification of muscle resulting in the formation of non-neoplasmic bone (Booth and Westers, 1989). It usually occurs in the proximal limb muscles, and is seen most commonly following contusion of the quadriceps femoris muscle (Jackson, 1975), although other regions include the elbow flexors and hip abductors.

Several aetiological theories have been suggested (Booth and Westers, 1989). Calcification of a muscle haematoma can occur following fibrosis, or intramuscular bone formation may result from periosteal detachment. Rupture of the periosteum may lead to the proliferation of osteoblasts and their escape into the surrounding muscle. Intramuscular connective tissue may undergo metaplasia into bone, and Urist et al. (1978) demonstrated that certain skeletal muscle cells, known as inducible osteogenic precursor cells (IOPC), have the capability of differentiating into osteoblasts. Certain individuals have been shown to have a predisposition to the condition (Rothwell, 1982).

Clinically, the patient presents with severe post-traumatic pain and limitation of movement. There is local swelling and erythema, and the area is warm and tender to palpation. Tenderness usually becomes more pronounced with time, and tissue signs do not respond to conservative management. The factor which should alert the practitioner to the possibility of MOT, is a reduction in movement range over time. Normally, an increasing range would be expected as a condition resolves. Radiological evidence of ossification is usually seen within two months following injury, and other investigations including computed tomography (Vas et al., 1981), and ultrasound scanning (Kramer et al., 1979) have been used.

Management of MOT is aimed at lessening any disability rather than affecting the bone mass. Initially, the soft tissue response to trauma, especially bleeding, is limited by the use of such regimes as rest, ice, compression and elevation (RICE). Rehabilitation is slower than with a normal muscle haematoma, isometric exercises being used 7–14 days following injury, but active exercises (within the pain-free range) are not used until 2–4 weeks after injury (Booth and Westers, 1989).

## Tendons

A variety of conditions may affect tendons, the most common in sport being tenosynovitis, tendinitis and tenovaginitis. Tendinitis is an inflammation and scarring of the tendon which can occur in varying degrees. Scarring may interfere with tendon function and/or cause persistent local inflammation.

Tenosynovitis is a lesion to the gliding surfaces of the outside of the tendon and the inside of its sheath, but not the sheath itself (Fowler, 1984). The lesion usually occurs as a result of overuse or compression. Pathological features are similar to those seen in rheumatoid arthritis (Williams and Sperryn, 1976), including an increase in the number of lining cells of the sheath, together with proliferation of local blood vessels, oedema and cellular changes. As the roughened surfaces of the sheath move against each other, pain and crepitus occur. The same condition, occurring to tendons which do not have a true sheath, is termed peritendinitis. Here, the paratenon thickens, and shows fibrinoid degeneration and dense fibrous adhesions (Snook, 1972). Local oedema is evident, sometimes with palpable crepitus, and pain may disappear with activity (Williams and Sperryn, 1976).

Tenovaginitis occurs when the tendon sheath is chronically inflamed and thickens. It is the fibrous wall of the tendon sheath rather than the synovial lining which is affected. Common sites include the flexor sheaths of the fingers or thumb. When the sheaths of extensor pollicis brevis and abductor pollicis longus are effected, de Quervain's syndrome is present.

## Skin

The initial reaction to mild skin injury is the classic triple response described by Lewis and Grant (1924). Making a firm mark across the skin with a pin, for example, causes an initial pallor, followed by a dull red line (flush) with a surrounding red area (flare). Local swelling (wheal) will occur if the skin marking was intense. This response is due mainly to the effects of histamines, and through the axon reflex.

The initial reduction in blood flow and consequent dramatic increase is the result of increases and decreases in muscle tone of the arteriole walls. The larger lumen of the vessels involved reduces peripheral resistance and a larger volume of blood enters the area. Local capillaries supplied by the affected arterioles are re-opened or dilated and the area is engorged with blood. The initial increase in blood flow will last for approximately one hour (Evans 1990), and then the blood flow gradually slows.

Blood slowing occurs by haemoconcentration, water and smaller molecules being lost through the capillary wall. The concentration of blood proteins give rise to rouleaux formation where the red cells clump together (Fig. 2.1). In addition white cells stick to the vessel walls further reducing the vessel lumen size.

### Skin wounds

Skin wounds may be divided into two categories, open and closed. Closed wounds occur when there is no penetration of the epidermis, and open wounds are those in which the epidermis has been pierced. Closed wounds encompass contusions, abrasions and friction burns, such as those caused by gravel. Open wounds in sport include lacerations and puncture wounds.

A contusion or bruise involves a direct blow to the skin surface. Bleeding occurs from torn blood vessels into the skin and subcutaneous tissues, forming a bruise or ecchymosis. Released blood will clot and degrade, producing superficial colour changes. An abrasion or graze occurs through a glancing injury, or repeated microtrauma to the skin surface. The skin surface breaks through, but the damage is not full thickness. Extensive areas of skin may be affected, and intense pain usually occurs as raw nerve endings are exposed. Bleeding may be extensive, but healing is rapid unless infection ensues. Extensive debriding injuries involving large areas of skin loss (for example from a motorcycle accident) may require grafting.

A laceration is a full thickness skin injury, which exposes the subcutaneous tissue. Clean lacerations may require stitching but heal well, jagged injuries involving skin tearing may leave more scarring.

Pressure or friction may cause an abrasion in which the skin surface is removed, or a blister, in which the epidermal surface skin layer is detached from the underlying tissue. The gap between the two layers is filled with lymph, exposing nerve endings to fluid pressure, and so causing pain. When pressure or friction is applied progressively, the epidermal skin layer may adapt to form a thickened callus (Williams, 1979).

Healing of an incised wound such as a cut, where the wound edges are in apposition, occurs by first intention. If the wound edges are separated and more major skin damage has occurred (or if infection has intervened), then healing is by second intention (Evans, 1990).

With healing by first intention, slight haemorrhage occurs and the cut is filled with a blood clot on the first day. By the second and third day the clot has become organized and epithelial cells from the two sides of the cut have joined. This single layer of covering multiplies to form stratified squamous epithelium, that is, normal epidermis. Fibroblasts lay down collagen in the granulation tissue and a band of scar tissue is formed by two weeks after the injury.

Healing by second intention takes longer, as the spread of epithelial cells over the larger area takes time. The large amount of granulation tissue results in more extensive scarring and likely contracture.

# References

Adams, A (1966) Effect of exercise upon ligament strength. *Research Quarterly*, **37**, 163–176.

Amis, A.A. (1985) Biomechanics of ligaments. In *Ligament Injuries and their Treatment* (ed. D. H. R. Jenkins), Chapman and Hall, London.

Apley, A.G. and Solomon, L. (1988) *Concise System of Orthopaedics and Fractures*, Butterworth, Oxford

Bassett, C.A.L. (1965) Electrical effects in bone. *Scientific American*, **213**,(4) 18

Bassett, C.A.L. and Pawlick, R.J. (1964) Effects of electric currents on bone in vivo. *Nature*, **204**, 652

Becker, R.O. and Murray, D.G. (1970) The electrical control system regulating fracture healing in amphibians. *Clinical Orthopaedics and Related Research*, **73**, 169

Becker, R.O., Spadaro, J.A. and Marino, A.A. (1977) Clinical experience with low intensity direct current stimulation of bone growth. *Clinical Orthopaedics and Related Research*, **124**, 75–83.

Blau. S.P. (1979) The synovial fluid. *The Orthopaedic Clinics of North America*, **10**, 21–35

Booth, D.W. and Westers, B.M. (1989) The management of athletes with myositis ossificans traumatica. *Canadian Journal of Sports Science*, **14**, (1) 10–16.

Bullough, P.G. (1981) Cartilage. In *Scientific Foundations of Orthopaedics and Traumatology* (ed. R. Owen, J. Goodfellow and P. Bullough), Heinemann Medical, Oxford

Burri, C., Helbing, G. and Spier, W. (1973) Rehabilitation of knee ligament injuries. In *The Knee*. Springer, New York

Cabaud, H.E., Chatty, A., Gildengorin, V. and Feltman, R.J. (1980) Exercise effects on the strength of the anterior cruciate ligament. *American Journal of Sports Medicine*, **8**, 79–86.

Crawford-Adams, J. (1978) *Outline of Fractures*, Churchill Livingstone, London

Cyriax, J. (1982) *Textbook of Orthopaedic Medicine*, Vol. one, 8th edn, Bailliere Tindall, London.

Cyriax, J. and Cyriax, P. (1983) *Illustrated Manual of Orthopaedic Medicine*, Butterworth, London, pp. 228

De Andrade, J. R., Grant, C. and Dixon, A. (1965). Joint distension and reflex muscle inhibition in the knee. *Journal of Bone and Joint Surgery*, **47**, A 313–322

De Domenico, G. (1982) Pain relief with interferential therapy. *Australian Journal of Physiotherapy*, **28**, (3) 14–18

Donaldson, C.L., Hulley, S.B. and Vogel, J.M (1970) Effects of prolonged bed rest on bone mineral. *Metabolism*, **19**, 1071–1084

Donley, P.B. and Denegar, C. (1990) Pain and mechanisms of pain relief. In *Therapeutic Modalities in Sports Medicine* (ed. W. E. Prentice), Times Mirror/Mosby College Publishing

Dyson, M. (1987) Mechanisms involved in therapeutic ultrasound. *Physiotherapy*, **73**, (3) 116–120

Ettinger, B., Genant, H.K. and Cann, C.E. (1987) Postmenopausal bone loss is prevented by low dosage oestrogen with calcium. *Annals of Internal Medicine*, **106**, 40–45

Evans, D.M.D. (1990) Inflammation and healing. In *Cash's Textbook of General Medical and Surgical Conditions for Physiotherapists*, 2nd edn, (ed. P.A. Downie), Faber and Faber, London, pp. 12–29

Evans, P. (1980) The healing process at cellular level: a review. *Physiotherapy*, **66**, (8), pp. 256–259

Fowler, J.A. (1984) Soft tissue injuries and sports injuries. In *Cash's Textbook of Orthopaedics and Rheumatology for Physiotherapists* (ed. P. A. Downie), Faber and Faber, London, pp. 512–552

Fox, J., Galley, F. and Wayland, H. (1980) Action of histamine on the mesenteric microvasculature. *Microvascular Research*, **19**, 108–126

Frank, G. Woo, S.L., Amiel O., Harwood, F. Gomez, M. and Akeson, W. (1983) Medial collateral ligament healing. A multidisciplinary assessment in rabbits. *American Journal of Sports Medicine*, **11**, 379–389

Freeman, M., Dean, M. and Hanham, I. (1965) The etiology and prevention of functional instability of the foot. *Journal of Bone and Joint Surgery (Br)*, **47**, 678–685

Garrett, W.E. (1990) Muscle strain injuries: clinical and basic aspects. *Medicine and Science in Sports and Exercise*, **22**, 436–443

Garland, J.J. (1987) *Fundamentals of Orthopaedics*, 4th edn, W.B. Saunders, Philadelphia

Gauffin, H., Tropp, H. and Odenrick, P. (1988) Effects of ankle disk training on postural control in patients with functional instability of the ankle joint. *International Journal of Sports Medicine*, **9**, 141–144

Glencross, D. and Thornton, E. (1981) Position sense following joint injury. *Journal of Sports Medicine*, **21**, 23–27

Gould, J.A. (1990) *Orthopaedic and Sports Physical Therapy* (2nd ed.), C.V. Mosby, St Louis, p. 108

Hedlund, L.R. and Gallagher, J.C. (1988). Estrogen therapy for post menopausal osteoporosis: current considerations of the menopause. *Annals of Clinical and Laboratory Science*, **15**, 219–228

Heikkinen, E. and Vuori, I. (1972) Effect of physical activity on the metabolism of collagen in aged mice. *Acta Physiologica Scandinavica*, **84**, 543–549

Hert, J. and Zalud, J. (1971) Reaction of bone to mechanical stimuli. (VI). Bioelectrical theory of functional adaptation of bone. *Acta Chirurgicae Orthopaedicae et Traumatologicae Cechoslovaca*, **38**, 280

Hertling, D. and Kessler, R. M. (1990) *Management of Common Musculoskeletal Disorders*, J.B. Lippincott, Philadelphia

Hettinga, D.L. (1990) Inflammatory response of synovial joint structures. In *Orthopaedic and Sports Physical Therapy* (ed. J. A. Gould), 2nd edn, C. V. Mosby, St Louis, pp. 87–117

Huddleston, A.L., Rockwell, D. and Kuland D.N. (1980) Bone mass in lifetime tennis athletes. *Journal*

of the American Medical Association, **244**, 1107–1109

Jackson, D.W. (1975) Managing myositis ossificans traumatica. *Phys. Sports. Med.*, October, 56–61

Keene, J.S. (1990) Ligament and muscle tendon unit injuries. In *Orthopaedic and Sports Physical Therapy*, 2nd edn (ed. J. A. Gould), C. V. Mosby, St Louis

Kellett, J. (1986) Acute soft tissue injuries – a review of the literature. *Medicine and Science in Sports and Exercise*, **18**, (5) 489–500

Kramer, F.L., Kurtz, A.B., Rubin, C. and Goldberg, B.B. (1979). Ultrasound appearance of myositis ossificans. *Skeletal Radiology*, **4**, 19–20

Krolner, B., Toft, B. and Nielsen, S. (1983) Physical exercise as a prophylaxis against involutional bone loss: a controlled trial. *Clinical Science*, **64**, 541–546

Lachman, S. (1988) *Soft Tissue Injuries in Sport*, Blackwell, Oxford

Laros, G.S, Tipton, C.M. and Cooper, R.R. (1971) Influence of physical activity on ligament insertions in the knees of dogs. *Journal of Bone and Joint Surgery*, **53A**, 275–286

Lentell, G.L., Katzman, L.L. and Walters, M.R. (1990) The relationship between muscle function and ankle stability. *Journal of Orthopaedics and Sports Physical Therapy*, **11**, (12) 605–611

Lewis, T. and Grant, R.T. (1924) Vascular reactions of the skin to injury. *Heart*, **11**, 209–65

Li, G., Zhang, S., Chen, G., Chen, H. and Wang, A. (1985) Radiographic and histological analysis of stress fracture in rabbit tibias. *American Journal of Sports Medicine*, **13**, 285–294

Low, J. and Reed, A. (1990) *Electrotherapy Explained. Principles and Practice*, Butterworth-Heinemann, Oxford

Lowden, A. (1986) Application of ultrasound to assess stress fractures. *Physiotherapy*, **72**, (3) 160–161

Lynch M.K. and Kessler, R.M, (1990) Pain. In *Management of Common Musculoskeletal Disorders*, 2nd edn (ed. D. Hertling and R. M. Kessler), J.B. Lippincott, Philadelphia

MacKinnon, J.L.(1988) Osteoporosis. A review. *Physical Therapy*, **68**, (10) 1533–1540

Maitland, G.D. (1991) *Peripheral Manipulation*, 3rd edn, Butterworth-Heinemann, Oxford

Mankin, H.J. and Conger, K.A. (1966) The acute effects of intra-articular hydrocortisone on particular cartilage in rabbits. *Journal of Bone and Joint Surgery*, **48A**, 1383–1388

Martin, A.D. and Houston, C.S. (1987) Osteoporosis, calcium and physical activity. *Canadian Medical Association Journal*, **136**, 587–593

Mazess, R.B. and Whedon, G.D. (1983) Immobilization and bone. *Calcified Tissue International*, **35**, 265–267

McArdle, W.D., Katch, F.I. and Katch, V.L. (1986) *Exercise Physiology. Energy, Nutrition, and Human Performance* (2nd edn), Lea and Febiger, Philadelphia

McBryde, A.M. (1985) Stress fractures in runners. *Cli-*

nics in Sports Medicine, **4**,(4) 737–752

Melzack, R. and Wall, P.D. (1965). Pain mechanisms: a new theory. Science, **150**, 971–979

Moss, A. and Mowat, A.G. (1983) Ultrasonic assessment of stress fractures. British Medical Journal, **286**, 1479

Nilas, L., Christiansen, C. and Rodbro, P. (1984) Calcium supplementation and post-menopausal bone loss. British Medical Journal, **289**, 1103–1106

Nilsson, B.E. and Westlin, N.E. (1977). Bone density in athletes. Clinical Orthopaedics and Related Research, **77**, 179–182

Noyes, F.R. and Grood, M.J. (1976) The strength of the anterior cruciate ligament in humans and rhesus monkeys: age-related and species-related changes. Journal of Bone and Joint Surgery, **58A**, 1074–1082

Noyes, F.R, DeLucas, J.L. and Torvik, P.J. (1974) Biomechanics of anterior cruciate ligament failure: an analysis of strain-rate sensitivity and mechanisms in primates. Journal of Bone and Joint Surgery, **56A**, 236–53

Noyes, F.R., Kelly, C.S., Grood, E.S. and Butler, D.L. (1984) Advances in the understanding of knee ligament injury, repair and rehabilitation. Medicine and Science in Sports and Exercise, **16**, (5) 427–443

Noyes, F.R., Grood, E.S., Nussbaum, N.S. and Cooper, S.M. (1977) Effect of intraarticular corticosteroids on ligament properties – a biomechanical and histological study in rhesus knees. Clinical Orthopaedics and Related Research, **123**, 197–209

Paget, S. and Bullough, P.G. (1981) Synovium and synovial fluid. In Scientific Foundations of Orthopaedics and Traumatology (ed. R. Owen, J. Goodfellow, and P. Bullough), Heinemann Medical, Oxford

Palastanga, N., Field, D. and Soames, R. (1989) Anatomy and Human Movement, Heinemann Medical, Oxford

Panush, R.S. and Brown, D.G. (1987) Exercise and arthritis. Sports Medicine, **4**, 54–64

Panush, R.S., Schmidt, C., Caldwell, J., Edwards, N.L. and Longley, S. (1986). Is running associated with degenerative joint disease? Journal of the American Medical Association **255**, 1150–1154

Pascale, M. and Grana, W.A. (1989) Does running cause osteoarthritis? The Physician and Sports Medicine, **17**,(3) 157–166

Puranen, J., Ala-Ketola, L., Peltokalleo, P. and Saarela, J. (1975). Running and primary osteosteoarthritis of the hip. British Medical Journal,**1**, 424–425

Radin, E.L., Eyre, D. and Schiller, A.L. (1979) Effect of prolonged walking on concrete on the joints of sheep. Abstract. Arthritis and Rheumatism, **22**, 649

Riegger, C.L. (1990) Mechanical properties of bone. In Orthopaedic and Sports Physical Therapy, 2nd edn (ed. J. A. Gould), Mosby, St Louis, pp. 3–47

Rothwell, A.G. (1982). Quadriceps haematoma. A prospective study. Clinical Orthopaaedics and Related Research, **171**, 97–103

Rzonca, E.C. and Baylis, W.J. (1988) Common sports injuries to the foot and leg. Clinics in Pediatric Medicine and Surgery, **5**, (3)

Salter, R.B. and Harris, W.R. (1963) Injuries involving the epiphyseal plate. Journal of Bone and Joint Surgery, **45A**, 587

Salter, R.B., Gross, A. and Hall, J.H. (1967) Hydrocortisone arthropathy – an experimental investigation. Canadian Medical Association Journal, **97**, 374–377

Smith, E.L., Smith, P.E. and Ensign, C.J. (1984) Bone involutional decrease in exercising middle-aged women. Calcified Tissue International, **36**, 129–138

Snook, G.A. (1972) Tenosynovitis in long distance runners. Medicine and Science in Sports and Exercise, **4**, 166

Steams, M.L. (1940) Studies on development of connective tissue in transparent chambers in rabbits ear. American Journal of Anatomy, **67**, 55

Stokes, M. and Young, A. (1984) The contribution of reflex inhibition to arthrogenous muscle weakness. Clinical Science, **67**, 7–14

Taunton, J.E. and Clement, D.B. (1981) Lower extremity stress fractures in athletes. Physician and Sports Medicine, **9**, 77–86

Threlkeld, A.J. and Currier, D.P. (1988) Osteoarthritis: effects on synovial joint tissues. Physical Therapy, **68**, (3) 364–370

Urist, M.R., Nakagawa, M., Nakata, N. and Nogami, H. (1978) Experimental myositis ossificans: cartilage and bone formation in muscle in response to a dissufible bone matrix derived morphogen. Archives of Pathology and Laboratory Medicine, **102**, 312–316

Van der Meulen, J.C.H. (1982) Present state of knowledge on processes of healing in collagen structures. International Journal of Sports Medicine, **3**, 4–8

Vas, W., Cockshott, W.P., Martin, R.F., Pai, N.K., and Walker, I. (1981) Myositis ossificans in haemophilia. Skeletal Radiology, **7**, 27–31

Videman T. (1982) The effect of running on the osteosteoarthritic joint: an experimental matched pair study with rabbits. Rheumatology and Rehabilitation, **21**, 1–8

Viidik, A. (1966) Biomechanics and functional adaptation of tendons and joint ligament. In Studies on the Anatomy and Function of Bone and Joints (ed. F. G. Evans), Springer, Berlin

Walter, J.B. and Israel, M.S. (1987) General Pathology, 6th edn, Churchill Livingstone, London

Weisman, G., Pope, M.H. and Johnson, R.J. (1980) Cyclic loading in knee ligament injuries. American Journal of Sports Medicine, **8**, 24–30

Wilkinson, P.C. and Lackie, J.M. (1979) The adhesion, migration and chemotaxis of leucocytes in inflammation. Current Topics in Pathology, **68**, 47–88

Williams, J.G.P. (1979) Injuries in Sport, Bayer (UK), Haywards Heath, England

Williams, J.G.P. and Sperryn, P.N. (1976) Sports Me-

*dicine*, Edward Arnold, London

Woo, S.L.Y, Gomez, M.A. and Akeson, W.H. (1981) The time and history-dependent viscoelastic properties of the canine medial collateral ligament. *Journal of Biomechanical Engineering*, **103**, 293–298

# 3 Psychological aspects of sports injury

## The injury-prone athlete

A variety of psychological variables may predispose an athlete to injury. General personality make-up, trait anxiety, locus of control and self-esteem have all received attention (Kerr and Fowler, 1988). Several authors have attempted to show that specific aspects of personality make an athlete more prone to injury. Some believe that certain personality traits, which are largely genetically determined, make some athletes more likely to be injured than their peers. Others argue that temporary (transient) mood states are more liable to have a significant effect.

Jackson et al. (1978) examined footballers using the Cattell 16PF (personality factor) test, and concluded that tender-minded players were more likely to be injured. In addition, the reserved and detached players suffered more severe injuries. Reilly (1975), using the same test with professional soccer players, found a relationship between apprehensiveness and injury. Personality factors, such as being over-protective, easily distracted, or attention-seeking, may also predispose to injury.

Anxiety, and the unconscious attempt to cope with it, can cause abnormal behaviour in the athlete (Sanderson, 1981) and may increase the likelihood of injury. Coping mechanisms for tension or anxiety can, in some instances, create a distortion of reality. An example is the overly-tense athlete who simply denies that he or she is anxious. This person may be emotionally vulnerable and will often lose composure easily, possibly becoming violent. Individuals of this type may harbour a sense of guilt which they try to reduce by self-punishment. Injury to these individuals may simply be a form of

'self destruction' which confirms their opinion of themselves as losers. A number of the visible psychological characteristics displayed by the injury-prone athlete are listed below, and these must be recognized by the sports injury practitioner (Sanderson, 1981).

1  Counter-phobia—athlete attempts to counter anxiety by being overtly aggressive and fearless, repeatedly testing his or her indestructibility.
2  Sign of masculinity—athlete uses injury as a mark of courage. Needs visible 'scars of battle' to show manhood. Continues to play despite injury, but exaggerates pain to seek admiration.
3  Masochism—punishes him or herself for feelings of guilt, often about failure to reach his or her own unrealistic targets.
4  Injury as a weapon—tries to punish others, for example the young athlete who is forced to play by over-zealous parents.
5  Escape—the 'training room athlete' who fears competition because of feelings of inferiority, but cannot opt out for fear of isolation.
6  Psychosomatic injury—no physical injury, or slight injury made worse by emotional factors.

Bramwell et al. (1975) investigated the effect of psychological states on injury. These authors studied stressful life events, and measured these as the accumulation of Life Change Units (LCU). Positive stressful life events included marriage, getting a better job, and passing an examination, while negative events referred to bereavement, redundancy, divorce, etc. These authors showed that injured players had amassed significantly more LCUs in both one and two year periods preceding injury. Categorizing athletes into low, medium and high risk depending on LCU, it was noticeable that 73% of the high risk category experienced significant time loss through injury.

Coddington and Troxell (1980) examined the effect of stressful life events on injuries in schoolchildren. They found that the risk of injury was five times greater when a major event, such as the death of a parent, or parents separating, had occurred. Kerr and Minden (1988) showed the number of injuries in gymnasts to be four times greater and the severity to be increased by 4.5 times when athletes had experienced recent stressful life events.

There are two possible explanations for the effect of stressful life events on sports injury. First, the athlete's attention may be affected, with life events somehow hindering concentration. The method for this may be explained in terms of the psychological information processing systems used by the athlete (Kerr and Fowler, 1988).

Skilled athletes rely on two information processing systems. One is fast, allowing automatic, and therefore seemingly effortless, actions, the other is slower and requires more conscious control. The slower process is used to monitor overall strategies and allows individual components of automatic actions to be pieced together (Schneider and Fisk, 1983). To perform well, an athlete must 'let go' and allow these automatic actions to 'flow' freely. Any attempt to control the natural rhythm of the action will hinder its automatic nature and result in a loss of efficiency. Stressful life events could lead to worry about performance, which in turn may prevent an athlete from 'letting go'. Additionally, inappropriate thoughts may prevent the slower secondary system from monitoring overall performance efficiently. If several stressful life events occur at the same time an athlete will have to adjust to many life changes in a short time period (Kerr and Fowler, 1988).

Kerr and Minden (1988) claimed that the majority of gymnasts in their study reported 'lack of concentration' and 'thinking of other things' as the major cause of their injuries. These statements would seem to lend support to the hypothesis that the type of information processing used may have an effect on sports injury.

Stressful life events may ultimately lead to mental fatigue and exhaustion. This may present externally as apathy and lassitude, where an athlete is 'not interested' and lacks concentration. Remedial action could involve a period of attention training, to enable the athlete to focus on a task or to shift attention between different tasks rapidly. Coaches and therapists must recognize that an athlete is vulnerable to injury after a stressful life event. Training should be modified by reducing its intensity and concentrating on basic skills rather than introducing new ones.

Life stress does not have a uniform effect on all people, and individual reactions will depend on the predictability and controllability of the event, as well as the individual's psychological make-up, and 'stress resistance'. Also important is the social support available to an athlete from peers, family and sports officials.

## Injury and rehabilitation

### Reaction to injury

The psychological reaction of an athlete to a sports injury is similar to a grief response, and will often evolve through a number of definite stages (Wiese and Wiess, 1987). Initially, injury is likely to be met with denial, which quickly turns into anger. With time, as the true significance of the injury becomes apparent to the athlete, depression sets in. Finally, acceptance is seen, and the athlete takes a more constructive attitude which assists the rehabilitation process. In a study examining the reported responses of athletes to sports injury, Gordon, Milios and Grove (1991) described both positive and negative aspects (Table 3.1).

The coping mechanism that an athlete uses with respect to injury is influenced by many different factors, including personality, previous history of injury, level of competition, social support systems, and how serious the injury is perceived to be (Andersen and Williams, 1988). A history of frequent injuries is likely to lead to bitterness and frustration, demotivating the athlete and leading to apathy during rehabilitation. A severe injury may at first lead to post-traumatic shock, in which the

**Table 3.1 Psychological response to injury: athlete behaviour**

| Negative behaviour | Positive behaviour |
| --- | --- |
| Failure to take responsibility for own rehabilitation | Asks questions of therapist in order to understand injury |
| Non-acceptance of injury | Listens well to advice |
| Non-compliance and non-co-operation | Co-operation and compliance with therapist |
| Denial of seriousness or extent of injury | Receptive to restrictions placed on athlete |
| Displays of depression | Initiates progression of rehabilitation at home |
| Bargaining with therapist over treatment and time out of competition | Early acceptance of injury |
| Missing appointments | Does not bargain |
| Displays of anger | |
| Overdoing rehabilitation, e.g. attempting too much too early | |

Adapted from Gordon, Milios and Grove (1991).

athlete is unaware of severe pain or disability, and the initial psychological effect is small. Later, however, the psychological effects of severe injury can be considerable, and personality factors are an important factor in determining the final outcome of rehabilitation.

The nature of a sport and the accepted stereotyped reaction of peers to an injured colleague is important. A severe injury in contact sports is often perceived as a sign of manhood for example, whereas a similarly severe injury in golf may be perceived as weakness. Because the latter game is not so physically demanding, to become injured is not so socially acceptable. Equally, the level of competition is of importance. A top level competitor has more to lose than the weekend athlete and so his or her reaction to injury is likely to be more traumatic.

Certain body parts produce a greater psychological affect than others when injured. Injury to the knee or back, for example, demands a higher degree of psychological adjustment than a hamstring or groin tear (Gordon, Milios and Grove, 1991). One possible explanation for this is the perception by an athlete that any injury to the knee or spine must be serious, whereas muscle injuries are often dismissed as 'just a pull'.

**Personality and reaction to injury**

Eysenck (1957) described two major factors of personality. These were extroversion–introversion and neuroticism–stability (Fig. 3.1). The competitive sportsperson is typically extrovert, being outgoing, assertive and optimistic. Extroverts crave excitement, and are generally less able than introverts to tolerate tasks of a mundane nature. They are more likely to find rehabilitation 'boring', and will be impatient to return to sport after injury. Extroverts are thought to have higher pain thresholds than introverts (Lynn and Eysenck, 1961).

The typical introvert is hesitant, reflective and pessimistic. Injury has greater psychological impact, and he or she has a lower tolerance of pain, making an injury appear more serious than it actually is. This athlete, often only goaded into physical action by colleagues, needs strong encouragement during rehabilitation, and later when returning to sport.

Stable individuals, whether introvert or extrovert, will generally be less problematic within the sporting context, being calm, even tempered and

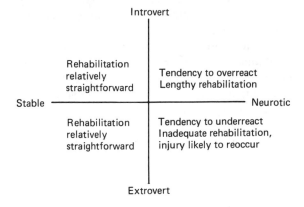

**Figure 3.1** Personality factors and reaction to injury.

emotionally stable. The highly neurotic athlete is more difficult to deal with because he or she is nervous, anxious and moody. The neurotic-introvert is more likely to develop phobias and anxiety, and is plagued by psychological conflicts which only make his or her anxiety worse (Sanderson, 1977). This type of individual tends to turn the neurosis in on him or herself, and the psychological trauma of injury is likely to be greater. In addition, this athlete is likely to be more apprehensive when returning to sport and this must be considered during the final stages of rehabilitation when the aim is to restore the athlete's confidence in a body part.

The extrovert generally has a strong self-esteem or self-concept, which is usually highly dependent on both physical appearance and physical function. The neurotic-extrovert will often perceive his or her self-esteem to be threatened by injury, and emotional problems may result. This leads to the phenomenon of 'playing through' an injury or 'working it off' in an attempt to maintain self-esteem.

### Response to rehabilitation

In addition to responses to injury, the response to rehabilitation itself can be both positive and negative. Those with a positive attitude to rehabilitation tend to work hard, be co-operative with the therapist, and ask constructive questions. A negative attitude to rehabilitation is shown by such things as an unwillingness to follow a home exercise programme, failure to keep appointments, continually questioning the therapist's judgement, and a reluctance to listen.

Athletes' reactions to injury and subsequent rehabilitation differ from those of the general public (Gordon, Milios and Grove, 1991). The competitively fit athlete wil have already experienced greater physical discomfort during training and so may be better able to adapt to the demands of a rehabilitation programme (Sanderson, 1981). An athlete will tend to be more 'body aware' and, especially in the case of experienced athletes, more likely to act quickly to promote healing by use of measures such as RICE. The general public tend to be more concerned with pain than with the conse-

quences of injury, the reverse being true for an athlete.

The therapist is in a better position to support and influence the injured athlete than is any other member of the rehabilitation team. This is because, by its very nature, physiotherapy creates a close patient/carer relationship. This affinity can be helped by developing a positive and dynamic atmosphere which is professional, relaxed and cheerful.

## Psychological aspects of pain

### Pain perception

The sensory threshold at which a person describes actually feeling a stimulus is roughly the same for everyone. But, if the stimulus intensity is gradually increased, the point at which a subject describes this sensation as pain (pain threshold) shows a wider variation. Individual and cultural differences exist, and each is influenced by a wide variety of psychological factors. The highest intensity of pain which can be endured (pain tolerance level) varies between individuals. Personality, lifestyle, situation, accepted behaviour, cultural and religious differences may all influence pain tolerance.

Eysenck (1967) showed extroverts to have higher pain thresholds than introverts, and argued that this could be explained in terms of increased cortical inhibition. In addition extroverts tend to express pain more freely, and are often more ready to accept the social disapproval which this can bring (Griffiths, 1980).

The situation in which the person experiences pain is also important. Injuries sustained by boxers are often not noticed until after their bout because their attention is focused elsewhere. Beecher (1959) observed that soldiers injured in battle requested less morphine than civilians with similar injuries. The social context was important here. The soldiers were grateful to be alive and looked forward to being removed from the battlefield, whereas to the civilians the injury was a depressing event.

The individual's past history is also relevant. As children, we learn how to respond to a painful stimulus by observing others, and Violon and

Giurgea, (1984) showed that family members respond to pain in a similar manner. Anxious subjects tend to complain of pain more, and if anxiety is reduced, pain intensity is also lowered. When a subject understands the cause of their pain, anxiety will reduce. For this reason, explanation forms an essential part of the rehibilitation process.

## Patient–therapist interaction

Pain inhibition may be achieved by creating positive emotional responses, which may facilitate control of nociceptor input by descending central control. During illness the body's sensory awareness may be lowered, and positive emotions can help restore the normal pain 'body image'. In this situation the physiotherapist may act as a 'treatment modality applied directly to the mind' (Charman, 1989) and affect the intensity and meaning of the patient's pain, both positively and negatively. Body language, voice and patient handling all give out signals which can change a patient's attitude to pain, making them a 'pain manager', rather than a 'pain victim'.

The concept of pain management by the patient was taken further by Williams (1989) with her 'school for bravery' approach. She emphasized the importance of changing from 'illness' to 'wellness' by behavioural modification. Patients were encouraged to participate in controlled exercise and recreational activities, despite being chronic pain sufferers. Combining fear reduction with confidence building she reported that over 80% of patients abandoned 'illness behaviour' illustrated by such signs as lack of facial expression, excessive slow movements, altered movement patterns, use of pain gestures and attention seeking.

These concepts, although originally described in hospital in patients, have a significant overflow to sports personnel, particularly those suffering from long-term or recurring injury.

## Anxiety and stress

### Anxiety

Two types of anxiety are generally recognized. State anxiety, which is temporary, occurs as a result of an individual's reaction to a particular situation. Trait anxiety, on the other hand, is a more persistent feature of a person's character or personality.

Whether a situation makes a person anxious will depend very much on his or her interpretation of the events which are occurring. This is often judged in the light of past experience, and in the context of sport, an individual's ability, or perceived ability, to perform a certain task. Anticipation is a key aspect here, a person's negative expectation of an event, rather than the event itself, causing the anxiety.

One underlying cause of anxiety in many people is fear of failure. This is often associated with loss of self-esteem and prestige within their peer group, leading to humiliation. The anxiety process often leads to greater physiological responses than does a purely physical threat.

Social factors are important in anxiety creation. For example, in a junior athlete, unremitting pressure from a well-meaning parent can lead to high levels of anxiety. The reverse is also true; good social support, where a parent lets a child know it is acceptable to fail can reduce anxiety and often lead to parallel improvements in performance.

### Stress

Individuals vary tremendously in their reactions to a particular situation, so it is more helpful to refer to perceived stress. Stress can be described from two perspectives, the stressful agent or 'stressor' and an individual's reaction to the stress.

Stress affects the body by producing an ergotropic response, primarily brought about by sympathetic nervous stimulation. Relaxation produces the opposite effect, through parasympathetic activity, of a trophotropic response. The ergotropic response is basically concerned with preparing the body for physical action, and represents the classical 'fight-or-flight' response. Conversely, the trophotropic response is designed to reduce the metabolic rate and restore the body to its natural resting state. It embodies the 'relaxation response'. A synopsis of each response is given in Table 3.2.

**Table 3.2   Effects of the ergotropic and trophotropic responses**

| Ergotropic response | Trophotropic response |
| --- | --- |
| Primarily sympathetic | Primarily parasympathetic |
| Excitement, arousal | Relaxation |
| Mobilization of body | Energy conservation |
| ↑Heart rate, blood pressure and respiration | ↓Heart rate, blood pressure respiration |
| ↑Blood sugar | ↑Gastrointestinal function |
| ↑Muscle tension | ↓Muscle tension |
| Pupil dilatation | Pupil constriction |
| ↑$O_2$ consumption | ↓$O_2$ consumption |
| ↑$CO_2$ elimination | ↓$CO_2$ elimination |

After Hertling and Kessler (1990).

### Stress reduction techniques

Stress management techniques fall broadly into two categories. First, there are those concerned with purely somatic (body) responses, and secondly, more mentalistic or cognitive (mind) techniques. The two categories are not distinct, but blend to form a variety of psycho-physiological responses.

A great diversity of approaches to stress management and relaxation techniques exist, but the four techniques most widely used in sport are progressive relaxation, autogenic training, visualization and biofeedback. These will be briefly described, but readers interested in pursuing these approaches further are referred to the texts listed in the further reading section at the end of this chapter.

With all the techniques, the reduction of initial stressors is important. Relaxation should be practised in a warm and quiet room, with low levels of lighting. The television, radio, or hi-fi should be switched off, and telephones taken off the hook. The subject should ask other members of the household not to disturb them while they are relaxing. Any restrictive clothing, such as tight belts, clasps, watches and jewellery should be removed. The body should be relaxed and supported. If the subject chooses to lie supine, the lumbar spine may be supported with a small rolled towel, and the head should rest on a small pillow or folded towel. The knees may be flexed over a pillow or roll to reduce the stretch on the popliteal structures.

### Progressive relaxation

This technique was first described by Jacobsen (1929). The procedure involves repeatedly tensing particular sets of muscles, and then relaxing them. The instructions for relaxation may be recorded on tape, although a live performance often gives better results. The sequence of muscle relaxation is shown in Table 3.3.

The advantages of this technique are, first, that it is easy for an athlete to practise alone, and does not involve concentrating the mind. Secondly, it teaches an athlete to recognize the difference between a tense and a relaxed muscle. This has obvious advantages, in that the athlete is then able to identify when physical stress is occurring throughout the day and reduce this. The same 'tense–release' methods can be used prior to competition with the specific muscles to be used in performance.

The disadvantage of this and any other purely physical approach is that it does not occupy the mind. Subjects often complain that they were thinking of something else or that their mind was elsewhere.

**Table 3.3   Muscle sequence for progressive relaxation**

Grip/straighten fingers
Flex/extend wrists
Flex/extend elbows
Rotate shoulders

Dorsiflex/plantarflex ankles
Flex (20°)/extend knees
Grip knees together
Tighten buttocks

Pull abdomen in
Arch back slightly
Brace shoulders
Shrug shoulders
Push head against floor

Grit teeth
Open mouth slightly
Frown
Raise eyebrows
Smooth forehead

*Autogenic training*

This method, first described by Schultz and Luthe (1959) uses a series of self statements designed to initiate physical and mental changes, and stems from work on self-hypnosis. The statements are designed to focus on warmth (vasomotor system) and heaviness of limbs (neuromuscular system).

Initially the training aims at inducing muscle relaxation. The subject begins by focusing his or her attention on the right arm and repeating the statement 'my right arm feels warm, heavy and relaxed' a number of times to him or herself. Once a feeling of warmth and heaviness is achieved, the attention is changed to the left arm, then the right and left legs. Some subjects find it more effective to split up the statements of warmth and heaviness, using 'my right arm is warm and relaxed', followed by 'my right arm is heavy and relaxed'.

Once muscle relaxation can be regularly achieved, the aim is then to reduce the heartrate with statements such as 'my heartbeat is slow and calm' or simply by passively observing the heartbeat. Then the breathing rate is reduced with statements such as 'my breathing is slow and shallow'. Attention is then turned to the trunk 'my stomach is warm and calm' and the head 'my forehead is cool and relaxed'.

The emphasis throughout the training is on 'letting go' and 'letting it happen' and not trying to force the body to relax. Different subjects will take longer or shorter periods to learn the technique, but most will achieve some results within six weeks.

*Visualization*

Visualization, or mental rehearsal (practice), is used both for relaxation and performance enhancement. The procedure first requires the athlete to reach a relaxed and more receptive state through one of the other relaxation methods. Within this state, various positive visual images are created by the athlete in his or her 'minds eye'. As many sensory stimuli as possible are used, sounds, feelings, pictures, smells and tastes merging into a total vision. If the athlete wishes to see him or herself winning or achieving a particular target, he or she should try to experience feelings of elation, sensations of physical exertion and the sounds of the crowd roaring.

The visualization is always positive, and may include positive statements or affirmations. Phrases such as 'I am full of energy' (positive) being used rather than 'I am not tired' (negative).

During the relaxation and visualization period, the athlete should remain alert, and in control of the images he or she uses. To facilitate this, the technique should be performed sitting rather than lying down, and the imagery should be purposeful rather than simply daydreaming. The visualization can be used either in the first person, or the third person. The athlete may imagine him or herself inside his or her own body, experiencing an ideal performance, or he may see him or herself from outside, as though on video playback.

Performance enhancement can be achieved by rehearsing an ideal model of a skill. After performing well, the athlete should replay the skill and review his or her performance. Again, the positive must be emphasized, and the athlete should not replay errors, but only successful outcomes for future reference. These images may be used to rehearse a skill before competition as part of a warm-up.

Another method of enhancing performance is for the athlete to imagine not the skill itself, but the feelings of winning, or the outcome of performance. He or she may imagine him or herself as a person or animal who demonstrates a particular trait which is required, such as strength, speed, bravery, etc.

Mental practice has been shown to benefit motor skill acquisition (Vandell et al., 1943; Clark, 1960; Fansler et al., 1985) and strength development (Cornwall et al., 1991), although this later effect is less certain.

*Biofeedback*

Biofeedback is the use of instrumentation to detect and display bodily processes, enabling an individual to then modify those processes. The basic requirements of a biofeedback system are a sensor which is capable of detecting a particular physiological reaction and a processor which creates an electrical impulse in response to the reaction, which is then displayed to the user.

The technique can be used to reduce autonomic effects, gain control over normally involuntary actions or re-educate voluntary movement after injury. A number of modalities can be used for biofeedback, including skin responses, cardiovascular measurements, electroencephalography and electromyography.

Electromyography (EMG) feedback is particularly valuable in the rehabilitation of muscle function. The electrical signal produced by motor unit firing is displayed visually or aurally. The subject then aims to reduce or increase motor unit recruitment to alter the feedback signal. This type of feedback may be used as motivation in rehabilitation strength training, or for postural re-education. The technique can also be used to re-educate muscle action sequences, for example in the treatment of shoulder instability (Beall, Diefenbach and Allen, 1987).

Skin reactions, such as galvanic skin response and skin temperature have been used extensively in relaxation training. The skin resistance is measured and amplified to give a feedback signal in galvanic skin response. As arousal or stress level is elevated, insensible sweating will increase, lowering the skin resistance and altering the signal. With temperature feedback, a thermistor is used to detect skin temperature changes occurring as a result of vasodilatation or vasoconstriction. With practice, the sympathetic activity controlling these changes can, to a certain extent, be controlled by the athlete.

Electroencephalogram (EEG) signals are useful when trying to initiate a relaxation response. When awake and alert, the brain emits electrical impulses in the beta frequencies (above 14 Hz), but when asleep, the frequencies reduce to the theta level (4–7 Hz) and still further to the delta level (below 4 Hz) during anaesthesia. Between the fully alert and sleeping states, there is a level of daydreaming or 'relaxed wakefulness' at the alpha level (7–14 Hz). This is the level of relaxation, and subjects can be trained using EEG biofeedback to stimulate the brain to produce waves at this level and so encourage relaxation. In addition, the mind is more susceptible to self-suggestion at the alpha level, and

EEG feedback can be used prior to visualization techniques.

## Motivation

Motivation is the desire that leads an individual to engage in, or sustain, a particular activity. Magill (1989) defined motivation as 'the causes of the initiation, maintenance and intensity of behaviour'. Factors which motivate often fulfil a need in an athlete, and needs will change and fluctuate with time. In order to motivate athletes to perform a particular task, and maintain the motivation, we must recognize the athletes' needs and act on them.

Both personal and social factors can act as motivators. Personal factors include such things as goals, physical sensations, and the way in which an athlete views him or herself. Social factors embrace considerations such as peer pressure, affiliation and rewards. The social and personal factors will merge to alter the meaning a situation has to an athlete, and it is this which will determine behaviours such as effort, persistence and performance (Lewthwaite, 1990).

Motivating factors may consist of both intrinsic and extrinsic rewards. An intrinsic reward relies on a person's own feelings, it is something internal. Athletes who train out of sheer enjoyment, or because they feel more competent when they do so are intrinsically motivated. Extrinsic motivation relies on a reward which is outside the person. Winning a medal or cup is an extrinsic reward.

One of the problems with extrinsic motivation, is that an athlete can feel manipulated by the reward system, and have a sense that continual striving removes their personal control (Rejeski and Kenney, 1988). To be effective, motivation must consist of a combination of both intrinsic and extrinsic rewards, which are carefully planned.

Three personal motivational factors, involving both intrinsic and extrinsic rewards, are important in the context of exercise and injury, and will be considered further. These are goal setting, belief in one's personal capability, and perceptual-affective experience (Lewthwaite, 1990).

# Goal setting

Goals may be classified according both to type and timescale. Two types of goal are generally used in the context of sport. The first, task-involved goals, rely on the need to improve a skill or performance of an activity. The second, ego-involved, focus on the necessity to prove oneself and be judged as competent or at least avoid being judged incompetent. Various social and situational factors will influence goals, such as age, cultural background, peers, coaches, and performance evaluation.

The timescale during which a goal is to be achieved is also important, and goals may be either long term or short term. Long-term goals are the things an athlete wants to achieve as the end result of all his or her training. These may be dreams or aspirations, such as a young athlete wanting to compete in the Olympic games, or end results, such as the injured athlete wanting to compete next season. Short-term goals are those which the athlete wants immediately and which will affect his or her immediate performance.

A number of features are important in the goal setting process. First, a goal should be difficult enough to stretch an athlete, but at the same time it should be achievable. To do this, a goal must take into account the capabilities of an athlete, and will require knowledge of past experience and personality characteristics. Secondly, goals should be specific, rather than general. For example, a goal to perform ten repetitions with a specific weight is better than simply telling an athlete to do their best. Feedback or knowledge of results is necessary to inform the athlete how he or she is performing with respect to the goal. Thirdly, a goal which is decided with the participation and agreement of the athlete is more effective. Often, when an athlete is instrumental in the goal setting process, goals will be set to a higher standard. Some guidelines for goal setting are listed below.

A goal should be:

1 Specific — specify a set number of repetitions or weight to be lifted for example rather than saying 'do your best'.

2 Meaningful — tell the athlete what the average score is and give them a reason for obtaining the goal.
3 Difficult — a goal must stretch an athlete. If it is too easily obtained there is no reason for performance to improve.
4 Obtainable — failure to achieve a short term goal over a number of trials will demotivate.
5 Measurable — the athlete must know if he or she is achieving the goal and will require knowledge of results.
6 Individual — personality factors and previous performance should be taken into account to 'tune' the goal to the athlete.
7 Agreed — participation in the goal making process is more effective.

A number of authors have demonstrated the benefits of goal setting to performance. Locke and Bryan (1966) showed specific goals to be better than a general goal to 'do your best' on a lighting pattern task. The specific goal group not only performed better, but had a faster rate of performance improvement. Harari (1969) assessed performance on a 750 yard running task, and found goals which were specific to an athlete's own performance (individual goals) and which were difficult, to be most effective. Nelson (1978) showed goal setting to be effective on an elbow flexion strength test. Of four groups tested, the one which was given an age norm (meaningful goal) performed the best.

# Belief in capability

The belief that one is capable of performing to a certain standard is an important intrinsic factor in determining an athlete's motivation. Bandura (1982) described two types of self-confidence or 'self-efficacy' in this context. First, efficacy expectation. This is the belief of an individual that they can achieve something because of their innate abilities. For example, someone may believe that they have the 'will power' to modify their eating habits and so lose weight, or the 'natural talent' to win a race. Secondly, Bandura referred to 'outcome expectations', or the belief that when one acts in a certain way, a particular result will follow. In the example of weight loss, the person displaying this characteristic would believe that changing eating habits will result in weight loss, whether they want them to or not.

Within the context of sports injury rehabilitation, it is not enough for an athlete undergoing rehabilitation to believe that a certain flexibility exercise will restore full range of movement (an outcome expectation). The athlete must also be encouraged to believe that he or she has the capacity to endure discomfort, and to persist with the exercise programme (efficacy expectation).

### Perceptual-affective experience

The perception of effort, and the emotion attached to that effort can act as a motivation. People naturally tend to persist with activities which are enjoyable and are resistant to uncomfortable or painful actions, but the subjective definition of what is enjoyable varies greatly between individuals.

The standard subjective measure of exercise intensity is the rating of perceived exertion (RPE) or Borg scale (Borg, 1982; Table 3.4). This runs from 6 to 20 and is based roughly on the difference between resting and maximal heartrates (60–200 b.p.m.). Various central (cardiopulmonary) and peripheral (biochemical) physiological cues enable

**Table 3.4   Rating of perceived exertion (RPE)**

| Original rating | Description |
| --- | --- |
| 6 | |
| 7 | Very, very light |
| 8 | |
| 9 | Very light |
| 10 | |
| 11 | Fairly light |
| 12 | |
| 13 | Somewhat hard |
| 14 | |
| 15 | Hard |
| 16 | |
| 17 | Very hard |
| 18 | |
| 19 | Very, very hard |
| 20 | |

After Borg (1982).

the athlete to rate his or her own exertion, but a number of psychosocial factors are also involved. Subjects tend to score lower on the RPE scale when exercising with others (Hardy, Hall and Prestholdt, 1986). Subjects appear to be influenced in the direction of another's response, perhaps to present themselves favourably. Studies with male subjects and female investigators have shown that the males tend to rate themselves lower at intense workloads than when tested by a male experimenter (Boutcher, Fleisher-Curtain and Giles, 1988), suggesting that they were concerned to 'appear fit'. Female subjects when tested by male experimenters did not show the same variation in rating.

Although two subjects may rate a particular work intensity similarly, their emotional response to this workload may be entirely different. Someone who has not exercised before is likely to find intense exercise unpleasant (negative), where as the athlete may find this same workload challenging (positive). Using an 11 point 'feeling scale' Hardy and Rejeski (1989) showed RPE to be directly related to the past level of physical activity, and to the belief that exercise is an integral part of a healthy lifestyle. Furthermore, it has been shown (Lewthwaite, 1990) that feelings of aversion to intense exercise in children are negatively correlated with attraction to and involvement in sport.

Clearly, the social context and the emotion attached to an exercise can act as a motivator. It is more likely that an athlete will work hard in an enjoyable group atmosphere than an isolated training session which he or she attends begrudgingly.

## Psychological effects of exercise

### Exercise and self-concept

Athletes and coaches usually associate exercise with the improvement of a number of physiological variables. In addition to these however, several psychological characteristics have also been shown to change as a result of participation in a regular exercise programme. Enhancement of self-confidence, self-esteem, and body image have been shown (Vincent, 1976; Sonstroem, 1984) and reductions in anxiety, depression, stress and tension have been demonstrated (Cooper, 1982). Of these variables, self-esteem, defined as 'the degree to which individuals feel positive about themselves' or a 'personal judgement of worthiness' would seem to be the one with the greatest potential for benefit from exercise (Sonstroem and Morgan, 1988).

## Enhanced wellbeing

Athletes often claim that exercise makes them feel good, and the 'runners high' is a widely-reported phenomenon. Reductions in stress and anxiety have been reported, lasting for between two and five hours after the cessation of training (Morgan, 1985), and decreased depression has been demonstrated as a result of 6–20 week exercise programmes (Greist et al., 1979). In addition, altered states of consciousness have been described following distance running (Mandell, 1979). Weight training programmes have been shown to enhance self-concept in both male (Dishman and Gettman, 1981; Tucker, 1982) and female (Brown and Harrison, 1986) athletes. Three theories exist to explain these phenomena, the distraction hypothesis, and the production of monamines and endorphins.

The distraction hypothesis proposes that participation in vigorous exercise distracts the athlete from stress. Comparison between exercise, meditation and distraction show similar reductions in state anxiety (Bahrke and Morgan, 1978), but the effect resulting from exercise appears to last longer (Morgan, 1985).

Depression is also affected by exercise. Reductions in the monoamine chemicals noradrenalin and serotonin (5–HT) are associated with depressed states in humans, and these same chemicals have been shown to increase in rats subjected to chronic exercise (Brown et al., 1979). Increases in the release of endorphins and enkephalins, or slowing of the dissociation rates of these chemicals has also been proposed (Pert and Bowie, 1979). By measuring plasma levels of these chemicals or using opiate antagonists to neutralize them, researchers have demonstrated some association between exercise and endorphins. Carr et al. (1981) reported significant rises in beta-lipotrophin and beta-endorphin levels in female subjects exercising at intensities up to 100 W. Farrell et al. (1983) showed increases in plasma leucine-enkephalin-like activity from mean values of 22.2 pmol/ml to 26.1 pmol/ml following a ten-mile road race. Anxiety, measured on a profile of moods states (POMS) test, was also shown to reduce.

It seems likely that these various physiological and psychological changes act synergistically in some way to produce the altered mood states associated with chronic exercise (Morgan, 1985).

## Exercise addiction

The experience of exercise for an athlete, and the way in which this fits into the rest of his or her life, is one factor which determines whether or not an exercise becomes addictive (Crossman, Jamieson and Henderson, 1987). Addiction is both physiological and psychological in nature and reflects that person's need for exercise. This need can be positive or negative. Positive addiction exists when an athlete receives some psychological or physical benefit from an activity, and is able to control the activity. The negatively addicted athlete is controlled by the activity and will experience severe negative affects (withdrawal) with a missed exercise bout. Addicted individuals often engage in an activity at the expense of their health or other factors, such as relationships and career prospects. The negatively addicted athlete may be failing to gain approval from significant others and may shelter feelings of inadequacy or unattractiveness. This type of athlete often exercises alone or in isolation from the group. They experience feelings of enhanced self-concept and even euphoria during and immediately after exercising. Importantly, this individual is more likely to ignore pain or injury and work through this to complete a workout. In the same vein, they tend to be anxious if a workout is missed and almost appear to suffer withdrawal symptoms. Some characteristics of exercise addiction are listed below. (Glaser, 1976; Anshel, 1991).

The athlete may:

1 Perform several bouts of exercise per week for up to an hour at a time.

2  Experience a high degree of positive effect after exercising.
3  Exercise alone or isolate themselves when in a group.
4  Be highly satisfied and less self-critical when exercising than at any other time.
5  Experience a state of euphoria when exercising.
6  Be more depressed/anxious/angry after missing a workout.
7  Tend to ignore physical discomfort/injury in order to complete an exercise regime.

# References

Andersen, M.B. and Williams, J.M. (1988) A model of stress and athletic injury: prediction and prevention. *Journal of Sport and Exercise Psychology*, **10**, 294–306

Anshel, M.H. (1991) A psycho-behavioral analysis of addicted versus non-addicted male and female exercisers. *Journal of Sport Behaviour*, **14**,(2) 145–154

Bahrke, M.S. and Morgan, W.P. (1978) Anxiety reduction following exercise and meditation. *Cognitive Therapy Research*, **2**, 323–333

Bandura, A. (1982) Self efficacy mechanisms in human agency. *American Psychologist*, **37**, 122–147

Beall, M.S., Diefenbach, G. and Allen, A. (1987) Electromyographic biofeedback in the treatment of voluntary posterior instability of the shoulder. *American Journal of Sports Medicine*, **15**, 175–178

Boutcher, S.H., Fleisher-Curtian, L.A. and Giles, S.D.(1988) The effects of self-presentation on perceived exertion. *Journal of Sport and Exercise Psychology*, **10**, 270–280

Beecher, H.K. (1959) *Measurement of Subjective Responses*, Oxford University Press, Oxford

Borg, G.A.V. (1982) Psychological bases of physical exertion. *Medicine and Science in Sport and Exercise*, **14**,(5), 377–381

Bramwell, S., Masuda, M., Wagner, N. and Holmes, T. (1975). Psychosocial factors in athletic injuries. *Journal of Human Stress*, **1**, 6–20

Brown, R.D. and Harrison, J.M. (1986) The effects of a strength training program on the strength and self-concept of two female age groups. *Research Quarterly for Exercise and Sport*, **57**,(4) 315–320

Brown, B.S., Payne, T., Kim, C., Moore, G., Krebs, P. and Martin, W. (1979) Chronic response of rat brain norepinephrine and serotonin levels to endurance training. *Journal of Applied Physiology*, **46**, 19–23

Carr, D.B., Bullen, B.A., Skrinar, G.S., Arnold, M.A., Rosenblatt, M., Beitins, I.Z., Martin, J.B. and McArthur, J.W. (1981) Physical conditioning facilitates the exercise-induced secretion of beta-endorphins and beta-lipotrophin in women. *New England Journal of Medicine*, **305**, 560–562

Charman, R.A. (1989) Pain theory and physiotherapy. *Physiotherapy*, **75**,(5) 247–254

Clark, L.V. (1960) Effect of mental practice on the development of certain motor skills. *Research Quarterly*, **31**, 560–569

Coddington, R. and Troxell, T. (1980) The effects of emotional factors on football injury rates – a pilot study. *Journal of Human Stress*, **6**, 3–5

Cooper, K.H. (1982) *The Aerobics Programme for Total Well-being*, Bantam, New York

Cornwall, M.W., Melinda, P.B. and Barry, S. (1991) Effect of mental practice on isometric muscular strength. *Journal of Orthopaedic and Sports Physical Therapy*, **13**, 5

Crossman, J., Jamieson, J. and Henderson, L. (1987) Responses of competitive athletes to lay-offs in training: exercise addiction or psychological relief? *Journal of Sport Behaviour*, **10**,(1) 28–38

Dishman, R.K. and Gettman, L.R. (1981) Psychological vigour and self-perceptions of increased strength. *Medicine and Science in Sports and Exercise*, **13**, 73–74

Eysenck, H.J. (1967) *The Biological Basis of Personality*. C.C. Thomas, Springfield, Illinois

Eysenck, H.J (1957). *The Dynamics of Anxiety and Hysteria*, Routledge and Kogan Paul, London

Fansler, C.L., Poff, C.L. and Shepard, K.F. (1985) Effects of mental practice on balance in elderly women. *Physical Therapy*, **65**, 1332–1338

Farrell, P.A., Gates, W.K., Morgan, W.P. and Pert, C.B. (1983) Plasma leucine enkephalin-like radioreceptor activity and tension-anxiety before and after competitive running. In *Biochemistry of Exercise*, (ed. H.G. Knuttgen, J.A. Vogel and J. Poortmans). Human Kinetics Publishers. Champaign, Illinois, pp. 637–644

Glasser, W. (1976) *Positive Addiction*, Harper and Row, New York

Gordon, S., Milios, D. and Grove, J.R. (1991) Psychological aspects of the recovery process from sport injury: the perspective of sport physiotherapists. *Australian Journal of Science and Medicine in Sport*, **23**, (2) 53–60

Greist, J.H., Klein, M.H., Eischens, R.R., Faris, J., Gurman, A.S. and Morgan, W.P. (1979) Running as treatment for depression. *Comprehensive Psychiatry*, **20**, 41–53

Griffiths, D. (1980) *Psychology and Medicine*, Macmillan, London

Harari, H. (1969) Levels of aspirations and athletic performance. *Perceptual and Motor Skills*, **28**, 519–524

Hardy, C.J. and Rejeski, W.J. (1989) Not what, but how one feels: the measurement of affect during exercise. *Journal of Sport and Exercise Psychology*, **11**, 304–317

Hardy, C.J., Hall, E.G. and Prestholdt, P.H. (1986) The mediational role of social influence in the perception of exertion. *Journal of Sport Psychology*, **8**, 88–104

Jackson, D.W., Jarrett, H., Bailey, D., Kausek, J., Swanson, J. and Powell, J.W. (1978) Injury prediction in the young athlete: a preliminary report. *American Journal of Sports Medicine*, **6**, 6–14

Jacobsen, E. (1929) *Progressive Relaxation*, University of Chicago Press, Chicago

Kerr, G. and Fowler, B. (1988) The relationship between psychological factors and sports injuries. *Sports Medicine*, **6**, 127–134

Kerr, G. and Minden, H. (1988) Psychological factors related to the occurrence of athletic injuries. *Journal of Sports Psychology*

Lewthwaite, R. (1990) Motivational considerations in physical activity involvement. *Physical Therapy*, **70**, (12) 808–819

Locke, E.A. and Bryan, J.F. (1966) Cognitive aspects of psychomotor performance. The effects of performance goals on levels of performance. *Journal of Applied Psychology*, **50**, 286–291

Lynn, R. and Eysenck, H.J. (1961) Tolerance for pain, extroversion, and neuroticism. *Perceptual and Motor Skills*, **12**, 161–162

Magill, R. A. (1989) *Motor Learning. Concepts and Applications*. WCB Publishers, Iowa

Mandell, A.J. (1979) The second wind. *Psychiatric Annals*, **9**, 57–69

Morgan, W.P. (1985) Affective beneficence of vigorous physical activity. *Medicine and Science in Sports and Exercise*, **17**,(1) 94–100

Nelson, J.K. (1978) Motivating effects of the use of norms and goals with endurance testing. *Research Quarterly*, **49**, 317–321

Pert, C.B. and Bowie, D.L. (1979) Behavioral manipulation of rats causes alterations in opiate receptor occupancy. In *Endorphins in Mental Health*. (ed. E. Usdin, W.E. Bunney, and N.S. Kline), Oxford University Press, Oxford, pp. 93–104

Reilly, T. (1975) *An Ergonomic Evaluation of Occupational Stress in Professional Football*. Doctoral Thesis, Liverpool Polytechnic

Rejeski, W.J. and Kenney, E.A. (1988) *Fitness Motivation. Preventing Participant Dropout*. Life Enhancement Publications, Champaign, Illinois

Sanderson, F.H. (1977) The psychology of the injury-prone athlete. *British Journal of Sports Medicine*, **11**, 56–57

Sanderson, F.H. (1981) The psychology of the injury-prone athlete. In *Sports Fitness and Sports Injuries* (ed. T. Reilly), Faber and Faber, London, pp. 31–36

Schneider, W. and Fisk, A. (1983) Attension theory and mechanisms for skilled performance. In *Memory and Control of Action* (ed. Magill), North Lolland, New York, pp. 119–143

Schultz, J.H. and Luthe, W. (1959) *Autogenic Training: a Psycho-physiologic Approach in Psychotherapy*, Grune and Stratton, New York

Sonstroem, R.J. (1984) Exercise and self esteem. *Exercise and Sports Science Reviews*, **12**, 123–156

Sonstroem, R.J. and Morgan, W.P. (1988) Exercise and self-esteem: rational and model. *Medicine and Science in Sports and Exercise*, **21**,(3) 329–337

Tucker, L.A. (1982) Effect of a weight training program on the self concept of college males. *Perceptual and Motor Skills*, **54**, 1055–61

Vandell, R.A., Davis, R.A. and Clugston, H.A. (1943) The function of mental practice in the acquisition of motor skills. *Journal of General Psychology*, **29**, 243–250

Vincent, M.F. (1976) Comparison of self-concepts of college women, athletes and physical education majors. *Research Quarterly*, **47**, 218–225

Violon, A. and Gilurgea, D. (1984) Familial models for chronic pain. *Pain*, **18**, 199–203

Wiese, D.M. and Wiess, M.R. (1987) Psychological rehabilitation and physical injury: implications for the sports medicine team. *The Sport Psychologist*, **1**, 318–330

Williams, J.I., (1989) Illness behaviour to wellness behaviour. *Physiotherapy*, **75**,(1) 2–7

## Further reading

Lewis, D. (1986) *The Alpha Plan*, Methuen, London

Mitchell, L. (1980) *Simple Relaxation*, John Murray, London

Selye, H. (1978) *The Stress of Life*, McGraw-Hill, Maidenhead

# 4 Assessment of sports injuries

## Assessing musculoskeletal injury

Physiotherapy which involves the application of modalities alone is of little value to a patient and may be of great harm. Physiotherapy is a complete system of healthcare which involves clinical examination, evaluation of the patient's problem, planning and treatment application.

Evaluation of the injured sportsperson may for convenience follow the SOAP format, a mnemonic for 'Subjective, objective, assessment and plan'. The subjective and objective examinations closely emulate the techniques of Cyriax (1982) and Maitland (1991). From this examination an assessment is made listing the problems and treatment goals, and, finally, a treatment plan is constructed.

## Subjective examination

Before the therapist touches a patient to examine signs, consideration should first be given to occupation, which sport is involved, physical training, and symptoms. A history is taken to establish the symptoms and development of the condition. History taking is a clinical skill which the sports therapist must master. Although the format will vary between patients, the communication skills required can be universal. These do not come easily to all practitioners, and training may have to be taken.

The aim of the practitioner is to understand the patient, almost to the extent that he or she feels what the patient feels (Maitland, 1991). The words and expressions the patient uses to describe his or her problem must be interpreted in the way in which the patient interprets them. Unfortunately, each of us describes what we experience in slightly

different ways. The way in which we interpret physical sensation in particular is governed by past experiences, genetic make-up, upbringing, ethnic background, and a whole host of other variables which together make up our personal frame of reference.

In order to break down the therapist–patient barrier, the practitioner must be able to accept the patient for what he or she is, without making value judgements. It is all too easy for the inexperienced practitioner to 'look down' on the patient and to appear superior in an attempt to cover up his or her own insecurity. The aim of the therapist is to relax the patient and gain his or her confidence, by creating an open, friendly and supportive atmosphere in the consultation.

Understanding the patient is rarely a simple matter, because many barriers can exist. The patient may be from a different ethnic background and have another language as their mother tongue (especially on the international sports scene). This will obviously affect the ease with which an athlete can describe what he or she feels, particularly in the highly stressful situation created by injury in competitive sport. People from different backgrounds will have different pain thresholds (see pp.52–3), and may have many preconceived ideas about an injury. Certain terms create horror on the face of an athlete (e.g. arthritis) while others are too familiar (e.g. cartilage).

It is a mistake for the therapist to assume anything during the consultation. At regular intervals throughout the examination, the therapist should stop and draw together the various aspects of what the patient is saying. The practitioner's interpretation of the situation up to that point should be put to the patient for confirmation. This process of continual confirmation rather than blind assumption is a great aid to accuracy in the subjective examination.

Phrasing questions and answers correctly is one way of aiding clarity, and Maitland (1991) recommended four methods of phrasing questions during the subjective examination. The first method is paralleling. This takes advantage of the patient's current train of thought, by following the previous question with one in a similar vein. To do this the therapist must have an overall idea of the information he or she wants to obtain, so that the subjective examination does not become stuck on one area. In addition, the therapist must be able to remember the answers to the previous questions for the paralleling process to continue. For example: patient, 'My heel hurts more when I run on hard surfaces'. *Question*, 'How far do you run?' *Answer*, 'Only three miles.' *Question*, 'What shoes do you run in?'

The use of key words or phases is another approach. During the patient's description of events or sensations, the patient may state things which have particular importance to the diagnosis, although he or she may not realize this. The therapist must stop the patient and confirm what is being said. For example: patient, 'I was just running slowly and I twisted my knee.' *Question*: 'So was your foot actually fixed to the ground as you twisted?' The third type of question is biasing. This is usually (but not always) detrimental to the subjective examination. The therapist asks a question which leads the patient to answer in a particular way. For example, the *question* 'Does that hurt?' suggests only pain, whereas 'How does that feel?' opens the question up to other sensations (burning, tingling, weakness, etc).

Finally, there are occasions on which an immediate response is required, often to confirm something when the answer given was ambiguous. For example: *question*, 'How does your knee feel now?' *Answer*, 'Not too bad'. *Immediate response*, 'Is it better or worse than before?'

In addition to question content, the tone in which the question is posed is important. Questions should be asked slowly and deliberately, aiming at clarity. They should be kept as succinct as possible (but not abrupt) and phrased in terms which the patient will understand. If the patient

uses particular terminology, the therapist should adopt the same phrases where appropriate. This is a useful way of emphasizing that the patient and the therapist are on the same communication level.

In addition to the answers given to specific questions, non-verbal communication or 'body language' is extremely important. Non-verbal signals often come out subconsciously before words have had time to form, and are usually more natural and less controlled (Maitland, 1986).

A general guide to some of the common questions asked during the subjective examination is listed below. These should obviously be phrased to suit the communication level of the patient.

1  Onset and development of condition:
   When did the condition start and what was the patient doing?
   Was there a sudden or insidious onset?
   Did the patient hear a click or 'feel something go'?
   How long has the condition lasted, is it acute or chronic?
   Is it the first episode, or a reoccurrence?
   Is the condition getting better or worse?
   Can the patient still work, is litigation pending?
2  Symptom location:
   Where are the symptoms felt and do they travel to other areas of the body?
   (use a bodychart to illustrate)
3  Symptoms behaviour:
   What are the symptoms?
   What makes the condition worse (aggravates) what makes it better (eases)?
   Do the symptoms occur at a specific time?
   Is there any diurnal variation?
   If there is more than one symptom, are they linked?
4  Other conditions/treatments:
   Have any medical tests been carried out?
   Has an X-ray been performed?
   Is the patient on any medication, if so what?
   Has the patient received treatment from another practitioner?
   Is there a relevant family history?
   Has eating or sleeping been affected?
   Has there been any recent weight loss?
   With spinal conditions – is there any change in

bladder or bowel habits?

Is there any history of dizziness, nausea or blackouts?

## Objective examination

For the experienced clinician, a detailed history can often create a surprisingly accurate picture of the condition. The aim of the objective examination is to clarify this picture and to focus on a specific body area, and accurately localize the anatomical site which has been affected.

### Inspection

The objective examination starts during the history taking with general observation. The patient's general appearance as he or she gets undressed, the posture both sitting and standing, how he or she walks and whether he or she guards the affected limb must all be observed. When the patient is undressed, before any physical tests are begun, a visual inspection is carried out, first of the whole body and then of the affected area. Bony alignment is assessed and any swelling noted. Muscle bulk is compared with the unaffected side of the body. The general skin condition in the area is examined and the patient questioned about any skin lesions.

### Examination of tissue tension

Physical examination itself involves active, resisted and passive movements. Willingness to move and a general assessment of range is obtained from active movements. In addition, active movements form an essential part of the examination procedure for mechanical therapy (see p. 140). McKenzie (1981) described a series of single and repeated spinal movements to indicate the presence of tissue dysfunction, discal derangement and postural abnormalities when dealing with spinal conditions. The range of movement and pain are assessed, and the alteration of these variables with repeated movements is an important indicator for prognosis.

Contractile structures are assessed by resisted tests and inert structures by passive movements (physiological and accessory). In each case, the examination is logical and methodical, comparing one side of the body with the other. If an abnormality is found the test is repeated for clarification.

During passive movements the feeling of a joint at the end of its movement range (end feel) is noted. When bone contacts bone (elbow extension) the end feel is hard, with soft tissue approximation (elbow flexion) the end feel is soft. When a normal joint capsule is stretched (external rotation of the shoulder) the end feel is abruptly springy, when muscles are put on stretch (straight leg raising) the end feel is rubbery and less abrupt. Abnormal end feels are created by abnormalities such as muscle spasm, swelling and tissue entrapment.

With passive movements, joints will exhibit specific configurations of movement limitation, known as capsular patterns, indicating that the entire joint capsule is inflamed (Cyriax and Cyriax, 1983). For example, when the shoulder capsule is inflamed, abduction is the movement most limited, followed by lateral rotation. Capsular patterns of the major joints are shown in Table 2.2.

Only when tissue function has been tested does palpation begin. Palpation is a skill which requires training, and great accuracy can be achieved. Maitland (1986) quoted a study by Evans (1982) in which experienced manipulative therapists were required to detect a subtle resistance within a 4.0 mm range of movement. The standard deviation for this task was 0.16 mm, and the therapists were able to perform grade I mobilization techniques with a mean amplitude of oscillation of 0.02 mm.

### Palpation

Accurate and clinically useful palpation demands a good knowledge of surface anatomy; without this, palpation simply becomes ineffective massage. When palpating, the examiner is especially interested in warmth, swelling, crepitus and pain (Corrigan and Maitland, 1983). Warmth indicates the presence of increased metabolic activity due to inflammation or haemarthrosis. Alteration in skin temperature (hot or cold) accompanied by sweating giving a 'clammy' feeling may indicate sympathetic involvement.

Swelling can be either extra-articular or intra-articular, and varies in consistency from hard to soft. Hard intra-articular swellings are usually due to bony abnormalities, such as osteophytes or osteochondrotic fragments. Soft intra-articular swelling may be either fluid from synovial effusion or synovial thickening. Synovial fluid is recognized on inspection and confirmed by fluctuance to palpation. Synovial thickening is best felt by rolling the fingers across the area of synovial attachment to the underlying bone.

Extra-articular swelling again varies in density, and can be the result of many factors, including calcification, oedema, haematoma, fatty deposits, scar tissue and synovial swelling of tendon sheaths and bursae. The size, shape, consistency and attachment of the swelling is noted.

To gain an accurate picture of what lies beneath the skin, the therapist should focus his or her attention on what is being palpated, and use just one finger where possible (Stoddard, 1982) for specific structures. Skin temperature can usefully be tested with the back of the hand, and skin rolling massage techniques will often indicate pathological changes in the subcutaneous tissue. Altering the palpation pressure will change the depth assessed, and again comparison is made with the unaffected side.

It is important to remember when assessing bony position that bone is felt through skin and subcutaneous tissues. If the condition of the soft tissue changes a 'palpatory illusion' may occur, giving the false impression that joint position has actually changed (Lewit, 1991).

In this book, details of the initial screening examination for each joint are given at the beginning of each particular chapter and draw mostly on the work of Cyriax and Cyriax (1983). More specific tests are described along with the structures which are injured, and represent the work of various authors. Where joint play is assessed prior to mobilization, the examination is derived mostly from the work of Maitland (1991).

## Assessment and plan

The information gained from the subjective and objective examination is now brought together in the assessment. This is an interpretation of the examination findings, with particular reference to the ways in which physiotherapy can relieve the signs and symptoms (Wood, 1984)

Within the assessment, short- and long-term goals are decided, and recommendations made for the treatment programme. A list of the major symptoms can be made, either separately or simply by highlighting the most important findings of the subjective and objective examinations. A general statement is then made of the impression that the therapist has gained during the examination.

A plan of the programme is made, to show how the treatment will develop. The type, duration and frequency of treatment is suggested (Saunders, 1990). The examination process is ongoing, and as the patient's reaction to treatment is known, irritability is assessed, and subsequent treatment modified accordingly. As new facts present themselves, further treatment modification is made.

## Clinical decision-making

During the assessment process, various decisions must be made concerning the most appropriate course of action. Should the patient be sent for X-ray? Should the patient be referred? Which modality is appropriate? Is immobilization called for? To help this procedure, structured decision-making techniques may be used (Wolf, 1985).

The first step in the decision-making process is to narrow down the problem and focus on a single area. Instead of trying to analyse all aspects of the decision at once, the process is taken step by step. Each decision should have a definite beginning and end point, to prevent an endless discussion which fails to come to a conclusion. For example, when dealing with an ankle injury we may want to decide whether to immobilize the joint or not. If this is the case, we must focus our attention just on this topic. We may also want to know which modalities to use, when to start exercise, when the athlete is fit to play, etc., but these are entirely separate decisions, the consideration of which will only cloud the issue at the moment.

The second step is to structure the problem as a logical sequence of decisions and represent this diagrammatically by a 'decision tree' (Fig. 4.1). At

Problem: With a grade II ankle sprain, should the ankle be immobilized?

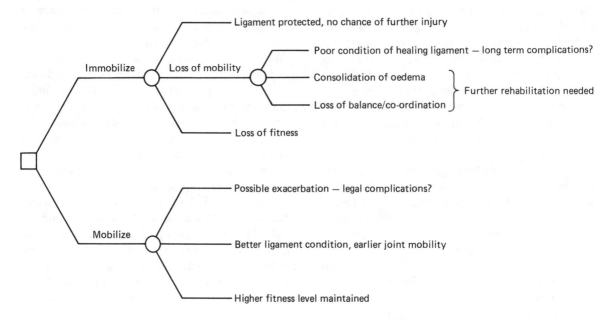

**Figure 4.1** The decision tree.

each stage the available options and the possible consequences which may occur if that option is chosen are listed. With the example in Fig. 4.1 we may have to decide whether or not to immobilize the ankle. If we do immobilize it, there are many negative consequences (loss of flexibility, strength and skill) and various positive ones (joint protection, ligamentous shortening).

These consequences, and many others, are all possible, but we need to know how likely it is that they will occur. This is step three. We now estimate the probability that the consequences we have listed in step two will actually occur in the clinical situation we are dealing with. This is done subjectively, using the clinical experience of one or a number of practitioners. The probability score given may not be mathematically accurate, but it does clarify the decision-making process. Using the example of the ankle once more, there is a high probability (100%) that immobilization in a cast will produce some loss of flexibility. However, there is a lower probability that skill will be reduced. Our estimate for this will be higher when returning an athlete to running (90%), but lower

with rifle shooting (30%).

The final step is valuation. We now estimate how important a particular outcome will be to the patient and, in terms of cost/benefit, the value to society as a whole. If the ankle is immobilized, there may be some loss of joint function in the short term, but joint protection is gained. This may have great value where we know an athlete will be unwilling to rest or use crutches, for example.

This whole process may seem long-winded, but the time taken can give great benefits in terms of patient welfare and financial savings. The ultimate aim is to choose the best treatment approach and in so doing obtain the best outcome with the minimum risk to the patient.

### Assessing strength and flexibility

Both strength and flexibility are important components of fitness and are essential for full function of a joint. Strength and flexibility are measured in their most basic forms by comparing the performance of the injured and uninjured sides.

## Strength

Strength assessment may be made more objective by recording the strength performance on the Oxford scale (Table 4.1).

Strength may be assessed with an isometric dynamometer, or by obtaining the 1RM (repetition maximum) or 10RM on weight training apparatus. Isometric dynamometers are portable and easily used clinically and the tests are accurate and repeatable. Their disadvantage is that isometric strength gains are joint angle specific (p.100). Measurements with weight training apparatus obviously relate well to performance in training, but do not necessarily reflect pure strength gains, as skill improvement, particularly when inexperienced users begin training, is largely responsible for performance enhancement (see p.99).

Isokinetic assessment is even more accurate still, and is increasingly used for the precise assessment of muscle function.

**Table 4.1  Oxford classification of muscle power**

| | |
|---|---|
| 0 . . . . . | No contraction present |
| 1 . . . . . . | Flicker only |
| 2 . . . . . | Contraction in gravity eliminated position |
| 3 . . . . . | Contraction against gravity |
| 4 . . . . . | Contraction against resistance (record value) |
| 5 . . . . . | Normal muscle function |

## Isokinetic assessment

### Muscle force
The measurement of torque during maximal concentric contraction is the most common method of isokinetic strength testing. Torque is measured for a single joint movement, the axis of the joint being aligned with that of the dynamometer. In some instances, a rapidly performed movement, such as a throwing action, may exceed the velocity limit of the dynamometer. Equally, extremely strong subjects, may produce movements in excess of the torque capacity of the isokinetic apparatus. Peak torque, either measured as an absolute value or expressed as a percentage of the subject's bodyweight, and angular velocity are all useful measures used in clinical assessment.

When measuring maximum torque, between two and six repetitions are usually performed before a stable measurement is achieved. The maximum torque is normally described as the highest single torque value recorded (Baltzopoulos and Brodie, 1989). However, some authors (Morris et al., 1983; Patton and Duggan, 1987) have used mean values of three or five repetitions respectively, and so the testing methods should always be defined.

The velocity of movement (degree per second or rads per second) is also recorded, and it must be remembered that torque will reduce as angular velocity increases (Fig.4.2).

Early dynamometers were only able to measure concentric activity, in both muscle sets of a group. With the development of a powered mode, eccentric muscle work may now be measured. This can be used in combination with concentric activity as with normal exercise (concentric/eccentric), or with both muscles in the group acting eccentrically (eccentric/eccentric). Again, the resistance is totally accommodating, and the powered mode has the additional advantage that it may also be used for continuous passive motion (CPM).

### Muscle endurance
Muscular endurance can be assessed using isokinetic dynamometry by computing a fatigue index. Various methods have been used to calculate this

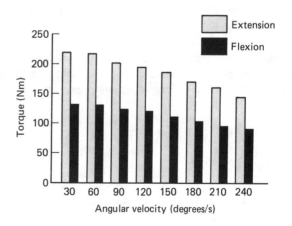

**Figure 4.2**  The maximum torque at different angular velocities of knee extension and flexion. From Baltzopoulos and Brodie (1989), with permission.

index. Probably the most common for knee extension is that described by Thorstensson and Karlson (1976). In this test, subjects perform 50 consecutive knee extensions at 180°/s. The decline in torque over the 50 repetitions is calculated as the percentage difference between the mean torque of the first and last three repetitions.

Patton et al. (1978) used time to muscular exhaustion, Barnes (1981) used the difference (as a percentage value) between the maximum torque and that obtained in the tenth maximal contraction. Norris (1987) used the time to 50% maximal torque, and Baltzopoulos, Eston and McLaren (1988) used the decline in maximum torque over time using a 30 second test period.

### Effects of inertia and gravity

Chart recordings of torque generated by subjects working at high velocities, may show an initial high peak known as the 'impact artefact' or 'torque overshoot', followed by oscillations which decrease in amplitude (Fig. 4.3). This occurs in the time from rest, to the limb catching up with the preset speed of the dynamometer. During this phase, the limb is accelerating towards the preset speed and is therefore not being exercised isokinetically.

The torque overshoot is greater during proximal joint testing due to the greater limb mass and longer distance between the limb's centre of gravity and the axis of rotation. If the overshoot is interpreted as the peak torque, the subject's muscular capacity will be overestimated (Baltzopoulos and Brodie, 1989).

With sagittal and frontal plane movements the effects of gravity must be considered. With small force outputs the effect of gravity may obscure

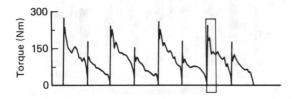

**Figure 4.3** Torque overshoot (boxed area) during knee extension-flexion movements. From Baltzopoulos and Brodie (1989), with permission.

results. The dynamometer will only record the force used against its internal resistance. It would normally not show the force used to overcome gravity in an upward movement, or the contribution made by gravity in a downward action. Nelson and Duncan (1983) determined the gravitational torque generated by the limb-lever system when it was allowed to fall passively at various angular positions. From this, a correction factor was calculated to be added to the maximum torque registered by the dynamometer. Using this method, results will only be valid if the limb is allowed to fall against the resistance of the dynamometer with the subject's muscles relaxed.

Various computer programs have been produced which correct for gravity and inertial effects. These replace the need for manual data analysis and increase the accuracy of isokinetic dynamometry.

### Flexibility

Once comparison with the uninjured side has been made, flexibility assessment can be made more objective by goniometry. Three types are generally used, the standard (lever) goniometer, the gravity goniometer and the electrogoniometers.

The standard goniometer is positioned with its two lever arms in line with the long bones forming the joint and the goniometer axis aligned to the joint axis. The joint angle is recorded in degrees. Measurements made with this instrument have the advantage of convenience and low cost, but difficulties can arise in identifying the joint axis, particularly with complex movements, and aligning the lever arms. The electrogoniometer has the same function, but a potentiometer is used to sense changes in joint angle, giving a digital readout. This unit has the advantage that it can measure changes in joint angle during movement, but positioning can still be a problem.

The Leighton flexometer (Leighton, 1942) is a gravity goniometer which measures joint angle with respect to the vertical, by comparing the limb position with that of a weighted arm. It has the advantage that the operator does not have to locate the joint axes, and has been shown to be reliable (MacDougall, Wenger and Green, 1982).

When general limb flexibility is to be assessed, rather than specific joint angles, field tests are useful. Some, such as the sit and reach test, measure actual values, while others represent performance on a pass or fail basis and are useful for screening. Some of the first tests were developed by Cureton (1941), who used trunk flexion and extension, shoulder extension in prone lying, and ankle flexibility. Later, Fleishman (1964) used a battery of tests to assess static and dynamic flexibility. Static flexibility was assessed by toe-touching, spinal extension and trunk rotation. Dynamic flexibility was assessed by combined movements, such as standing from a squatting position, twisting, and touching a point on the wall behind the subject.

Watson (1983) described nine useful tests for static flexibility which can be used as part of a pre-season screening programme, as listed below. The movements are performed slowly, with the final position being held for three seconds. Scores are expressed in relation to body height to make comparison between subjects more useful.

1  Stand and reach/sit and reach. The knees are kept straight throughout the movement.
2  Spinal hyperextension — either performed against a wall with the subject's hips held, or in a lying position.
3  Spinal rotation in a sitting position.
4  Side bending — the subject stands with his or her back on a wall, the hips are held, and the feet must stay on the ground. The distance the fingers reach down the thigh is measured.
5  Horizontal shoulder movement — no vertical movement is allowed, and the arms should stay straight.
6  Straight leg raise — both legs should remain straight.
7  Hip extension — this can be performed actively by the athlete or passively by a partner.
8  Ankle flexion and extension.
9  Hip abduction — the subject should keep his or her heels 15 cm from the groin throughout the movement.

### Assessing fitness to play

As the patient progresses with rehabilitation, more fitness aspects will need to be developed and assessed. Eventually, a stage is reached at which the question must be asked 'Is the athlete fit to play?', and the physiotherapist must be able to make an objective decision about this. A number of factors must be considered, including the nature of injury, stage of tissue repair, the sport, the player's position and his or her level of involvement (Wright, 1981). The physiotherapist must use his or her knowledge to analyse the various movements involved in a sport, and equate these with the functional anatomy of the injured body part. This will enable him or her to assess the stress an athlete will be placing on the injured area.

Clinical assessment may begin in the treatment room with the various tests outlined in this chapter, but functional testing must be carried out in the gymnasium and eventually on the sports field. The athlete must not be allowed to return to competitive sport until he or she has full painless active and passive range of motion, full strength in balance with other body parts, sufficient endurance, and normal movement patterns (Reid, 1982).

The aim is to progress through the various tests, moving from rehabilitation exercises to movements which mimic sports tasks but at a lower level. Eventually a stage is reached at which the test is harder than the task to be performed in competition and full confidence is regained. Performance in late stage rehabilitation exercises can be used as an indicator of strength, flexibility, power, endurance and skill.

Functional testing for the upper limb includes varieties of push-ups and dips with a gradually increasing range of movement. When these can be performed without pain, the athlete is asked to take his or her body weight through the arms at speed. Initially, the hands are in contact with the ground and the feet are kicked up. When confidence is gained and no pain is experienced this is progressed to dropping onto the hands and kicking the legs into the air simultaneously. Gymnastic movements, such as forward rolls and handstands, are also useful measures (Fig. 4.4). Lower limb tests include hopping forwards, backwards and side to side, deep hopping, bench stepping of various kinds, leg thrusts, striding, jumping and plyometric exercise (Fig. 4.5).

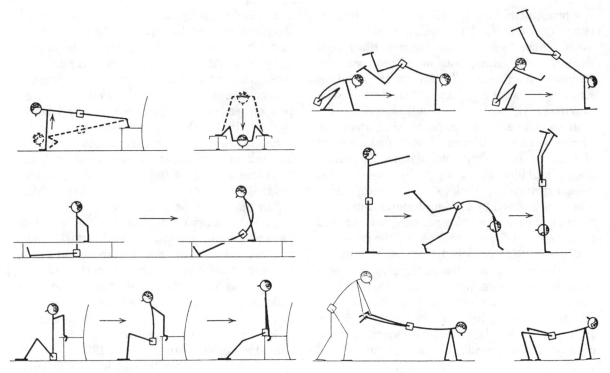

**Figure 4.4**   Functional testing of the upper limbs.
From Reilly (1981), with permission.

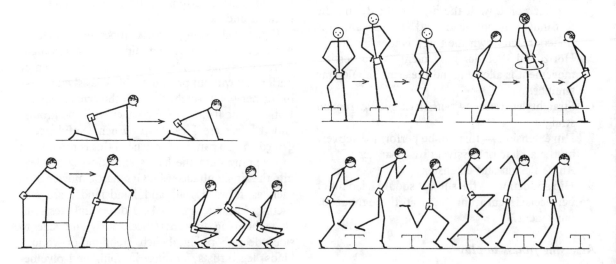

**Figure 4.5**   Functional testing of the lower limbs.
From Reilly (1981), with permission.

# References

Baltzopoulos, V. and Brodie, D.A (1989) Isokinetic dynamometry. Applications and limitations. *Sports Medicine*, **8**,(2) 101–116

Baltzopoulos, V., Eston, R.G. and McLaren, D. (1988) A comparison of power outputs on the Wingate test and on a test using an isokinetic device. *Ergonomics*, **31**, 1693–1699

Barnes, W. (1981) Isokinetic fatigue curves at different contractile velocities. *Physical Therapy*, **60**, 1152–1158

Corrigan, B. and Maitland, G.D (1983) *Practical Orthopaedic Medicine*, Butterworth, London

Cureton, T.K. (1941) Flexibility as an aspect of physical fitness. *Supplement to Research Quarterly*, **12**, 381–390

Cyriax, J. H. (1982) *Textbook of Orthopaedic Medicine*, Vol. 1, 8th edn., Bailliere Tindall, London

Cyriax, J.H. and Cyriax, P.J. (1983) *Illustrated Manual of Orthopaedic Medicine*, Butterworth, London

Fleishman, E.A. (1964) *The Structure and Measurement of Physical Fitness*, Prentice Hall, New Jersey

Leighton, J.R. (1942) A simple objective, and reliable measure of flexibility. *Research Quarterly*, **13**, 205–216

Lewit, K. (1991) *Manipulation Therapy in Rehabilitation of the Locomotor System*, 2nd edn, Butterworth-Heinemann, Oxford

MacDougall, J.D., Wenger, H.A. and Green, H.J. (1982) Physiological testing of the elite athlete. *Mutual Press*, Canada

Maitland, G.D. (1986) *Vertebral Manipulation* (5th edn), Butterworth–Heinemann, London

Maitland, G.D. (1991) *Peripheral Manipulation* (3rd edn), Butterworth-Heinemann, Oxford

McKenzie, R.A. (1981) *The Lumbar Spine. Mechanical Diagnosis and Therapy*, Spinal Publications, Waikanae, New Zealand

McKenzie, R.A. (1990) *The Cervical and Thoracic Spine. Mechanical Diagnosis and Therapy*, Spinal Publications, Waikanae, New Zealand

Morris, A., Lussier, K., Bell, G. and Dooley, J (1983) Hamstring/quadriceps strength ratios in collegiate middle-distance and distance runners. *Physician and Sportsmedicine*, **11**, 71–77

Nelson, S. and Duncan, P. (1983) Correction of isokinetic torque recordings for the effect of gravity. *Physical Therapy*, **63**, 674–676

Norris, C.M. (1987) *The Assessment of a Novel Physiotherapy Technique – Combined Vacuum and Pressure*. MSc Thesis, University of Liverpool

Patton, J. and Duggan, A. (1987) An evaluation of tests of anaerobic power. *Aviation, Space and Environmental Medicine*, **3**, 237–242

Patton, W.R., Hinson, M., Arnold, B.R. and Lessard, M.A. (1978) Fatigue curves of isokinetic contractions. *Archives of Physical Medicine and Rehabilitation*, **59**, 507–509

Reid, D.C. (1982) Sports medicine: functional assessment and return to game fitness. In *Proceedings of the VII Commonwealth and International Conference on Sport, Physical Education, Recreation and Dance*. (ed. M.L. Howell and M.I. Bullock). Department of Human Movement Studies, University of Queensland

Reilly, T. (1981) *Sports Fitness and Sports Injuries*, Faber and Faber, London

Saunders, H.D. (1990) Evaluation of a musculoskeletal disorder. In *Orthopaedic and Sports Physical Therapy* (ed. J.A. Gould), C.V. Mosby, St Louis

Stoddard, A. (1982) *Manual of Osteopathic Technique*, Hutchinson, London

Thorstensson, A. and Karlson, J. (1976) Fatigability and fibre composiiton of human skeletal muscle. *Acta Physiologica Scandinavica*, **98**, 318–322

Watson, A.W.S. (1983) *Physical Fitness and Athletic Performance*, Longman, Harrow

Wolf, S.L. (1985) *Clinical Decision Making in Physical Therapy*, F.A. Davis, Philadelphia

Wood, P.M. (1984) Examination and assessment of the spine and peripheral joints. In *Cash's Textbook of Orthopaedics and Rheumatology for Physiotherapists*, (ed. P.A. Downie), Faber and Faber, London, pp. 188–202

Wright, D. (1981) Fitness testing after injury. In *Sports Fitness and Sports Injuries* (ed. T. Reilly), Faber and Faber, London, pp. 266–273

# 5 First contact management

## Injury prevention

Injury prevention should perhaps be the most important topic in the field of sports medicine. The term 'prevention' is normally used in the context of sports injuries to refer to any measure which can stop an injury occurring. But the processes of prevention also play an important role in arresting the exacerbation of a current injury and ensuring that the same injury does not recur.

The causes of sports injuries are many and varied. Williams and Sperryn (1976) implicated failure in technique, faulty sports equipment, poor physical fitness, inadequate warm up and psychological factors. Taimela, Kujala and Osterman (1990) divided injury risk factors into intrinsic and extrinsic groups, as shown in Table 5.1.

Some factors will clearly affect athletes differently, and certain elements are more important in one sport than another. However, in general the more risk factors an athlete shows, the more likely

**Table 5.1  Injury risk factors**

*Extrinsic*
Organization and management
Type of sport
Training errors
Environment
Equipment

*Intrinsic*
Age
Gender
Somatotype
Local anatomy and biomechanics
Fitness
Physical symmetry
Joint integrity
Motor control (skill)
Psychological/psychosocial factors

Adapted from Taimela, Kujala and Osterman (1990).

he or she is to be injured. Consequently, the aim of the coach or practitioner should be to reduce these risk factors to a minimum.

## Warm up

The subject of warm up is dealt with in depth in Chapter 6. A general warm up, intense enough to induce mild sweating without causing fatigue, is important for injury prevention. The general activity should be followed by a specific warm up designed to produce a suitable arousal level in the athlete, and to rehearse any complex skills which will be used later in competition.

Joints, muscles and other soft tissues should be extended through their full physiological range before competition. However, it is important that flexibility training in itself is separate to, and follows after, a warm up.

It is also important that vigorous exercise does not end abruptly, but slows gradually during a cool down period. This period allows the cardiopulmonary system to return to resting levels without placing undue stress on the body. In addition, delayed onset muscle soreness (DOMS) may be reduced by flushing fresh blood into the muscles previously worked during exercise.

## Fitness

All the components of fitness are required for injury prevention, and importantly, a balance should exist between each. For example, increased flexibility without a similar increase in strength may compromise joint integrity. Similarly, strength and muscle bulk increases without adequate flexibility and skill can leave an athlete 'muscle bound' and lacking agility.

Symmetry of muscle development and range of motion is also important. Athletes who exercise unilaterally, for example throwers, must take care that they redress the imbalance caused by their sport with a suitable strength-training programme.

It is also important that training accurately reflects the physical demands of a sport, and that exercise is specific to the physiological adaptations that the sport requires (SAID principle see p.89). Sports requiring speed and power, for example, will suffer if only strength is included in training. The 'strong' athlete who has trained exclusively with heavy weight training is open to injury when rapid explosive actions are used in sport. This is because the skills involved in the two actions are very different.

### Psychological factors

Athletes of a certain psychological type may be more predisposed to injury, and the sports coach must recognize this. Equally, during particularly stressful periods, or when life pressures outside the sporting context are great, athletes who do not normally get injured may start to have problems. These concepts are dealt with in Chapter 3, but all coaches and practitioners working with sports teams must get to know their athletes. Realizing that a player is having problems with his or her spouse, or has recently had a family bereavement is vital to 'total player management'.

### Equipment and environment

All athletes are under pressure to buy particular sportswear. Professional athletes may receive sponsorship, and amateur athletes are fashion conscious. It is important to emphasize to the athlete that sports equipment should be comfortable and functional. If a particular shoe or item of clothing does not fit correctly, another should be tried, the fit being more important than the type.

The field of play should also be the focus of attention, particularly in amateur sport. Before training, both the environment and equipment should be inspected by the coach. If, for example, a child falls on a broken bottle that no one realized

was there, part of the responsibility lies with the coach for not checking the area beforehand.

Another aspect of 'environment' that warrants attention is the other players. In youth sport, players should be matched for size and maturity. Where the age group of players covers a wide range, there can be a great difference in body size due to the premature development of some youngsters. Clearly a 14-year-old athlete who is 1.8 m tall and weighs 76 kg should not be playing opposite a ten-year-old who is 1.5 m tall and weighs 45 kg, especially in contact sports.

### Rules

In professional sport, rule changes have had a dramatic effect, particularly with head injuries (see p. 260). However, the local youth club under-12 team must also have a firm policy of sports regulation. Where children are involved, it is important to lay down firm rules concerning safety and equipment. The coach who tries to be popular by allowing a 'free-for-all' is really being irresponsible and is likely to be the cause of injury.

### Screening

The subject of physical screening of youngsters in sport is one which attracts much discussion. A variety of anatomical abnormalities may develop largely unnoticed to the layperson. However, these can often be readily identified by the sports medicine practitioner with a series of annual screening tests. Posture (p. 232), flexibility (p. 69) and strength (p. 67) can all be measured using fairly simple field tests. These can be incorporated into a training session and educational period for youngsters, at the beginning of a season.

### First aid

First aid treatment marks the beginning of the rehabilitation process. Correct management at this stage can reduce the severity of an injury and so shorten the time an athlete is away from sport. More importantly, effective first aid can save lives. In this section, a number of first aid methods relevant to the injured sportsperson are described. All therapists involved with sports injuries management are recommended to obtain certification in cardiopulmonary resuscitation (CPR) and basic first aid.

### The unconscious athlete

Unconsciousness is the result of an interruption of normal brain activity. The most common cause in sport is concussion. The first decision to be made with an unconscious athlete is whether he or she is still breathing. If not, resuscitation must be started *immediately*.

If the athlete is breathing, the severity of loss of consciousness should be assessed. Response of the eyes, body movements and speech all give clues to the level of consciousness. Table 5.2 shows a number of responses which may be tested. In addition, pulse and respiratory rate and depth should be noted, as any sudden change is important.

### *Concussion*

Concussion occurs when the brain is rapidly 'shaken', and the condition can be present even though the patient is still conscious. Often, the period of unconsciousness is so brief that it may go unnoticed, and there is only transient memory loss. This is frequently the case with contact injuries, in which one athlete collides with another and hits his or her head.

**Table 5.2   Response testing in the unconscious athlete**

Do the eyes open:
  spontaneously
  to speech
  to pain

Does the athlete move:
  to verbal command
  to painful stimulus

Is the athlete's speech:
  normal
  confused
  inappropriate
  incomprehensible

After such an incident, an athlete should be allowed to continue only if he or she did not lose consciousness. Tests such as the ability to stand up without assistance, to stand alone with eyes closed, and to run to a mark and change direction rapidly are all useful (Walkden, 1981). Even then, the athlete should be regularly checked.

Caution must always be exercised with concussion injuries. Unfortunately, the practitioner or coach who has to decide whether to allow an athlete to continue playing has no way of knowing if secondary brain damage is going to develop. At the time of injury, bleeding may have occurred which could accumulate and give rise to sub-dural haematoma.

If the athlete remains unconscious, he or she should be placed in the recovery position until an ambulance is available to take him or her to hospital. If there is bleeding or discharge from an ear, the athlete should be turned so that the affected ear is dependent. Nothing should be given by mouth, and the athlete should not be left unattended. Testing for responses should continue regularly (every 10 minutes or less) and any changes in the athlete's condition should be recorded.

### *Epilepsy*

If an epileptic athlete loses consciousness, he or she may fit. Rigidity may last for a few seconds and cyanosis of the mouth and lips can occur. The athlete should be protected by clearing a space around him or her. Any tight clothing around the neck should be loosened, and something soft should be placed under his or her head.

No attempt should be made to move or restrain the athlete, and nothing should be given by mouth until he or she has fully recovered. If the subject is in danger of biting his or her tongue, a gag may be placed between the teeth. The handle of a spoon or other implement covered with a thick cloth can be useful.

### *Diabetic coma*

In diabetes mellitus, both hyperglycaemia and hypoglycaemia may give rise to unconsciousness. Hyperglycaemia usually develops gradually and so is rarely a first aid problem.

With intense unaccustomed exercise, the blood sugar level may fall, and hypoglycaemia can then result. An athlete may initially feel faint, dizzy or light-headed, and may be confused or disorientated. The skin becomes pale, the pulse rapid, and sweating occurs. Breathing often becomes shallow, and muscle tremor may be apparent. The level of consciousness drops rapidly.

If the athlete is conscious a sugary drink will help, but if he or she is unconscious nothing should be given and hospital treatment should be sought. If the coma is due to hypoglycaemia, the response to sugar is usually rapid and the danger of secondary symptoms is averted. If hyperglycaemic coma is present, slightly more sugar will not harm the patient (Sperryn, 1985).

## Resuscitation

With an unconscious subject who is not breathing, or in whom no heartbeat can be detected, it is vital that these processes be restored or sustained until hospital treatment is available. A basic mnemonic usefully describes the course of action: ABC — airway, breathing, circulation.

### Airway

If breathing is noisy, or not present, the airway may be blocked. This can occur if the tongue has fallen back and is covering the airway, or if the airway is narrowed due to the position of the head. Absence of the gagging reflex may allow saliva or vomit to accumulate at the back of the throat and block the airway. The subject's chin should be pulled forwards and the head tilted back (Fig. 5.1a). This will open the airway. If breathing is still noisy, the head should be turned to one side, keeping the head well back.

Foreign matter may be cleared from the mouth by sweeping two fingers around the inside the mouth (Fig. 5.1b). The practitioner should look, listen and feel for signs of respiratory movements (Fig. 5.1c). If these are not present, artificial ventilation is required.

### Breathing

When the airway is cleared, the subject should be laid supine, and mouth-to-mouth, or mouth-to-nose ventilation given. In small children the nose and mouth may be used together. The subject's mouth is opened wide and his or her nose pinched closed, at the same time keeping the subject's head well back (Fig. 5.2a). The practitioner breathes out directly into the subject's mouth, making sure a good seal is maintained between his or her own lips and the subject's mouth. The chest should be observed to assess lung inflation (Fig. 5.2b). If this does not occur, the airway may still be blocked, in which case the head should be readjusted and artificial ventilation resumed. If no chest movement occurs this time, the subject should be treated with an abdominal thrust as though choking (see below).

After two lung inflations, the carotid pulse should be tested (Fig. 5.2c). If a pulse is present, but breathing has not commenced, artificial ventilation should be continued at a rate of 12–16 inflations per minute. If the pulse is not detected, external chest compression is required.

In cases of facial injury, or if the subject is trapped face down, manual techniques, such as the Holger–Nielsen method, may be more suitable. However, description of this technique is beyond the scope of this book, and the reader is referred to the *First Aid Manual* (1989), (pp. 216–217).

### Circulation

For external chest compression, the subject should be supine on a firm surface. The practitioner kneels to one side, and places the heel of one hand, reinforced by the other, over the subject's lower sternum (Fig. 5.3a). Keeping the elbows locked, a downwards pressure is exerted onto the patient's sternum by the practitioner leaning downwards and pushing through straight arms (Fig. 5.3b). The force used should be sufficient to depress the sternum by 4–5 cm. The pressure is released and the procedure repeated 15 times. Following this, attention is again focused on the mouth and two breaths of artificial ventilation are given. This sequence of 15 repetitions of external chest compression and two breaths of artificial ventilation

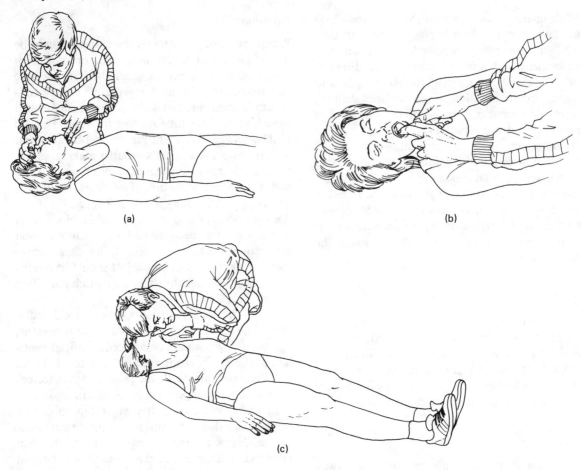

(a)

(b)

(c)

**Figure 5.1** Opening the airway. (a) Pull the athlete's chin forwards and tilt the head back. (b) Clear away foreign matter by turning the head to the side and sweeping two fingers around inside the mouth. (c) Look, listen and feel for signs of respiratory movements.

continues until hospitalization is available, or the subject recovers. The carotid pulse is checked after one minute and then after each third minute. When the pulse returns, chest compression is stopped. If breathing returns and is sustained, the subject is placed into the recovery position.

If an assistant is available, resuscitation may be carried out with one person performing chest compression and the other artificial respiration. The rate is then five compressions to one inflation (Fig. 5.3c).

A number of resuscitation aids are available. Some consist of a plastic sheet, mouthpiece and valve which covers the face of the subject and holds the mouth open. Plastic airways themselves are helpful to hold the tongue away from the back of the throat, and airways with a valve to stop the passage of saliva to the practitioner are also available. All airways have the potential to damage the soft palate and should only be used after appropriate training.

### Recovery position

When an unconscious athlete is breathing and shows a regular pulse, he or she should be placed into the recovery position. This will ensure that the airway remains open, by stopping the athlete's

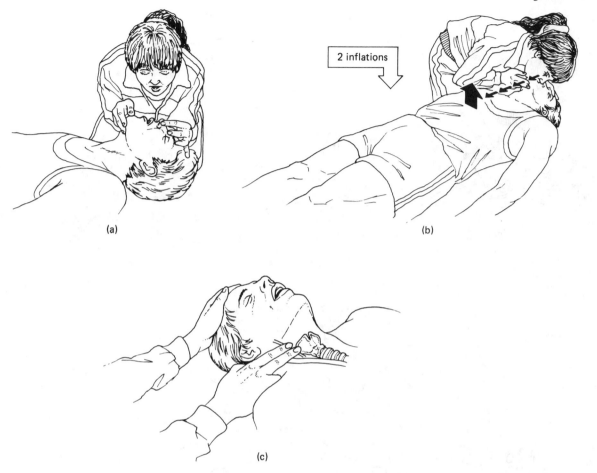

(a)

2 inflations

(b)

(c)

**Figure 5.2** Breathing. (a) Open the athlete's mouth, pinch his nose closed and tilt the head back. (b) Breathe directly into the athlete's mouth and observe his chest movements. (c) Test the carotid pulse.

tongue from falling back, and by keeping the neck extended.

The subject's head is protected, and the open airway maintained. His or her nearest arm is placed under his or her hip and the subject is rolled towards the practitioner. The uppermost arm and leg are flexed to 90°, to maintain the modified side-lying position (Fig. 5.4).

If the limbs cannot be bent, the side-lying position may be maintained by placing a rolled blanket or similar item below the athlete along one side of his or her body.

**Skin wounds**

Skin wounds are common injuries in sport, especially when athletes train on hard surfaces. As discussed in Chapter 2 wounds may be either open or closed, depending on whether the epidermis has been completely penetrated. With closed wounds, such as abrasions and gravel burns, the aim is to prevent infection and remove any foreign material. The injured area is cleaned with 0.5% chlorhexidine or a mixture of chlorhexidine and cetrimide, and grit or other material is removed with sterile

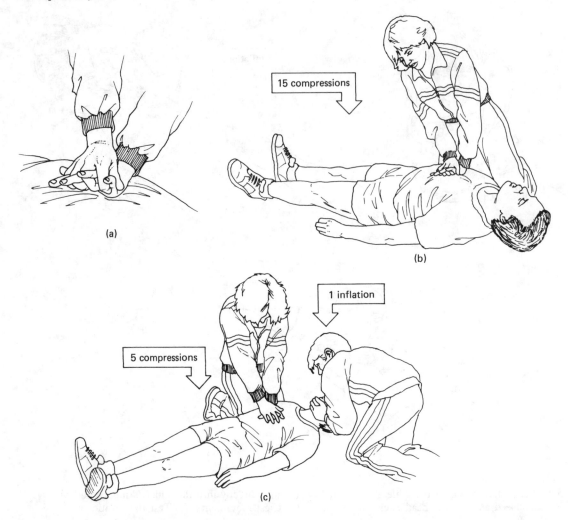

**15 compressions**

**1 inflation**

**5 compressions**

(a)

(b)

(c)

**Figure 5.3** Circulation. (a) One hand, reinforced by the other, is placed over the athlete's sternum. (b) Keeping the elbows locked, a downwards pressure is exerted to depress the sternum by 4–5 cm. (c) With an assistant, one person performs chest compression, and the other artificial respiration.

forceps. The area is left to dry, and then may be painted with an aqueous solution of gentian violet or mercurochrome.

Exposed areas may be left without a dressing, as air will assist healing. If an abrasion cannot be left exposed, it should be dressed with a single layer of petroleum jelly, gauze and a dry dressing. The area should be checked every 48 hours, to ensure infection has not started and that healing is progressing. When a practitioner decides that a player must continue until the end of a match, a wound may be sprayed with sterile talcum powder, or thin strips

of adhesive dressing may be applied at right angles to the cut, and the area bandaged to protect it.

Open wounds, such as lacerations and puncture wounds, are more serious. The amount of bleeding which occurs is dependent on the site of the injury and the depth of the wound, arterial damage will obviously cause profuse bleeding. The first priority is to stop bleeding with direct pressure over the wound and elevation of the injured limb. Pressure should be given with a sterile (or at least clean) dressing, or the patient's/practitioner's hand.

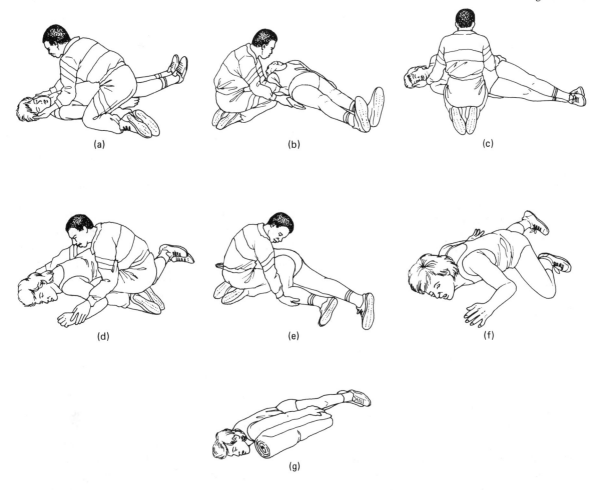

**Figure 5.4** The recovery position. (a) Protect head, open airway. (b) Place nearest arm under hip. (c) Roll athlete towards practitioner. (d) Bend uppermost arm. (e) Bend uppermost leg. (f) Final position. (g) Modification if limbs cannot be bent.

Minor lacerations may be cleaned and closed with sterile adhesive strips or dumb-bell sutures. These have the advantage that no local anaesthetic is needed for their application, and they avoid the risk of stitch marks and suture tearing of the skin.

More extensive wounds may require suturing. When deeper tissues have been damaged, suturing in layers may be required. The deep layers being sutured with catgut and the skin closed with silk. Because of the risk of infection, all but the most minor open skin wounds should be managed in a hospital casualty department. If bleeding is pro-fuse, the patient may need to be treated for shock by lying him or her flat and elevating the lower limbs, until he or she can be removed to hospital.

All skin wounds run the risk of tetanus infection, so an athlete who sustains a major injury may require a full course of tetanus prophylaxis. This consists of three injections of 0.5 ml tetanus toxoid. The first is given at the time of injury, the second 6 weeks later and the third 6 months after the first. If an athlete is not sure of the time interval since his or her last tetanus injection, a booster dose of 0.5 ml toxoid if often given after injury as a precaution.

## Soft tissue injury

The initial aim with a soft tissue injury is to protect the area from further harm and slow the inflammatory process. A simple mnemonic for first contact treatment is RICE: rest, ice, compression, elevation.

### Rest

The immediate first aid concern (assuming a life-threatening situation does not exist) is to protect the injured body part from further injury. This may simply mean rest, or splinting/strapping in the case of an injured joint to limit movement. Inflatable splints are invaluable here for fast immobilization to permit safe removal to hospital. Details on strapping are given in Chapter 8.

During the acute phase of inflammation, the athlete should rest. However, rather than complete rest, 'functional rest' is to be preferred. Here, any activity which stresses the injured tissue is avoided, but other activities are allowed. In the sub-acute phase, the injured tissues themselves should be allowed to move gently, to produce a strong mobile scar, and to allow collagen fibres to align in the direction of stress (Sterns, 1940; Burri, Hebling and Spier, 1973; Cyriax, 1982). Total rest of an injured body part may lead to increased adhesions. In addition, a haphazard arrangement of collagen fibres within the newly formed scar will result in a reduction of tensile strength.

More vigorous general exercise is to be encouraged, with the injured body part still protected. This will help maintain general cardiopulmonary fitness and the condition of the non-injured tissues.

### Ice

Ice, or cold application, is used to slow the metabolic rate of the injured tissue and reduce hypoxic tissue damage (Knight, 1989). Furthermore, the production of cold-induced analgesia is desirable. An ice pack should be kept on for 15–20 minutes and reapplied every two hours for the first two days following injury.

If no ice is available, cold water is of use, but the tissue temperature changes are not as great as with ice, and so hypoxic damage is not prevented as efficiently. The use of ice is covered in detail in Chapter 7.

### Compression

Compression is used in combination with cold to reduce swelling. Compression should be sufficient to limit the formation of oedema but not to compromise the blood flow to the area. The circulation distal to the compression should be checked by observing skin coloration. In addition, a finger-nail or toe-nail should be squeezed on the injured limb which has been compressed. The subungual skin will go white with compression and the normal pink coloration should return a few seconds after pressure is released, illustrating that adequate circulation is reaching the nailbed.

### Elevation

Gravity will pull swelling into a dependent limb, so elevation should be used to aid lymphatic drainage. The limb need only be elevated above the level of the heart. Athletes with lower limb injuries, particularly to the ankle should be encouraged to keep the leg elevated on a stool when sitting throughout the day. In addition, gentle isometric or short range isotonic exercise is useful to stimulate the muscle pump and aid venous return and lymphatic drainage.

A combination of the above treatment techniques will produce the best results. Cold compresses can easily be applied with lint soaked in iced water and wrapped around the limb. A polythene bag covers the wet lint and an elastic tubular bandage covers both. The compress is reapplied every 5 or 10 minutes as its temperature rises. The limb is elevated and isometric exercise performed at a rate of one contraction every three to five seconds. Various cryogel impregnated bandages are commercially available which perform a similar job. Flaked ice in a towelling bag may be applied flat with an elastic bandage over the top. Again, elevation and muscle pump exercise is required.

## Fractures

Fractures should only receive treatment after breathing has been restored and bleeding stopped. If a fracture is present, squeezing the area, or gentle limb movements, will usually cause pain. If the accident was not seen, and the athlete has not moved, a screening examination is required. The 'squeeze technique' is used. This procedure, in which a body area is compressed to assess pain and bony contour, starts at the head, and then moves to the neck, shoulders and arms and so on until the whole body has been assessed. The experienced practitioner can carry out such an examination in 30–60 seconds.

If a fracture is found, the injured bone should be immobilized by splinting. A number of options exist. Several emergency splints are on the market, and sports clubs should be encouraged to have these available. The various types include inflatable splints, cardboard splints, backslabs and slings. If none of these are available, improvisation is the order of the day. Broom handles, hockey sticks and ski poles are all useful splints, and with lower limb fractures, using the other leg, is also effective. In each case the limb should be gently straightened (if pain is not intense) and immobilized.

Injuries to the shoulder/clavicle, or forearm fractures are best immobilized across the chest in a sling. If the elbow cannot be bent, the straight arm is fixed at the side of the chest, by straps around the pelvis, waist and chest.

The question of whether an injury is a fracture or not often arises in sport. Observation will show any obvious deformity, and palpation by squeezing will usually elicit intense pain, considerably more than with a soft tissue injury. In addition, bleeding is normally more profuse. However, the only way to be totally sure is to view a radiograph of the affected limb.

## Dislocations and subluxations

The most common joints dislocated in sport are the fingers and shoulder. No attempt should be made to reduce a shoulder dislocation, because of the danger of damage to the axillary nerve (but see p. 286). Finger dislocations may be reduced after the application of cold spray to produce some temporary anaesthesia. Traction is applied along the length of the bone. The advantage of reducing the dislocation immediately is that muscle spasm will not have developed fully. If left, the finger may have to be reduced under anaesthetic. However this advantage must be weighed against the danger that a fracture has occurred near the joint line which will only reveal itself on X-ray. For this reason, even if the joint is successfully reduced, an X-ray is desirable (Walkden, 1981).

## Genital injury

Injury to the genitalia is common in men, and a suitable box should be worn to offer some degree of protection. Bruising to the scrotum may occur by direct contact with another player or apparatus. The pain from such an injury is often incapacitating. Application of a cold sponge or ice may give some relief. If blood occurs in the urine after this injury, the player should seek medical attention.

Torsion of the testicles may occur in cycling, particularly in teenagers, and priapism (persistent erection) has been reported due to vascular obstruction (Sperryn, 1985). In both cases, medical advice is required.

Injury to the female genitalia may similarly occur through direct trauma causing contusion and possible pubic fracture, especially after a fall onto gymnastic apparatus. In addition, water-skiing may cause vaginal injury through forced douching. Female water-skiers are well-advised to protect the pudendal region by wearing a wet-suit and not a bathing costume. Immediate gynaecological assistance is required.

## Choking

Choking occurs when the act of swallowing forces something over the entrance to the trachea rather than into the oesophagus. Two first aid procedures may be used. Initially, the athlete should be bent forwards and firmly slapped between the shoulder blades three or four times. If this fails to dislodge the item, an abdominal thrust (Heimlich manoever) may be used. Here, sharp pressure is placed over the upper abdomen in an attempt to rapidly increase abdominal pressure and simulate a cough.

The victim may be lying supine, in which case the thrust can be through the straight arms of the practitioner. In standing, the practitioner wraps his or her arms around the victim and forces the heels of his or her hands up and into the victim's abdomen. The manoeuvre must be sharp and hard, and may be repeated three or four times (Fig.5.5).

## Cramp, stitch and winding

A sudden blow to the solar plexus may affect the autonomic nerve centre in this region. A momentary paralysis of the diaphragm may occur with spasm of the abdominal muscles, causing the player to be 'winded' (Fowler, 1981). Respiration is impaired and nausea may ensue. The player will almost always fall to the ground if the blow was

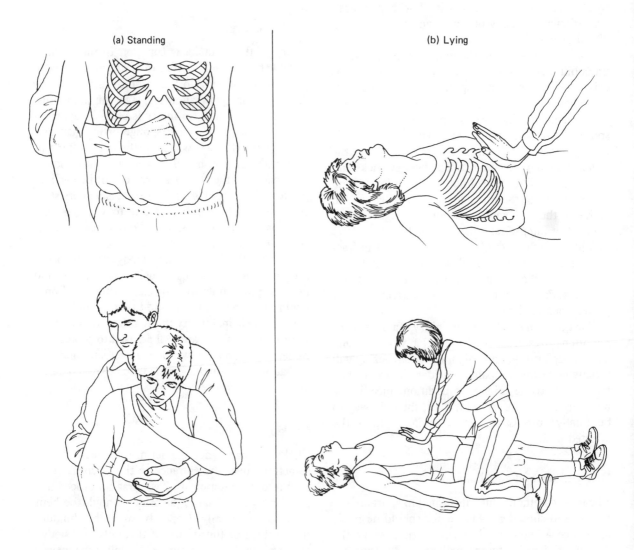

**Figure 5.5**   Abdominal thrust technique for choking (Heimlich manoever). (a) Standing position, (b) lying position.

severe, and should be left in the side lying position until recovered. Reassurance is all that is required and a cold sponge to the nape of the neck may sometimes help.

Cramps can be a particular problem to athletes because they are so unpredictable. The terms cramp or spasm are used to imply a painful, sustained and involuntary muscle contraction. It is important to realize that cramps are symptoms of some underlying fault. They may be the result of nerve entrapment, or metabolic disorder, and so, if persistent, the athlete should seek medical attention.

A number of possible causes of cramps have been suggested (Benda, 1989). Fluid loss, low glucose, electrolyte imbalance, training faults and fatigue have all been implicated. Cramps affect many different categories of people. Well-conditioned athletes are at risk, as are sedentary individuals who often complain of cramps in bed at night. The unfit individual who suddenly embarks on a vigorous keep-fit routine is particularly at risk.

Fluid loss will occur with profuse sweating, and athletes are best advised to take small amounts of water throughout a training period. Large amounts taken when cramp has occurred are not generally as effective, and lead to a bloated feeling.

Electrolyte imbalance altering the excitability of motor units is another possible cause (Fowler, 1981), and both potassium and salt may be involved. Some athletes use electrolyte drinks, but those containing a lot of sugar should be avoided, as should salt tablets. Salt will draw fluid out of the circulatory system, and sugar will slow fluid absorption. If salt or potassium is to be taken, it should be incorporated into the diet as a preventive measure. Potassium-rich foods, such as bananas and oranges, and salty foods are suitable.

Pain relief and reduction of muscle spasm may be achieved by the use of ice and stretching. Ice is used to produce cold analgesia, and then slow stretching is carried out. Contraction of the antagonist muscle will help to relax the cramped muscle through reciprocal inhibition. Direct pressure over the pain trigger point of the muscle, and deep massage using kneading techniques can both be effective with some athletes.

Stitch is pain which occurs in the upper abdomen. It occurs more often after a heavy meal and is common in runners. It is generally made worse by expiration and relieved slightly by inspiration. A number of possibilities exist as to its cause. After a heavy meal, the mesentery must bear excessive weight. This may give rise to minor internal bleeding. A reduction in oxygen supply to the diaphragm, or alterations in blood flow to the spleen and liver have also been suggested (Peterson and Renstrom, 1986).

Diaphragmatic breathing should be encouraged, allowing the abdominal wall to protrude during inspiration. Some athletes report obtaining relief by squeezing a hard object in their hand, but the mechanism for this effect is puzzling.

### Spinal injury

Sport accounts for 10–15% of severe spinal injuries, and unfortunately a significant number of these are made worse by incorrect management. Descriptions exist of patients who became quadriplegic after being able to move their limbs at the time of accident, and of individuals presenting with unstable neck fractures two weeks after injury (Garrick and Webb, 1990). A lack of neurological signs does not rule out spinal injury, and the safest approach is to assume that any player who has sustained substantial head or neck trauma has an unstable fracture until this has been disproven radiologically. Even with more minor trauma, unless the athlete is alert and able to demonstrate full range pain-free neck motion without neurological signs, he or she may still have sustained bony injury. The advice is clear; when in doubt immobilize the neck and refer the athlete for further investigation.

Where severe trauma to the spine has occurred, the athlete should not be moved unless he or she is in a life-threatening situation. If movement is necessary the aim is to prevent further injury to the spine. The position in which the athlete is found should be maintained unless priorities of airway or circulation demand otherwise. Initial treatment follows the ABC protocol, and if movement is required the head and body should be fully supported and moved as one. The therapist maintains the head position by placing his or her hands over the patient's ears. Three assistants kneel at one side of the athlete and two at the other side. The patient may be rolled in one piece (log roll) onto his or her side into the recovery position.

If an athlete is wearing a helmet (motorcycle or football) it should only be removed if there is airway obstruction or fire (Meyer and Daniel, 1985). An assistant stabilizes the head by placing his or her hands around the athlete's neck. The practitioner unfastens the chin strap and grips the helmet at either side of the rim, spreading this outwards. The helmet is slowly removed by applying traction from below as the assistant continues to stabilize the athlete's neck. When the helmet has been removed, traction is reapplied to the head and maintained until a backboard is in place (Fig. 5.6).

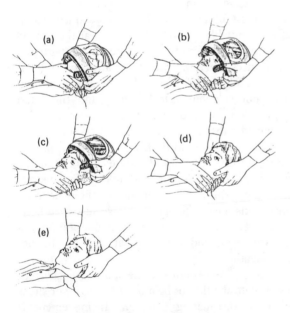

**Figure 5.6**  Helmet removal during airway obstruction. (a) One person stabilizes the patient's head, while the other spreads the helmet. (b) Traction is applied to spread helmet. (c) Helmet is removed with continued stabilization and traction from below. (d) Traction is reapplied from above. (e) Traction is maintained until backboard is in place. From Meyer and Daniel (1985), with permission.

## Environment and injury

### Thermal stress

The human body functions best at temperatures between 36.5 and 40.0°C (Astrand and Rodahl, 1986), and the body will try to keep itself within this region, to maintain equilibrium in the body core. When the external temperature rises, sweating occurs to try to lower body temperature, and when the external temperature is lower than the ideal, shivering starts in an attempt to increase body temperature through metabolic activity.

Heat is exchanged between the body and external environment through convection, conduction and radiation, and through the evaporation of water from the skin surface and respiratory passages. Heat loss through radiation occurs without contact between the body and the object receiving the heat, providing the environment is cooler than the body. In situations in which the temperature of the environment exceeds that of the body, radiant heat energy is absorbed from the surroundings, and heat loss must occur by evaporation. Conduction involves direct contact between objects, and is particularly important in water sports. The rate of heat loss by convection is largely dependent on the rate of movement of air (or water) over the body surface. Accidental immersion in cold water will result in rapid heat loss. This will be made worse by attempts to swim rather than waiting for help, as the moving water passing the body results in greater heat loss through convection. The cooling effect of temperature and wind speed combined is represented by the wind chill factor. When it is cold and windy, air touching the body surface becomes warmed by body heat, but is immediately taken away to be replaced by cold air once more. Table 5.3 shows the wind chill index at various temperatures and wind speeds. It can be seen that a temperature of 10°F is equivalent to −25°F when the wind is blowing at 20 mph. This speed can easily be achieved on a blustery winter's day by running at 8 mph into a 12 mph headwind. In addition, when more body surface is exposed, heat loss is greater. Thirty to forty percent of the total loss of body heat occurs through the head, so it is essential to wear a hat in a cold windy environment.

**Table 5.3  The wind chill index**

| Wind Speed (mph) | Ambient temperature (°F**) | | | | | | | | | | | | | | |
|---|---|---|---|---|---|---|---|---|---|---|---|---|---|---|---|
| | 40 | 35 | 30 | 25 | 20 | 15 | 10 | 5 | 0 | −5 | −10 | −15 | −20 | −25 | −30 |
| | Equivalent temperature (°F) | | | | | | | | | | | | | | |
| Calm | 40 | 35 | 30 | 25 | 20 | 15 | 10 | 5 | 0 | −5 | −10 | −15 | −20 | −25 | −30 |
| 5 | 37 | 33 | 27 | 21 | 16 | 12 | 6 | 1 | −5 | −11 | −15 | −20 | −26 | −31 | −35 |
| 10 | 28 | 21 | 16 | 9 | 4 | −2 | −9 | −15 | −21 | −27 | −33 | −38 | −46 | −52 | −58 |
| 15 | 22 | 16 | 11 | 1 | −5 | −11 | −18 | −25 | −36 | −40 | −45 | −51 | −58 | −65 | −70 |
| 20 | 18 | 12 | 3 | −4 | −10 | −17 | −25 | −32 | −39 | −46 | −53 | −60 | −67 | −76 | −81 |
| 25 | 16 | 7 | 0 | −7 | −15 | −22 | −29 | −37 | −44 | −52 | −59 | −67 | −74 | −83 | −89 |
| 30 | 13 | 5 | −2 | −11 | −18 | −26 | −33 | −41 | −48 | −56 | −63 | −70 | −79 | −87 | −94 |
| 35 | 11 | 3 | −4 | −13 | −20 | −27 | −35 | −43 | −49 | −60 | −67 | −72 | −82 | −90 | −98 |
| *40 | 10 | 1 | −6 | −15 | −21 | −29 | −37 | −45 | −53 | −62 | −69 | −76 | −85 | −94 | −101 |

Little danger | Danger | Great danger

* Convective heat loss at wind speeds above 40 mph have little additional effect on body cooling.
**°C = 0.556 (°F − 32)
From McArdle, Katch and Katch (1986), with permission.

Evaporation provides the most effective means of heat loss from the body. For each litre of water lost by the evaporation of sweat and moisture from the respiratory passages, 580 kcal is lost from the body (McArdle, Katch and Katch, 1986). The total amount of sweat lost will be determined largely by the amount of skin exposed, the air temperature and humidity, and the speed of air currents surrounding the body. The rate of water loss through sweating can be as much as two litres per hour. This must be compensated for by fluid intake, but during vigorous exercise only about 800 ml of fluid can be emptied from the stomach (McArdle, Katch and Katch, 1986), so the replacement of fluid is never complete. In addition, various factors can affect the ability of the body to take fluids up. A 10% glucose solution, for example, will reduce the rate of fluid uptake by 40%, so the use of glucose drinks to replace fluid alone is not logical. When glucose loss, rather than fluid loss, is the concern, these drinks may be of use, but it should be noted that it can take as much as 30 minutes for the ingested glucose to reach the working muscle. The use of complex (polymerized) sugars may be of greater value in this respect.

**Heat illness**

Heat illness occurs in the form of cramp, exhaustion and, finally, heat-stroke. Heat cramps occur after exercise in the particular muscles worked, probably due to electrolyte imbalance. Adding salt to meals in the periods before heat exposure is a useful precaution, but taking salt once cramp has occurred is not effective. Furthermore, ingestion of large amounts of salt is not well tolerated unless accompanied by large amounts of water which in turn results in a bloated feeling.

In those not acclimatized to hot weather, heat exhaustion can occur. This is thought to occur by ineffective adjustment of the circulation, combined with excessive fluid loss, which in turn results in lowered blood volume (McArdle, Katch and Katch, 1986). Blood pooling results, usually in the periphery, leading to a reduction in cardiac output. Symptoms include a weak rapid pulse, low blood pressure, headache, dizziness and general malaise. The athlete will recover if exercise is stopped and he or she is moved to a cool environment. Fluids should be given.

Heat-stroke is a more serious condition, requiring medical attention. It is a failure of the thermoregulatory systems of the body, causing sweating to cease, and the skin to become dry and hot. The body temperature rises to dangerous levels, and death can result. Body core temperature must be lowered, and treatment includes ice application and whole body immersion in cold water.

## Cold illness

In water, athletes with greater body fat percentages perform well, as they have additional insulation, as witnessed by the endomorphic tendencies of most cross-Channel swimmers. However, most humans do not acclimatize well to cold, and the response is usually one of avoidance, by producing a warmer microclimate with clothing and local environmental changes. Heat loss can be reduced by shunting blood from the periphery (shell) to the central area (core) of the body. However, prolonged peripheral vasocontriction during cold causes circulatory deprivation to the exposed parts and can cause severe tissue damage through ischaemic cold injury. Early sensations include numbness, tingling and burning sensations in the fingers, toes, nose and ear lobes. Neuromuscular function deteriorates, so that motor performance is impaired, as witnessed by a loss of finger strength and dexterity.

Frost-bite may occur when ice crystals form in the peripheral tissues, causing ulceration. First degree frost-bite affects the superficial layer of the skin, while second degree frost-bite involves the formation of skin blisters filled with exudate. Third degree frost-bite results when the deeper areas are frozen, including the subcutaneous tissues and muscle. Rapid freezing causes ice crystals to form within the cells, resulting in cellular damage and, ultimately, necrosis. Slow freezing occurs to the tissue fluids, but solutes are not involved in the freezing process. This increases the osmotic pressure of the extracellular fluid, and draws liquid out from the cells, causing exudate formation (Astrand and Rodahl, 1986).

If first and second degree damage has occurred, gentle re-warming is required, with any blisters being left untouched. The athlete should be sheltered, any restricting clothing should be loosened, and warm drinks given. Activity to increase metabolic heating is useful. Third degree frost-bite requires urgent hospitalization.

In addition to general cold injury, damage to the eyes may occur in events such as cross-country skiing and downhill skiing, with the combination of severe cold and wind. The blinking reflex may be impaired, reducing the nourishment to the cornea, and causing transitory damage (Kolstad and Opsahl, 1979).

Hypothermia occurs when the body core temperature drops below 35°C (Astrand and Rodahl, 1986), the body core temperature is measured rectally. Initial exposure to cold causes shivering, an autonomic response to generate heat through muscular activity. As the temperature drops further the athlete may become disorientated and may hallucinate. Further temperature reduction can cause loss of consciousness, with weak pulse and respiration. Reflexes are lost, pupil dilation occurs, and cardiac arrhythmias can occur.

Management in the field is by gradual body re-warming. Rapid re-heating can cause the core temperature to fall further, due to the return of cold venous blood from the extremities to the core.

## Clothing and temperature regulation

As the body temperature rises with exercise, sweating should be aided by wearing loose clothing which encourages air circulation around the body, and by clothing which allows the passage of moisture through it and away from the body (wicking). In addition, dark clothing radiates and absorbs heat well, whereas light clothing reflects heat.

In a cold climate, the athlete should wear fibrous materials and a number of layers of clothing to try to trap an insulating layer of air within the material of the garment. A hat should be worn to reduce heat loss from the head. As clothing becomes wet, it can lose as much as 90% of its insulating properties, because water conducts heat much more effectively than air. Cold weather clothing should ideally permit the passage of water vapour, but not of air.

Sports clothing can be combined effectively in three layers. The inner layer usually consists of shorts and a vest made of a fibre which is water permeable but non-absorbent. The seams of the inner layer must be positioned so that no abrasion is caused between the clothing and the athlete's skin.

The intermediate layer offers greater heat insulation properties, and is usually fibrous (wool or cotton) or fleecy. Modern materials have removed the need for bulk to provide insulating properties, and the intermediate layer should not restrict movement. The outer or 'shell' layer is waterproof, but should preferably still allow the passage of moisture from the body. This layer should also be strong enough to resist tearing, and should be convenient to remove. Zips or other fasteners around the ankles facilitate the removal of the shell garment without the need to remove sports shoes.

## Pressure stress

### Gas pressure

The pressure exerted on a diver when underwater can cause injury. Water is largely non-compressible, and so the weight of the mass of water on top of the diver combines with the atmospheric pressure at the surface. At surface level, the pressure is normally 760 mmHg, but as the diver descends the pressure increases by this value (one atmosphere) every 10 metres. Consequently, a diver at a depth of 20 metres is subjected to three atmospheres pressure (two from the water, one from the air). The body tissues are themselves largely non-compressible, but the air-filled cavities are at risk. These include particularly the lungs and respiratory passages, sinuses and middle ear.

Boyle's law dictates that the volume of a gas is inversely proportional to the pressure exerted on it. Thus, the volume of air in the lungs, for example, is halved as the pressure is doubled by descending underwater to a depth of two atmospheres. Underwater breathing systems supply air or a mixture of gases to the diver at high enough pressures to compensate for the effect of water depth.

However, the gas pressure itself can cause problems as the diver ascends and the gas expands. If the diver takes a deep breath and ascends without breathing out, the inspired gas will expand as the pressure upon it reduces. This can occur when a novice diver panics, takes a deep breath, and swims rapidly to the surface. Expansion of the gas can cause lung tissue to rupture, and air bubbles to be forced into the pulmonary venous system, causing an air embolus. This will pass into the systemic circulation and eventually to the brain, causing symptoms of confusion and blurred vision if mild, and unconsciousness or death if severe.

If the lung tissue ruptures and air bursts through the pleural sac, a pneumothorax will occur. Between the chest cavity and lung, an air pocket is formed which will expand as the diver ascends. This gas expansion will cause lung collapse. Pressure damage to the eye and ear is covered in Chapter 18.

### Gas concentration

Alteration in gas pressure will also change the partial pressures of each of the gases in a diver's compressed air tanks. Nitrogen, for example, increases in partial pressure by 600 mmHg for every 10 metres that the diver descends. The net flow of nitrogen through the alveolar membranes increases, and at a depth of 20 metres the body tissues will contain roughly three times as much nitrogen as they did on the surface (McArdle, Katch and Katch, 1986). This increase in quantity of nitrogen can give rise to nitrogen narcosis. Here, the diver first enters a state of euphoria similar to being drunk; later, numbing sensations are produced in the limbs, and the condition may prove fatal (Astrand and Rodahl, 1986). For this reason the time and depth of a dive are generally limited to about one hour at depths of 30 metres.

Nitrogen diffuses and leaves the body tissues very slowly. If pressure is suddenly reduced, by a diver ascending too rapidly, or by decompression in an aircraft, nitrogen is released from the tissues as gas bubbles. These build up in the small blood vessels and restrict blood flow, causing muscle and joint pain and even paralysis — a condition known as 'the bends'. Avoidance is through slow ascent, or replacing nitrogen with helium and allowing the diver to breath a nitrogen–helium gas mixture. This mixture will also prevent nitrogen narcosis, and is the choice for deeper diving.

### Altitude

At high altitudes the situation is reversed, as the air density reduces with increased height. At a height of 5500 m the air pressure is about half that at sea level, and this gives a corresponding reduction in partial pressure of oxygen ($PO_2$). The amount of oxygen carried by the blood reduces, and exercise performance is impaired.

The body's immediate response to the thinner air at altitude is an increase in respiratory drive, causing hyperventilation and an increase in blood flow, witnessed by an increased cardiac output (especially heart-rate) by as much as 50% above resting sea-level values.

During the first few days of training at altitude, mountain sickness may occur. The symptoms are headache (most common), dizziness, nausea and vomiting (less common). Appetite can become suppressed, and a diet low in salt but high in carbohydrate is best tolerated. The cool dry air of mountainous regions can cause mild dehydration, resulting in soreness and drying of the mouth, lips and throat.

Acclimatization periods to high altitudes are largely dependent on the altitude itself. Improvements may be seen within a few days, but total acclimatization may take between 4–6 weeks. Two weeks is normally sufficient for altitudes up to 2300 m, with an additional week added for every 610 m increase (McArdle, Katch and Katch, 1986).

## References

Astrand, P-O. and Rodahl, K. (1986) *Textbook of Work Physiology*, (3rd edn), McGraw-Hill, Maidenhead

Benda, C. (1989) Outwitting muscle cramps – is it possible? *Physician and Sportsmedicine*, **17**,(9), 173–178

Burri, C., Helbing, G. and Spier, W. (1973) Rehabilitation of knee ligament injuries. In *The Knee*, Springer, New York

Cyriax, J. (1982) *Textbook of Orthopaedic Medicine*, Volume one, 8th edn, Baillière Tindall, London

*First Aid Manual* (1989), 5th edn, Dorling Kindersley, London

Fowler, J.A. (1981) First aid in sport. In *Sports Fitness and Sports Injuries*, (ed. T. Reilly) Faber and Faber, London, pp. 253–258

Garrick, J.G. and Webb, D.R (1990) *Sports Injuries: Diagnosis and Management*, W.B. Saunders, Philadelphia

Knight, K.L. (1989) Cryotherapy in sports injury management. In *International Perspectives in Physical Therapy*, **4**, (ed. V. Grisogno), pp. 163–185

Kolstad, A. and Opsahl, R. (1979) Cold injury to the corneal epithelium, a case of blurred vision in cross-country skiers. *Acta Ophthalmologica*, **48**, 789

McArdle, W.D., Katch, F.I. and Katch, V.L. (1986) *Exercise Physiology. Energy, Nutrition, and Human Performance*, Lea and Febiger, Philadelphia,pp. 47–4

Meyer, R.D. and Daniel, W.W. (1985) The biomechanics of helmets and helmet removal. *Journal of Trauma*, **25**, 329–332

Peterson, L. and Renstrom, P. (1986) *Sports Injuries*, Martin Dunitz, London

Schuller, D.E., Dankle, S.K., Martin, M. and Strauss, R.H. (1989) Auricular injury and the use of headgear in wrestlers. *Archives of Otolaryngology—Head and Neck Surgery*, **115**, 714–717

Sperryn, P.N. (1985) *Sport and Medicine*, Butterworth, London

Sterns, M.L. (1940) Studies on development of connective tissue in transparent chambers in rabbits ear. *American Journal of Anatomy*, **67**, 55

Taimela, S., Kujala, U.M. and Osterman, K. (1990) Intrinsic risk factors and athletic injuries. *Sports Medicine*, **9**,(4) 205–215

Walkden, L. (1981) Immediate post-injury considerations in games. *In Sports Fitness and Sports Injuries* (ed. T. Reilly), Faber and Faber, London, pp. 247–252

Williams, J.G.P. and Sperryn, P.N. (1976) *Sports Medicine*, Edward Arnold, London

# 6 Physical training and injury

## Principles of training

In any form of physical training the body is exposed to a workload or physical stress at an intensity, duration and frequency sufficient to cause physical change. To achieve a training effect, the body must be overloaded, that is, exposed to a physical stress which is greater than that encountered in everyday living. The response to this training stress is catabolism, the breakdown of metabolic fuels or tissues. Following the catabolic response, an excessive tissue adaptation occurs, anabolism, causing the tissues affected to increase (Astrand and Rodahl, 1986).

As fitness improves, the intensity of the load which is required to produce a training effect will increase. Adaptation to the load occurs, and so further improvement will only occur if the training intensity is increased. Physical activity in itself is therefore not synonymous with physical training (Astrand and Rodahl, 1986). A training effect will only occur if an activity is sufficiently demanding.

In addition to a minimum intensity, the training load must be continued for a certain duration. High intensity training which is too brief may not allow time for the physical adaptations required by the body to occur. The frequency of training, that is, how often it is carried out, is also important. Training is a stimulus which causes an anabolic adaptation. This adaptation will take time, and so adequate recovery must be allowed between training sessions for the body tissues to modify themselves.

When training for aerobic (cardiopulmonary) fitness or stamina, exercise intensity may be assessed by measuring the heart-rate or maximal oxygen uptake ($VO_2$ max). The American College of Sports Medicine (1978) recommended the quantity and quality of exercise required to develop and maintain aerobic fitness and body composition. A training frequency of three to five days per week is required, at an intensity of 60–90% of the maximum heart rate reserve, or 50–85% $VO_2$ max. This should be carried out for a duration of 20–60 minutes, and be continuous or rhythmical in nature. These recommendations were later updated (ACSM, 1990) to include the provision of resistance training. One set of 8–12 repetitions was recommended with 8–10 exercises for the major muscle groups, for two days per week.

### Specificity

Any form of training follows the SAID principle, that is 'specific adaptation to imposed demands'. The change that occurs in an athlete's body (adaptation) as a result of training (the imposed demand) will be determined by the type of training which is used, and will be specific to it.

Specificity applies to strength and power development, but also to the energy systems used while exercising. A particular cardiopulmonary training programme will cause specific training adaptations. Aerobic fitness developed on a cycle ergometer, for example, will differ slightly from that obtained whilst running.

It is important therefore that training matches, as accurately as possible, the action which the athlete will use in a sport, in terms of joint range, muscle work, energy system and skill.

## Components of fitness

Two types of fitness are generally accepted, health related and task (performance) related. These include various components which can be described as 'S' factors for convenience. Health related fitness includes components which are considered to be beneficial to health, and are therefore included in preventive health care programmes.

In this context the term stamina is used to encompass both cardiopulmonary and local muscle endurance. Cardiopulmonary endurance is associated with a reduced risk of coronary heart disease (Ashton and Davies, 1986), and local muscle endurance is a factor in any sustained activity. Suppleness (flexibility) and strength (see below) are concerned with the health of the musculoskeletal system to maintain both range of movement and joint integrity.

Stamina, suppleness and strength are also essential to sports performance, but fast movements (speed and power) are also required, as are motor skills in general and the particular skills required for the execution of a sport. Injury will be more likely if the fitness components become unbalanced (see p. 72).

# Warm up

Many athletes conscientiously warm up in the belief that they will protect themselves against injury, and enhance their sporting performance. Whilst neither of these beliefs have been conclusively proven, there is mounting evidence in the literature to suggest that both may contain elements of truth. This section does not attempt a full review of the subject, but will draw on some of the many studies concerning warm up to illustrate important points.

### Warm up types

Warm up may be either passive, involving an external heat source, or active, involving body heat. An active warm up, in turn, may be general, using the whole body, or specific, working only those body parts to be used in competition.

Many external heat sources are suitable for a passive warm up. Common types used by athletes include hot baths or showers, and saunas. Clinically, physiotherapists use a number of modalities, including hot packs, whirlpool baths, and electrotherapy (shortwave diathermy in particular). Bene-

fits are claimed to result from the increase in tissue temperature, and physical performance has been improved using this type of warm up.

Carlisle (1956) showed improvements in swimming times after hot showers (8 minutes at 40°C). Davies and Young (1983) warmed the triceps surae muscle group with hot water baths, and showed increases in peak power output with cycling and jumping tasks. Sargeant (1987) also used water baths, and showed increases in peak force and power of 11% after heating, and reductions of up to 21% after cooling.

With a passive warm up, no significant active body movement is used, and little energy is expended. Subsequent physical work will not therefore be impaired due to depletion of energy stores (Shellock and Prentice, 1985). This type of warm up can be useful clinically, when active movement is either not desirable or not possible.

General warm ups are the type most commonly used in sport. The overall body temperature is raised by active exercise, increasing the temperature of the deep muscles and body core. Richards (1968) compared different durations of stool stepping as an active warm up, before a vertical jump task. Short, 1 and 2 minute, warm ups improved performance by 23%, while a 4 minute period had no effect. A 6 minute warm up reduced performance by 27%, presumably through fatigue.

Specific warm up involves movements which are to be used in actual competition, but at a reduced intensity. Rehearsal of body movement takes place, and the specific tissues directly involved in the activity are heated. This type of warm up would seem especially appropriate for events requiring highly skilled and co-ordinated actions, and some research is available to support this view. DeVries (1959) compared passive (hot showers and massage), active (callisthenics) and specific (swimming) warm up prior to a swimming task and showed significant improvement in performance only after the specific warm up.

### Effects of warm up

The effects of warm up seem to be physiological, psychological and biomechanical. Physiological effects are largely due to increases in tissue temperature, while psychological effects are mainly due to practice. Biomechanical effects are achieved by alterations in the tissue response to mechanical strain.

## Cardiovascular changes

The change from a relaxed resting state to a higher training level should be gradual, to avoid suddenly stressing the cardiovascular system. Equally, stopping training quickly, and thus reducing cardiac output too rapidly can compromise venous return.

A warm up of sufficient intensity will cause an alteration in regional blood flow. When resting, only 15–20% of the total blood flow goes to the skeletal muscles, but after about 10 minutes of general exercise this figure is increased to 70–75% (Renstrom and Kannus, 1992). During a warm up, blood flow is increased to active muscles, and reduced to visceral tissues earlier than would occur without a warm up. Increased blood flow causes the delivery of nutrients and removal of metabolic wastes to be enhanced (Karvonen, 1978).

Barnard et al. (1973) examined the effects of sudden strenuous exercise on men with no symptoms of cardiac problems. Each subject ran vigorously on a treadmill for 10–15 seconds without a warm up. In 70% of these subjects, abnormal changes were seen on an electrocardiogram trace, indicative of subendocardial ischaemia. These changes were reduced or even abolished when a warm up was performed before activity. Similarly, the effect of sudden onset exercise on blood pressure was improved. Average systolic blood pressures of 168 mmHg were seen without warm up and these reduced to 140 mmHg when warm up preceded exercise.

One of the reasons for these changes is that the adaptation of the coronary blood flow to strenuous exercise is not instantaneous. The cardiac output is unable to increase quickly enough to meet the demands of sudden high intensity work (Astrand and Rodahl, 1986), and a warm up gives the cardiovascular system time to respond, making myocardial ischaemia less likely at the start of vigorous exercise (Safran et al., 1989).

## Tissue temperature

The ability to perform physical work is improved by elevated temperature (Bergh and Ekblom, 1979). Warm up prior to maximal exercise will enable the adaptations necessary for these changes to occur sooner.

Oxygen dissociation from haemoglobin is more rapid and complete, and oxygen release from myoglobin is greater at higher temperatures (Astrand and Rodahl, 1986). The critical level of various metabolic processes is lowered, causing an acceleration in metabolic rate and more efficient use of substrates. Muscle contraction is more rapid and forceful (Bergh, 1980). The sensitivity of nerve receptors and speed of transmission of nervous impulses are both increased as temperature rises (Astrand and Rodahl, 1986). This more rapid transmission of kinaesthetic signals is particularly important when complex highly skilled movements are used. These temperature dependent changes are summarized as follows:

1 Increased speed of contraction and relaxation of muscle.
2 Increased force of muscle contraction.
3 Greater mechanical efficiency due to lowered viscous resistance within the muscles.
4 Haemoglobin releases oxygen more easily at higher temperature, therefore oxygen utilization by muscle is improved.
5 Similar effects with myoglobin.
6 Nerve and muscle metabolism is improved. If a specific warm up is used, motor unit recruitment for maximum activities is facilitated.
7 Dilation of local vascular bed leads to increased blood flow through active tissues.
8 Lower critical level of metabolic reactions.

## Mobilization hypothesis

In the initial period of intense exercise, the local energy supplies within the muscle (ATP and phosphocreatine) are quickly used up. To continue to supply energy the body must work anaerobically with resultant formation of lactic acid. This initial inability to meet the body's energy demand through aerobic metabolism is called the oxygen deficit. When exercise finishes, further energy is still required to metabolize the lactic acid which has been produced. This extra amount of energy is called the oxygen debt.

Gutin and Stewart (1971) argued that a function of warm up is to mobilize the body's cardiovascular system to reach a steady state. After the warm up, a brief rest period before competition started would allow the oxygen debt to be repaid, without allowing the cardiovascular system to return to normal resting levels. When competition commenced, the oxygen deficit would be smaller, and some anaerobic energy would be available to the athlete at the end of exercise.

Gutin et al. (1976) asked subjects to pedal a cycle ergometer at an intensity sufficient to produce a heart rate of 140 b.p.m., a rate which they claimed equated with a 50–60% $VO_2$ max. The subjects' performance in a subsequent exercise task was significantly better than a control group who did not undertake a warm up; a result possibly due to the mechanism described above.

A rest period is essential after the warm up, to allow the oxygen debt to be repaid. But, following rest, the body must be kept warm to maintain the warm up effects until the athlete competes. As an illustration, Andzel and Gutin (1976) used bench stepping both as a warm up and an exercise task. A 30 or 60 second rest after the warm up resulted in improved performance, but when no rest period followed the warm up, performance remained unchanged.

How long should a warm up last, and what intensity of exercise should be used? A number of papers have addressed these questions. Andzel (1982) compared warm up periods at an intensity sufficient to produce a heart rate of 120 and 140 b.p.m., followed by a 30 second rest period. Performance was significantly better with the 140 b.p.m. group. Richards (1968) argued that while some warm ups would enhance performance, others could interfere with performance if fatigue set in. By varying the length of stool stepping, she concluded that a 1 or 2 minute warm up was superior to a 4 or 6 minute period in her study, Bonner (1974) saw similar effects by alternating warm up periods with a static cycle task. Where performance was reduced in these examples, the workload was obviously too high. Sargeant and Dolan (1987) compared warm up periods with changing intensity assessed by percentage of $VO_2$ max, and concluded that a 39% $VO_2$ max intensity was superior to a warmup at 56% $VO_2$ max.

Unfortunately there are no hard and fast rules to guide the athlete in terms of the duration and intensity of warm up, but, generally, once the heart rate has reached about 140 b.p.m., this should be sustained for 2–3 minutes. This workload should be sufficient to induce light sweating, and is appropriate for the cardiopulmonary part of the warm up. Obviously, the time taken to achieve this heart rate will depend on exercise intensity and fitness level, so the total warm up period will be considerably longer.

### Biomechanical effects

Safran et al. (1988) showed that a greater force and length of stretch was required to tear isometrically preconditioned muscles than muscles which had not been preconditioned. They claimed that the rise in temperature occurring during the warm up period could alter the viscosity of the connective tissue within the muscle, and that isometric contractions caused a stretch at the musculotendinous junction. LaBan (1962) showed a 1.5% increase in the length of a stretched tendon following a temperature increase to 42.5°C. Warren, Lehmann and Koblanski (1971) demonstrated increases of 5.8% in length and 58% in force to failure for tendons heated to 45°C.

Shellock and Prentice (1985) argued that muscle elasticity is dependent on blood saturation. They claimed that cold muscles with lower blood saturation levels were therefore more susceptible to injury. Fluids exhibit higher viscosity at lower temperatures, so joint inertia will be greater when the synovial fluid of a joint is colder.

### Psychological effects

The psychological aspects of warm up fall broadly into two categories. First, there are psychological effects of a physical warm up which will be dealt with below. Secondly, aspects of sports psychology, such as visualization and imagery, which are dealt with in the section on sports psychology related to injury.

Two psychological factors are important in the context of warm up, these are rehearsal and arousal. Rehearsal will only take place when an athlete performs a specific warm up, with actions relevant to the sport to be performed in competition. During the warm up, the athlete is re-familiarizing him or herself with the skilled movements required by a sport. Confidence is improved, and the athlete may be more relaxed following this practice.

When an athlete is performing a skilled task, if he or she rests and then resumes the same task, his or her performance may suffer. This phenomenon is called warm up decrement (WUD), and is well documented (Adams, 1961; Nacson and Schmidt, 1971; Schmidt, 1982).

A number of explanations have been suggested to account for WUD. At a basic level it is seen as simply forgetting an aspect of the motor skill. Nacson and Schmidt (1971) suggested that WUD results from a loss of 'activity set'. They claimed that a number of variables, such as arousal level and attention, had to be adjusted (tuned) to a specific task. With practice, the adjustments reach an optimal level, which is reduced with rest. They showed that WUD could be reduced if, during the rest period, a completely different movement was practised. This second movement could not contribute to the memory of the first task, but did require a similar activity set to the original skill.

So far, we have dealt with skills which were practised during the warm up period to improve subsequent sporting performance. When the practice of one task improves performance on another, positive transfer is occurring. However, if during a warm up skills are practised which are different to those needed for competition, they may interfere with the learning process and negative transfer can occur. Here, performance suffers because a slightly different skill, with a different activity set, is remembered. An example would be practising tennis strokes with a racquet of different weight and size to that of the one used in competition.

The second psychological effect of warm up is that of arousal. The relationship between level of arousal and performance is demonstrated by the

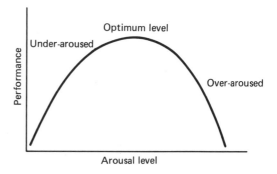

**Figure 6.1** Relationship between arousal and performance.

inverted-U hypothesis (Fig. 6.1). In a plot of arousal level against performance, it can be seen that increased arousal correlates initially with improved performance. But, as arousal continues to increase, an optimum level is reached. Above this point, further arousal is detrimental to performance.

The point of optimum arousal is related to the psychological profile of the athlete, and the complexity of the task to be performed. Gross motor activities involving strength, endurance and speed usually respond better to higher levels of arousal. Complex skills, involving fine muscle movement, balance and co-ordination are generally performed better at lower levels of arousal.

The function of warm up must therefore be to prepare the athlete psychologically, and place him or her at the level of arousal appropriate to the task to be undertaken. A highly motivated (aroused) athlete may need to be relaxed prior to a complex activity. Conversely, a poorly motivated athlete due to compete in a strength event may need his or her arousal level to be increased, by 'psyching' up.

## Warm up technique

The intensity and duration of the warm up period will depend on the type of activity to be undertaken and the athlete's fitness. A fitter athlete competing at a high level will take longer to warm up, as his or her thermoregulatory system will be more efficient.

During cold weather it will take longer for the body's core temperature to increase, and so the warm up should be longer or more vigorous.

Hogberg and Ljunggren (1947) showed a 15 minute warm up to be more effective than a shorter five minute period, but found the effects were not improved when the warm up period was increased to half an hour. DeVries (1980) suggested a warm up of sufficient intensity and duration to raise the body's core temperature by 1–2°C. This, he argued, was enough to induce mild sweating. Warm up effects may persist for 45–80 minutes, the time variation is dependent on the rate of heat loss.

General warm up exercises include jogging, light aerobics, and callisthenics. Each must be intense enough to cause mild sweating, but not so intense as to exhaust the athlete. These should be followed by specific warm up movements mimicking the actions to be carried out in competition. Examples for squash would be gentle flowing arm actions holding a racquet, gradually building up to full forearm and backhand movements.

At the beginning of the warm up, joints are only moved in the mid-range. As warm up continues, a greater range of movement is sought until the limb moves freely through the full range. The exercises are progressive and should always feel comfortable and without strain.

Flexibility training (see below) should not be practised at the beginning of a warm up (Sapega, et al., 1981). The benefits of elevated tissue temperature on flexibility make it more productive to perform stretching exercises after a warm up period.

## Warm down

On cessation of exercise it is important to reverse the processes which occurred during the warm up. The heart is no longer helped by the rhythmic contraction and relaxation of the leg muscles. Consequently, to stop intense exercise immediately will increase the demand on the cardiovascular system, causing the heart rate to rise. Metabolic waste products formed during exercise, such as lactic acid, will no longer be carried away from the working area with so much vigour. Instead they will remain in the area causing pain. This is thought to be one possible cause of delayed onset

muscle fatigue (Byrnes and Clarkson, 1985). Flushing the area with fresh blood by performing a gentle warm down can reduce this effect.

## Flexibility training

Flexibility is the range of movement possible at a specific joint or series of articulations and, the general absence of stiffness (Reilly, 1981).

Two types of flexibility are generally recognized, static and dynamic. Static (or extent) flexibility refers to the amount of movement obtained by passively moving a limb to a maximum degree. Dynamic flexibility is concerned with the amount of active movement possible as a result of muscle contraction. The concern here is not so much the degree of movement present, as the ease with which it is obtained. This type of flexibility is probably more important in speed events (Hardy and Jones, 1986).

Dynamic flexibility must not be confused with agility, which can be defined as the ability rapidly to change the direction of either the whole body or individual body parts without loss of balance (Borms, 1984).

### Effects of flexibility training

Flexibility training is generally thought to achieve effects in two broad areas, performance enhancement and injury prevention; and these two will be addressed.

### *Improved performance*

To achieve maximum performance, a limb must be able to move through a non-restricted range of motion (Shellock and Prentice, 1985). In sprinting, for example, lack of adequate dynamic flexibility could result in a reduced stride length with possible reductions in sprinting speed. In addition, greater resistance to movement through increased joint inertia at the end of movement range is more energy consuming.

Good flexibility is associated with good sporting performance in all activities where a maximal amplitude of movement is required to achieve the best technical effects. Similarly, a limited range of movement can reduce work efficiency in these situations (Borms, 1984). In addition, if flexibility is increased, force may be applied over an increased distance (Reilly, 1981), thus facilitating acceleration of an implement.

### Injury prevention

Cureton (1941) suggested that flexibility training may condition muscles, ligaments, and fascia to greater tensile strength and elasticity, leading to injury prevention. Holt, Travis and Okita (1970) proposed that increased flexibility of the hip extensors and low back muscles could result in fewer injuries with activities of daily living (but see also Muscle imbalance, p. 250.

DeVries (1962) argued that the maintenance of adequate joint mobility helps to prevent or relieve soft tissue pain, and Wilmore (1981) cited a study in which 82% of patients with low back pain benefited from an exercise programme which increased strength and flexibility.

Ekstrand and Gillquist (1982), and Ekstrand et al. (1983) asserted that muscle tightness may predispose athletes to certain injuries, and suggested that the type of training programmes undertaken can affect the number of injuries suffered. They went further to suggest that alterations in training methods may alter the risk of injury.

Many sports injury practitioners, coaches and trainers would agree that stretching exercises should be included in a training programme after a warm up period.

### Muscle reflexes

Flexibility may be limited by either contractile or inert (non-contractile) structures. Inert structures, including the muscle infrastructure itself, will respond to mechanical factors which influence the stress–strain curve (pp. 6–8). When trying to influence the flexibility of the contractile elements of the muscle, the consideration is not so much 'stretching' the muscle as encouraging it to relax.

Three muscle reflexes are important when using flexibility training, the stretch reflex, autogenic inhibition, and reciprocal inhibition.

When a muscle is stretched, elongation is detected by the muscle spindle afferent nerve fibres. These receptors send impulses to the dorsal roots of the spinal cord, causing a reflex which contracts the extrafusal fibres of the same muscle, in opposition to the original stretching force.

In addition to the muscle spindle, the Golgi tendon organ (GTO) in the muscle tendon will also register stretch. Both of these receptors are affected by changes in muscle length, but the GTO is also receptive to changes in muscle tension (Bray et al., 1986).

When a muscle is stretched, there is a corresponding stretch of the muscle spindle. But, if the stretch lasts for longer than six seconds, the GTO registers not only the change of length of the muscle, but also the alteration in tension in the muscle tendon. The GTO will then cause a reflex relaxation of the muscle, a process known as autogenic inhibition. This has a protective function, causing the muscle to relax and allowing it to stretch before it is damaged.

Stretching which involves short jerking movements will tighten the muscle through the stretch reflex, while movements lasting for longer than 6 seconds will allow the muscle to relax again through stimulation of the GTO, which will override the stretch reflex. When a muscle is tensed, a reflex relaxation of the antagonist will occur, a process known as reciprocal inhibition. If, for example, the biceps muscle contracts to flex the elbow, its antagonist, the triceps, must relax to allow the movement to occur.

### Techniques of flexibility

Four methods of stretching are generally recognised, static, ballistic and two proprioceptive neuromuscular facilitation (PNF) techniques.

During static stretching, a muscle is stretched to the point of discomfort and held there for an extended period. Ballistic stretching involves taking the limb to its end of movement range, and adding repetitive bouncing movements, usually for a period of about 30 seconds (Hardy and Jones, 1986). This method is no longer as popular as it was, because of the suggestion that injury may result from abrupt stretching of soft tissues (Etnyre and Lee, 1987).

PNF techniques have been adopted by the sporting world from neurological physiotherapy treatments. These techniques use alternating contractions and relaxations of muscles and capitalize on the various muscle reflexes to achieve a greater level of relaxation during the stretch.

Two PNF techniques are used, contract-relax (CR) and contract-relax–agonist-contract (CRAC), as described below. The CR technique involves lengthening a muscle until a comfortable stretch is felt. From this position, the muscle is isometrically contracted, and held for a set period. The muscle is relaxed, and then taken to a new lengthened position until the full stretch is again felt by the subject. The rationale behind the CR method is that the contracted muscle will relax as a result of autogenic inhibition, as the GTO fires to inhibit tension.

With the CRAC method, the muscle is stretched as above, but in the final stages of the stretch, the opposing muscle groups are isometrically contracted as the stretch is applied, to make use of reciprocal inhibition of the agonist, and reduce its tension. Of these techniques, PNF stretches have been shown to be more effective (Holt, Travis and Okita, 1970; Cornelius and Hinson, 1980; Holt and Smith, 1983; Etnyre and Abraham, 1986), and CRAC methods are generally better than CR.

These various procedures may be illustrated with a common hamstring stretch. A ballistic stretch could involve keeping the leg straight and vigorously reaching for the toes with a bouncing action, for example repeated toe touching in standing or long sitting. The rapid action may tighten the muscle, but stretches other soft tissues including the non-contractile muscle elements, muscle tendons, and ligaments surrounding the hip, knee and spine. In addition, repeated spinal flexion, in this particular exercise, may increase intradiscal pressure within the lumbar discs, placing the athlete in danger of discal migration (McKenzie, 1981) or discal herniation.

A static stretch performed in this position would involve reaching towards the toes, holding the movement, and allowing the muscle to relax and 'give'. Various authors have given guidelines for

the optimum holding period, and Borms et al. (1987) suggest a ten second duration is optimal for improving coxa-femoral flexibility.

The CR technique for the hamstrings could be performed with an athlete lying on his or her back. The athlete's leg is lifted by a training partner, keeping the knee straight. After holding the stretch for ten seconds, the athlete contracts his or her hamstrings by pulling the straight leg down towards the floor against the partner's resistance. The tension is kept on for 10–20 seconds, a sufficient time to allow the GTO to override the stretch reflex. The tension is then released, and the stretch reapplied by the training partner.

This stretch is taken further by applying the CRAC procedure. This time, as the stretch is applied, the athlete tries to increase the stretch him or herself by pulling the straight leg up towards his or her head, tensing the hip flexors. In so doing, the hamstrings are relaxed still further through reciprocal inhibition, and the stretch becomes more effective. A variety of general flexibility exercises is illustrated in Fig. 6.2. The stretching techniques are summarized as follows (Etnyre and Lee, 1987):

1  Ballistic—rapid jerking actions at end of range to force the tissues to stretch.
2  Static stretching (SS)—slowly and passively stretching the muscle to full range, and maintaining this stretched position with continual tension.
3  Contract relax (CR)—isometrically contracting the stretched muscle, and then relaxing and passively stretching the muscle still further. This action is usually performed by a partner.
4  Contract-relax–agonist-contract (CRAC)—the same as CR, except that during the final stages of the stretching phase the muscle opposite the one being stretched is contracted.

### Factors affecting flexibility

The amount of movement present at a joint during a stretch (amplitude) is affected by internal (body) and external (environmental) factors. Internal factors include the bony contours of the joint. These will differ between individuals, and in certain pathologies such as arthritis, movement will

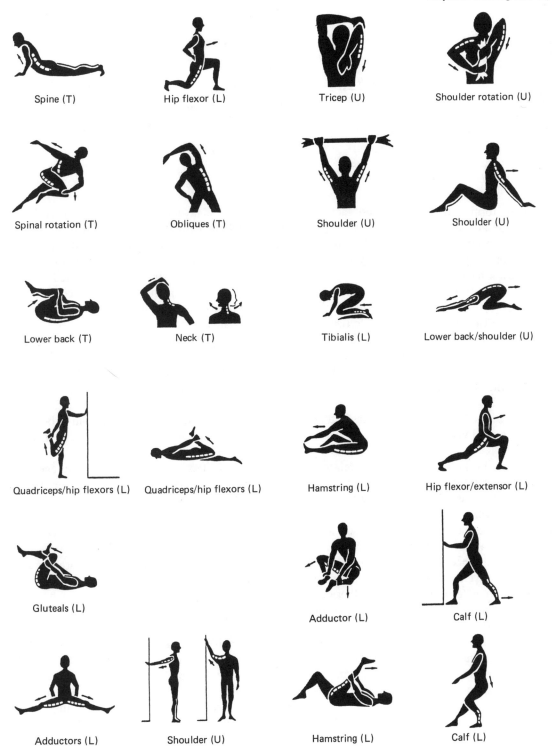

Spine (T)          Hip flexor (L)          Tricep (U)          Shoulder rotation (U)

Spinal rotation (T)          Obliques (T)          Shoulder (U)          Shoulder (U)

Lower back (T)          Neck (T)          Tibialis (L)          Lower back/shoulder (U)

Quadriceps/hip flexors (L)          Quadriceps/hip flexors (L)          Hamstring (L)          Hip flexor/extensor (L)

Gluteals (L)          Adductor (L)          Calf (L)

Adductors (L)          Shoulder (U)          Hamstring (L)          Calf (L)

**Figure 6.2**   Stretching exercises. T, trunk; U, upper limb; L, lower limb.

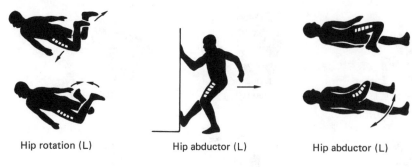

Hip rotation (L)　　　　Hip abductor (L)　　　　Hip abductor (L)

**Figure 6.2**  *continued.*

decrease as bone formation changes. These factors cannot readily be affected by flexibility training, but must be taken into consideration when prescribing stretching programmes, especially for the elderly and during rehabilitation.

Other internal factors include the volume of surrounding tissue, an obese individual frequently being less flexible than a lean one. Muscle tissue, tendons, and joint capsules are other internal factors which may be involved in movement limitation. Johns and Wright (1982) indicated that 47% of mid-range stiffness is due to the joint capsule, 41% due to muscle fascial sheaths, 10% due to the tendon, and 2% due to the skin. Other factors include cartilage, and viscosity of joint fluid (Holland, 1968).

Sapega et al. (1981) argued that the relative contributions of various soft tissues to passive resistance vary between joints. However, they pointed out that when a muscle is relaxed, it is the connective tissue framework of the muscle and not the myofibrillar elements themselves which provide passive resistance. Consequently they concluded that connective tissue is the major structure limiting joint motion (especially where adhesions are present) and should therefore be the target for stretching procedures.

Temperature is one external factor which affects flexibility, and we have seen that increases in tissue temperature can result in reductions in synovial fluid viscosity and increased soft tissue extensibility.

At a temperature of approximately 40°C a thermal transition of collagen occurs, allowing a greater plastic deformation when stretched (Rigby, 1964). Elastic (recoverable) deformation of con-

nective tissue is favoured by high-force short duration stretching with tissue at normal body temperature or slightly cooled, while plastic deformation (permanent lengthening) is greater with lower-force, longer-duration stretching at elevated temperatures. If the tissue is then allowed to cool in this stretched position, the results are noticeably better (Sapega et al. 1981).

Individual variations in body structure can have apparent affects on flexibility. Individuals with long slender limbs are likely to be more flexible than shorter individuals with thicker musculature. However, good flexibility in one joint does not guarantee similar attributes in other joints, because flexibility has been shown to be joint specific (Harris, 1969).

In general, flexibility decreases with age, although between individuals this trend is very much dependent on activity levels and other lifestyle factors (Borms, 1984). A general belief is that girls are more flexible than boys, but it is not clear whether this is due to body structure or social and environmental influences (Goldberg, Saranita and Witman, 1980).

**Therapeutic stretching**

When stretching is used as a manual therapy to mobilize a joint after injury or surgery, the various techniques will be combined. If muscle spasm is the limiting factor, ice may be used to limit the pain and this may be combined with PNF stretching (cryo-stretch procedures). However, to stretch connective tissue effectively, higher than normal temperatures are required, so heat is the modality of choice, where muscle spasm does not limit movement.

The ability of the heat source to reach the tissue to be stretched must be considered, and this will largely depend on the tissue depth and vascularity. In the forearm, temperature elevations of 7°F have been produced by 20 minutes of hot water immersion (Barcroft and Ebholm, 1943), and ultrasound produced a mean temperature elevation of 9°F in muscle near the femoral shaft in the human thigh (Lehmann, DeLateur and Silverman, 1966). Intra-articular knee temperatures have been effectively raised in both canine and human subjects by hot water immersion, shortwave, and microwave diathermy (Sapega et al., 1981).

After heating, pulley systems and weights may be used to apply a passive stretch to an immobile joint in which adhesions limit movement.

Sapega et al. (1981) recommended a stretching period of 20–60 minutes for the knee joint, with several 30 second breaks, during which full-range movements are carried out. In addition, they used biofeedback from an audible electromyographic device over the quadriceps to encourage maintenance of muscle relaxation. Following passive stretching, the joint was cooled for 15 minutes with crushed ice while maintaining the stretching force.

## Strength training

Strength is the ability to overcome a resistance, it is the maximum tension which a muscle can produce (McArdle, Katch and Katch, 1986). However, it is important to define the type of strength by prefacing the term with the category of muscle contraction which was used. We should therefore talk of isometric or isotonic strength, rather than simply strength alone.

### Adaptation to resistance training

Muscular contraction involves a combination of physiological and neurological processes, and consequently adaptations to resistance training are both myogenic and neurogenic in nature.

One of the most noticeable myogenic adaptations to resistance exercise is increased muscle size or hypertrophy. Increased cross-sectional area has been found to result from an increase in size of individual muscle fibres. Luithi et al. (1986) found an increase of 8.4% in cross-sectional area of the vastus lateralis following a six week period of resistance exercise.

The increase in size occurs in both type I (slow twitch) and type II (fast twitch) fibres, but selective hypertrophy occurs, altering the ratio between the two fibre types. In normal adults the ratio is about 1:1 or 2:1, but in competitive bodybuilders ratios as high as 6:1 have been found, compared with 0:1 in sprinters (Astrand and Rodahl, 1986). In addition, heavy resistance training has been shown to increase the proportion of type IIA (fast oxidative glycolytic) fibres (Bandy, Lovelace-Chandler, and McKitrick-Bandy, 1990). Of greater dispute is the possibility of muscle fibre splitting (hyperplasia) in humans. A greater number of muscle fibres is seen in competitive bodybuilders, but this is thought to be a congenital feature of the more successful athletes (MacDougal, 1992). Most authors agree that the increase in cross-sectional area following resistance training is the result of hypertrophy rather than hyperplasia.

In addition to the increase in fibre size which occurs with hypertrophy, connective tissue proliferation is also seen (McArdle, Katch and Katch, 1986). Thickening of the muscle's connective tissue support, and that of the musculo-tendinous junction may reduce the risk of soft tissue trauma.

Endurance training has long been known to increase the number of mitochondria and the capillary density (number per square millimetre of tissue). However, resistance training is thought to lead to hypertrophy without a significant increase in the number of capillaries (Astrand and Rodahl, 1986). As the number of capillaries stays the same, but the size of the muscle tissue increases, the capillary density is reduced. Each capillary must now supply a greater fibre area with oxygen and nutrients, a factor which may account for the relatively poor aerobic capacity of athletes who train solely for strength.

Alterations in muscle energy stores have been reported following resistance training programmes. Increased intramuscular stores of adenosine triphosphate (ATP) and creatine phosphate have been reported (MacDougall et al., 1977). Similarly, increases in two of the enzymes of anaerobic glycolysis (phosphofructokinase and lactate dehydrogenase) have been reported (Costill et al. 1979). Increases in phosphogen stores and the enzymes of anaerobic glycolysis could be expected to prolong the maintenance of a maximal muscle contraction (Bandy, Lovelace-Chandler and McKitrick-Bandy, 1990).

Significant strength gains may be made at the beginning of a strength training programme without noticeable changes in muscle size. The increase in strength is thought to be the result of more efficient activation of the motor units (Astrand and Rodahl, 1986). As Sale (1988) stated 'strength performance is determined not only by the quantity and quality of the involved muscle mass, but also by the extent to which the muscle mass has been activated'.

Increased EMG activity occurs during maximal muscle contraction following a resistance training programme, indicating an increased recruitment of motor units and a greater firing rate. Alterations in the nature of the EMG signal also suggest an improvement in the elastic properties of the trained muscle (McArdle, Katch and Katch, 1986). Furthermore, increased reflex potentiation (comparing the response of a muscle to nerve stimulation at rest with that during maximal contraction) has been noted following strength training (Sale et al. 1983) suggesting neural adaptation. Motor unit synchronization (groups of motor units being activated together) has been shown to be greater in strength athletes than control subjects, and to increase as a result of a resistance training programme. Sale (1988) argued that this would not produce a greater peak force, but may increase the rate of force development.

One possible mechanism for neural adaptation is increased activation of prime movers, as a result of improved skill and co-ordination. Activation of the prime mover may be limited by insufficient motivation, or inhibition. During new strength tasks, excessive co-contraction may occur to stabilize and protect the moving joints. Simultaneous contraction of the antagonist will reduce the force output of the agonist through reciprocal inhibition. Training could reduce the co-contraction and allow greater activation of the agonist muscle group resulting in a greater force output (Sale, 1988).

Graded inhibition of the motor neurones involved may occur, with disinhibition resulting from training (Astrand and Rodahl, 1986). Increased strength could then be seen as an increase in nerve impulses to a muscle group.

Increases in load may occur in resistance training without substantial elevations in strength. Rutherford (1988) cited an example of subjects training on a leg extension exercise. Improvements of 200% in the load lifted were accompanied by strength increases of only 11%. He argued that increased co-ordination of muscles used as 'fixators' in the leg extension movement could account for the improved weight training ability.

Whatever the exact mechanisms involved, it seems clear that neural adaptation is largely responsible for the initial strength gains following a resistance training programme. Gains made later on are more likely to result from muscle hypertrophy. In addition, neural adaptation is likely to be one of the factors leading to specificity of strength training.

### Specificity of strength training

Maximum force production from a muscle is then a result of a blend of myogenic and neurogenic adaptations which are specific to a particular movement pattern. Improvements in contractile properties, such as maximum force, velocity of shortening and rate of tension development, can vary with the type of contraction used in training (McArdle, Katch and Katch, 1986). Training a muscle to perform in a particular movement is not simply a question of overloading it against a resistance. For example, strengthening the leg muscles with a squatting exercise will not increase the performance on a leg extension movement to the same degree as training the same muscles on a leg extension bench. To strengthen a muscle for a specific movement, an exercise must mimic the movement as closely as possible. Similarly, strength gains resulting from isometric training will be specific to the joint angle at which the training was carried out.

Training a muscle at a specific velocity will result in strength gains at speeds close to, or less than, the training velocity (Rutherford, 1988), a phenomenon known as velocity specificity. One explanation of this principle is that before training, subjects are unable to produce maximal contractions at all velocities, and through practice they learn fully to activate their prime movers only at the velocities used during training.

Another possibility is preferential hypertrophy of one fibre type. There is little evidence for transformation of one fibre type to another, except following electrical stimulation. Preferential hypertrophy of type II fibres does occur, but at both fast and slow velocities, so the neural explanation seems more likely.

## Muscle work

Muscle contractions may be categorized into two types, static (isometric) where the limb segments do not move, and dynamic (isotonic) where movement does occur. The term isotonic (same tension) is confusing however, because as the limb segments move, leverage forces change and the muscle tension varies continually.

Dynamic contractions may be subdivided into either concentric (muscle shortening) or eccentric (muscle lengthening). Isokinetic contractions are dynamic (and may be concentric or eccentric), but the speed of contraction is held constant, by continually varying the resistance. Isokinetic systems do not permit acceleration, but recently the term 'isoacceleration' has been introduced (Westing, Seger and Thorstensson, 1991). This type of muscle work is performed when the subject works against a preset acceleration (concentric) or deceleration (eccentric) on a dynamometer.

The term 'isotonic' has come to be used to describe a concentric or eccentric contraction performed using free weights or a machine which offers a fixed resistance, and this convention is used in this book for clarity.

### Concentric training

During concentric contractions, alterations in leverage of the limb throughout the movement mean that the resistance imposed can be no greater than the weakest part of the muscle force curve. If the resistance exceeds the weakest point, the move-

ment is not completed, and the subject reaches a 'sticking point'. The force generated with concentric exercise cannot therefore be maximal throughout the range.

### Eccentric training

During an eccentric contraction the muscle is lengthening under active tension. Eccentric contractions are frequently used to resist gravity, the muscles being used as a 'brake'. Tensions developed during eccentric contractions are greater than those of concentric or isometric contractions, leading some authors to argue that the training effect is superior (Darden, 1975).

Greater strength increases have been demonstrated using eccentric training in comparison with concentric activity. Subjects working eccentrically for 6 repetitions at 120% of the concentric 1RM have been shown to produce equivalent strength gains to those performing 10 repetitions at 80% of 1RM (Johnson et al., 1976). However, the amount of muscle soreness (DOMS) encountered with pure eccentric work makes it more appropriate to start a training period with concentric contractions and progress to eccentric contractions in the final stages. In addition, training specificity and safety considerations make isolated eccentric training less desirable.

Greater force is produced when concentric contractions are immediately preceded by eccentric contractions, due to the recovery of elastic energy from the series and parallel elastic components of the muscle (see p. 15). In running, for example, as the speed increases, the amount of force produced by muscle contraction itself will proportionally reduce (force–velocity trade off). To compensate, the part played by elastic recoil of the muscle increases (Cavagna, 1977; Stanton and Purdam, 1989) giving the athlete 'spring in his or her step'.

### Plyometrics

Rapid eccentric contraction used immediately before an explosive concentric action forms the basis of plyometric training. This type of training was first used in Eastern bloc countries in the development of speed (Verhoshanski and Chornonson,

1967). The movements involve a pre-stretch of a muscle, followed by a rapid contraction causing the athlete to move in the opposite direction. Effects are achieved in both the contractile and inert structures of the muscle.

The rapid stretch of the muscle stimulates a stretch reflex, which in turn generates greater tension within the lengthening muscle fibres. In addition to increased tension, the release of stored energy within the elastic components of the muscle makes the concentric contraction greater than it would be in isolation.

Increased tension will in turn stimulate golgi tendon organ (GTO) activity, inhibiting excitation of the contracting muscle. Desensitization of the GTO has been suggested as a possible mechanism by which plyometrics allows greater force production (Bosco and Komi, 1979).

The use of muscle contraction involving acceleration in the concentric phase and deceleration in the eccentric phase more closely matches the normal function seen in sport, and therefore has advantages in terms of training specificity. However, the rapid movements involved are not suitable in early stage training as they can be relatively uncontrolled. Machinery is becoming available which offers a combination of the safety inherent in an isokinetic system and the functional advantages of positive and negative acceleration (Seger et al. 1988, Westing, Seger and Thorstensson, 1991). In addition, the use of 'inertial training' apparatus (Voight and Draovitch, 1991), in which the weight resistance travels horizontally, makes acceleration followed by deceleration more convenient.

### Practical considerations of plyometric training

Plyometric exercise is only effective when the concentric contraction occurs immediately following the pre-stretch cycle. If there is a pause in activity, some of the benefits are lost as elastic energy is wasted, and the effect of the stretch reflex is altered (Voight and Draovitch, 1991). This type of training is intense, and should only be used after a thorough warm up, and usually at the end of an exercise programme. To perform plyometrics the athlete needs a good strength base, and his or her proprioceptive activity should be tested using single leg standing and single leg half squats (eyes closed, position maintained for 30 seconds) before training commences. Any detriment in proprioception may cause the athlete to fall as fatigue sets in. Safety considerations including proper clothing and footwear, and a firm non-slip sports surface are essential.

Three types of exercises are normally used, in-place, short-response, and long-response. In-place activities include such things as standing jumps, drop jumps and hopping. Short-response actions are those such as the standing broad jump, standing triple jump, and box jumps. Long-response movements include bounding, hopping, and repeated hurdle jumps. Various plyometric exercises are shown in Fig. 6.3.

Although plyometric activity is primarily used for lower limb training, it does have an important place in training the upper limb and trunk. Overhead throwing actions using a medicine ball, and throwing and catching from a bent-knee sit up position are examples of this.

Resistance may be added to increase the overload on the working muscles as the plyometric activity is used. Vertical jumps may be performed using light dumb-bells, or a squat/leg press machine, and horizontal movements (lateral jumps, side hops) can be overloaded using an elastic cord.

Plyometrics has its use in late stage rehabilitation, and functional pre-competitive testing following injury. The adaptations produced by this type of activity within a previously injured muscle are likely to make it more capable of withstanding explosive effort as encountered in sprinting and jumping activities for example. This, in turn, may reduce the risk of re-injury. Using heavy resistance exercise in late stage rehabilitation of the injured athlete may allow the limb to regain lost strength, but without plyometric activity it is likely that the limb could still break down in a competitive situation, because the strength activity does not match the speed and power of the action to be used on the field of play.

### Isometric training

The term isometric literally means the same or constant (iso) length (metric). Tension is developed, but no change occurs in the external length

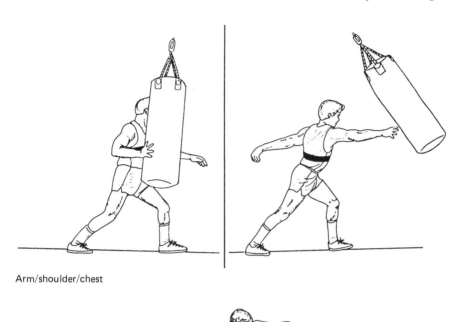

Arm/shoulder/chest

Legs

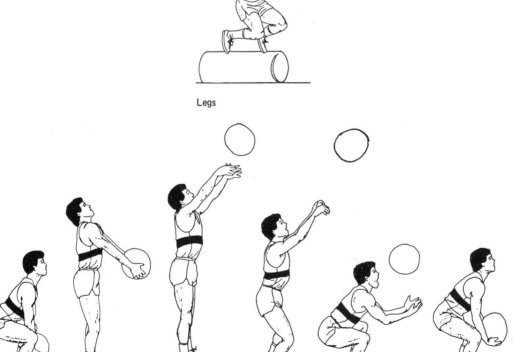

Shoulders

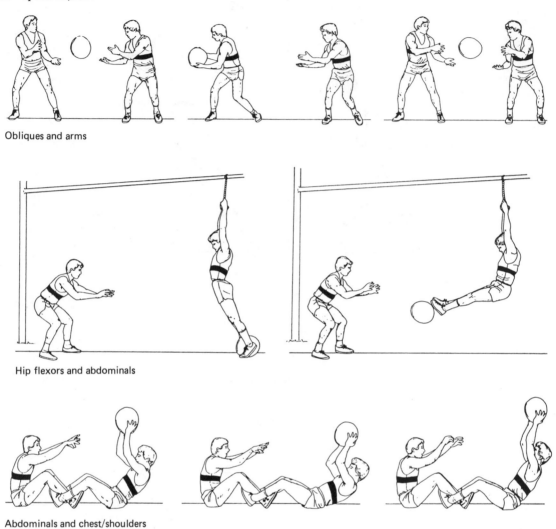

Obliques and arms

Hip flexors and abdominals

Abdominals and chest/shoulders

**Figure 6.3** Examples of plyometric exercises.

loped, but no change occurs in the external length of the muscle, and there is no movement of the object or limb segment. The external resistance can therefore be equal to the maximum tension the muscle can generate.

Isometric contractions will increase strength, but only at the joint angle at which the training is carried out (Fleck and Schutt, 1985). For more general strength training, a variety of joint angles must be used. It takes approximately four seconds

for the muscle to reach maximal tension, and this contraction should be maintained for six seconds (Astrand and Rodahl, 1986).

The use of purely isometric training would seem to be more appropriate at the start of a rehabilitation programme, when a patient's range of movement has to be limited. As soon as dynamic muscle work can be performed safely and effectively, this should form the mainstay of the strength training programme.

## Isokinetics

The fundamental feature of an isokinetic contraction, is the lack of acceleration. Speed is held constant, the name isokinetic literally meaning, iso (constant) kinetic (speed). The resistance encountered from an isokinetic system will equal the force generated by the muscles of the exercising limb. Consequently, the tension developed by a muscle exercising isokinetically can be maximal at all joint angles throughout the range of movement, providing a resistance which is totally accommodating.

Strength gains will be velocity specific (see pp. 100–101), and gains made at slow speeds do not carry over to movements faster than the training velocity. The faster movements used in isokinetics can reduce training time. In addition, muscle soreness following this type of exercise is minimal. The effort a subject produces can be difficult to judge, unless an accurate feedback system is available. The feedback system is also essential to maintain extrinsic motivation to perform at maximum levels.

A number of authors have indicated that strength gains using an isokinetic resistance system are superior to those from an isotonic system. However, this type of comparison is difficult because of the number of variables involved, and the results are inconclusive.

## Resistance training methods

### Exercise progression

As with exercise in general, strength training requires a muscle to be 'overloaded' or worked at a resistance greater than that normally encountered. This may be achieved in a number of ways, the most common of which in the context of sports injuries is weight training.

To increase the overload placed on a muscle, and progress in the exercise, a number of methods may be employed, as listed below.

1  Resistance
2  Leverage
3  Isolation
4  Gravity
5  Sets/repetitions
6  Rest interval
7  Frequency of training
8  Speed of movement
9  Range of motion
10  Duration of exercise
11  Type of muscle work
12  Group action of muscles
13  Starting length of muscle
14  Momentum/inertia

Increasing the resistance, exercise duration, and frequency will make the exercise harder, as will reducing the rest interval. Altering the effect of gravity, by inclining or declining a bench will affect the point of maximum leverage. Changing the length of the lever arm will also alter the resistance, for example arm abduction performed in the standing position will be more difficult with a weight bag in the hand than with one fastened to the elbow.

The relationship between length–tension and force–velocity (see p. 14) means that altering the starting length of a muscle or the speed of movement will change the overload. For example, when performing a sit-up exercise the hip flexors and abdominal flexors will work. By bending the hips, the work of the hip flexors will be reduced, increasing the overload of the abdominal flexors.

As the speed of movement increases, the force output from the muscle is reduced. In addition, more rapid actions have more momentum and are therefore harder to stop (a safety consideration) and are performed with ballistic muscle actions.

The type of muscle work (isometric or isotonic) and the function of the muscle (agonist, fixator, etc.) can be used to great effect, as can the range of movement. Initial rehabilitation exercises, in which the range of movement is limited tend to be isometric in nature, progressing to isotonic and increasing the range of motion. The motor skill involved with group muscle action makes it vital that a muscle is not simply worked as a prime mover, but as a fixator and synergist as well.

The combination of repetitions (number of complete executions of an exercise) and sets (number of repetitions grouped together) in weight training is the subject of considerable debate. In general, low numbers of repetitions have been traditionally used to increase strength while higher numbers have been favoured for endurance.

Research evidence to support this practice is conflicting. Berger (1962) found that athletes who trained for four, six and eight repetitions showed significantly greater gains in strength than those training for two, ten or twelve repetitions. Clarke and Stull (1970) and Stull and Clarke (1970) showed that both types of training produced gains in both strength and endurance. However, if both types of training produce an equal gain in strength and endurance, clearly using low numbers of repetitions is more economical in terms of time.

A number of combinations of sets and reps have been developed, the most widely used probably being that of DeLorme and Watkins (1948).

## Weight training programmes

### DeLorme and Watkins

This method requires the user to first discover the maximum weight which can be lifted ten times — the 10 repetition maximum (10RM). The programme then consists of three sets of ten repetitions at percentages of this maximal value, as follows:

1   1st set, 10 repetitions at 50% of 10RM.
2   2nd set, 10 repetitions at 75% of 10RM.
3   3rd set, 10 repetitions at 100% of 10RM.

The DeLorme and Watkins programme enables the movement to be rehearsed before a maximal contraction is required, perhaps recognizing the importance of neurogenic factors in strength performance.

### Pyramid system

In this routine, the number of repetitions performed with each set is reduced as the weight increases, the subject working on a 'light to heavy' system. This results in the athlete performing a few repetitions to fatigue when the muscle is thoroughly warm. An example is given below:

1   1st set, 12 repetitions at 50% maximum
2   2nd set, 8 repetitions at 65% maximum

3   3rd set, 6 repetitions at 75% maximum, or to fatigue.

### Oxford technique

This is the reverse of the pyramid system, now the user adopts a 'heavy to light' system starting by performing 10 repetitions at their 10RM and reducing to 75% and 50% of this value.

1   1st set, 10 repetitions at 100% 10RM
2   2nd set, 10 repetitions at 75% 10RM
3   3rd set, 10 repetitions at 50% 10RM

The Oxford technique (Zinovieff, 1951) works on the principle that as the muscle fatigues, the weight should be reduced to take account of the reduction in force output.

### DAPRE technique

Knight (1979) recommended that the resistance to be lifted should be based on recent performance. The technique of daily adjusted progressive resistance exercise (DAPRE) determines when, and by how much, to increase the weight, and allows for individual differences in the rate of strength development as shown below.

1   1st set, 10 repetitions at 50% working weight
2   2nd set, 6 repetitions at 75% working weight
3   3rd set, maximum number of repetitions with working weight
4   4th set, maximum number of repetitions with adjusted working weight

Four sets are performed, as indicated above, the first two sets being ten and then six repetitions with one half and then three quarters of the 'working weight'. This is roughly a 6RM, and is determined from previous performance. In the third set, the weight is adjusted depending on the number of repetitions which could be performed. For example, if in the third set the athlete is able to lift the weight only five times, the weight used in the fourth set will be the same. If he or she were able to perform ten repetitions in the third set, the weight is increased by 2.5 to 5 kg. The number of repetitions performed during the fourth set with this adjusted weight determine the new working weight to be used in the next training session (Table 6.1).

### High intensity strength training

For a muscle to work maximally, during the final set an athlete should not stop training simply because a certain number of repetitions have been performed, but only when no more can be performed. In this way volitional fatigue rather than number of repetitions determines the extent of the set.

If maximum work can be performed in a single set, multiple sets may not be necessary. Various authors (Hurley et al., 1984 a and b, Messier and Dill, 1985; Braith et al., 1989) have shown that high intensity weight training using a single set of seven to ten repetitions performed to volitional fatigue can produce strength gains comparable to traditional multiset systems.

Braith et al. (1989) found that a single set of high intensity exercise was effective in developing isometric strength. A training programme consisting of one set of 7–10 repetitions, with maximum effort resulted in isometric strength gains greater than those achieved by other authors (O'Shea, 1963; Smith and Melton, 1981), with traditional multi-set programmes.

Hurley et al. (1984) showed strength increases of 33% for the lower body and 50% for the upper body, when using a single set of 8–12 repetitions performed to volitional fatigue. Silvester et al. (1982) found that one set of arm curls performed to volitional fatigue was as effective at increasing biceps strength as three sets at maximal weights.

Messier and Dill (1985) also showed that a single set performed to volitional fatigue produced greater mean values of amount of weight lifted, than three sets at sub-maximal weight. The duration of training in this study was 20 minutes, compared with 50 minutes required for a multiple set programme.

Braith et al. (1989) argued that:

> the time required for increasing muscular strength may be substantially less that traditionally thought to be necessary

### Circuit training

Circuit training (Morgan and Adamson, 1962) consists of a series of exercises performed in a continuous sequence, with a minimum rest period between them. Initially, an individual carries out a performance test on each exercise to his or her maximum capacity. The score obtained determines the number of repetitions to be performed during training. In this manner individuals of differing fitness levels are able to train together, each performing the same exercises but at different levels of difficulty.

A variety of free exercises or apparatus may be used, incorporating different fitness components. Exercises for strength (push-ups, chins) may be interspersed with flexibility (straight leg raise), stamina (jogging), speed (throwing a medicine ball) and skill (flamingo balance). Specificity of training may be enhanced by mimicking the actions involved in a particular sport. For example, a circuit may be set up on a football pitch involving short sprints, zig-zag running, dribbling skills and shooting skills, in addition to upper body and trunk work. The circuit may be progressed by altering

**Table 6.1  Guidelines for adjusting weight in the DAPRE technique**

| Number of repetitions performed in third set | Adjusted working weight (fourth set) | Next session |
| --- | --- | --- |
| 0–2 | Deduct 2.5–5 kg | Deduct 2.5–5 kg |
| 3–4 | Deduct 0–2.5 kg | Same weight |
| 5–6 | Same weight | Add 2.5–5 kg |
| 7–10 | Add 2.5–5 kg | Add 2.5–7.5 kg |
| 10–11 | Add 5–7.5 kg | Add 5–10 kg |

the frequency (number of complete circuits), intensity (resistance, percentage of VO₂ max, range of motion) or duration (number of repetitions) of the various exercises. Either the number of repetitions may be dictated, in which case the aim is to complete the circuit as quickly as possible, or the time is specified with the aim of performing the greatest number of repetitions. An example of a typical circuit is given in Fig. 6.4.

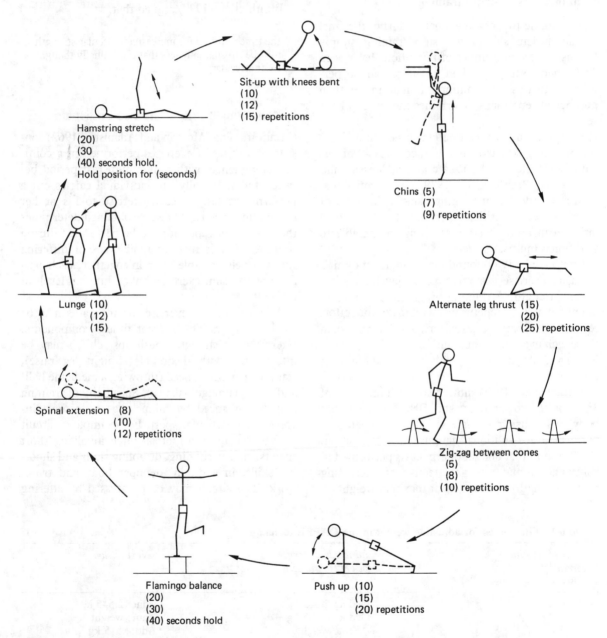

**Figure 6.4**   Circuit training. Example of a general circuit, with values for beginners (top), intermediates (middle) and advanced (bottom) athletes.

One specific type of exercise may be used, as with circuit weight training using only resistance training apparatus. Less emphasis is placed on heavy overload or a single muscle group, and instead a more general fitness programme is obtained. Circuit weight training involves alternating the bodypart worked (arms/legs/trunk) to prevent fatigue of one muscle group. Various types of work-rest ratio may be used. Typical combinations would be eight or more exercises, with a weight of 40–55% 1RM. As many repetitions as possible should be performed for 30 seconds, with a rest of 15 seconds (McArdle, Katch and Katch, 1986).

Increase in cardiopulmonary fitness has been shown to occur with circuit weight training, but it is dependent on rest period, exercise intensity, exercise type and total work. Allen, Byrd and Smith (1976) failed to show significant changes in $VO_2$ max using 30 second work and 60 second rest periods, the long rest period allowing too much recovery. A programme using a shorter rest period (15 seconds) showed an increase of 11% $VO_2$ max in women but no significant change in men (Wilmore, Parr and Girandola, 1978). Here, the rest period was short enough, but the exercise intensity for the men was not adequate. The women worked at 87.6% of their $VO_2$ max, but the men at only 78.2% of theirs. Longer training programmes have been shown to produce better results in terms of $VO_2$ max improvement (Pollock et al. 1969), and Gettman, Ayres and Pollock (1978) showed a 3.5% increase in $VO_2$ max after a 20 week circuit weight training programme. Subjects performed at 50% of their maximum strength in a 30 minute programme, which progressed from 10 to 20 repetitions, with a rest period which was reduced from 30 to 20 seconds.

Slow speed (60°/s) isokinetic circuit weight training has been shown to be better than high speed (120°/s) training at increasing cardiopulmonary fitness (Gettman and Ayres, 1978). This reflects the importance of the total work performed during the circuit. Athletes using slow speed training worked for a longer period than those using the high speed programme.

Improvements in $VO_2$ max are not as great with circuit weight training as with running. Average values after a 20 week programme were 3.5% for circuit weight training, compared with 35% for running (Gettman and Pollock, 1981). However, the real value of circuit weight training is to maintain cardiopulmonary fitness when an athlete is unable to run or perform other cardiopulmonary fitness activities due to lower limb injury. In a study comparing circuit weight training with running, Gettman et al. (1979) examined subjects who worked for eight week periods firstly at circuit weight training, then on a running programme, and finally on either running or circuit weight training. Improvements in $VO_2$ max obtained by running were preserved with circuit weight training, and both groups maintained cardiopulmonary fitness to the same levels. Increases in lean body mass, reductions in bodyfat, and strength improvements have all been shown with circuit weight training (Gettman and Pollock, 1981).

### Kinetic chain exercise

Movement of the limbs occurs as a kinetic chain. Several joints arranged in sequence move together to produce a complex motor action. If the terminal joint in the kinetic chain can move freely, the chain is open. If this same joint is unable to move independently because it faces a significant resistance, the action constitutes a closed kinetic chain. Most functional activities involving the lower limb in sport are performed using a closed kinetic chain. Walking, running, jumping, and rising from a sitting position are all examples of closed kinetic chain activities. The only open kinetic chain activity of the lower limb normally used in sport is kicking.

We have seen the importance of exercise specificity in terms of muscle work and energy system, but the exercise must also be specific to the type of kinetic chain action used. To exercise the quadriceps on a leg extension bench (open chain) does not accurately reflect the demands placed on the lower limb with running and jumping (closed chain). As many of the adaptations produced during resistance training, particularly in the first four weeks of training, are neurogenic in nature the mismatch in movement patterns could detrimentally affect the athlete's performance (Palmitier et al., 1991).

A common open chain movement used in knee training is the seated leg extension exercise. The muscles primarily responsible for this action are the quadriceps. Contrast this to the closed chain movement of the squat. When the leg extends to raise the body from the squatting position the hamstrings extend the hip and assist in knee extension as the foot is stabilized. This co-contraction (co-activation) greatly reduces the anterior shear forces acting on the knee, and is of particular importance in the rehabilitation of anterior cruciate ligament repairs (see pp. 174–177).

Several additional differences exist between open (single joint or 'isolation') and closed chain (multi-joint or 'general') exercises in resistance training. In an open chain action, movement occurs mainly distal to the joint axis, whereas with a closed chain action motion is both proximal and distal to the joint. An open chain action primarily emphasizes concentric work, but a closed chain movement brings a more balanced action of concentric, eccentric and isometric contractions into play.

## Proprioceptive neuromuscular facilitation

This technique uses mass movement patterns to more closely simulate normal activity. Proprioceptive neuromuscular facilitation (PNF) techniques combine movements in diagonal patterns utilizing one of each of the following, flexion/extension, adduction/abduction and internal/external rotation. The various combinations for the upper and lower limbs are summarized in Fig. 6.5.

Each diagonal movement takes advantage of the anatomical position of the major muscles involved in the action, enabling them to shorten completely from a fully stretched starting position (Voss, Ionta and Myers, 1985). For example, flexion-adduction-external rotation of the leg is accomplished primarily by those muscles which are anteriorly and medially positioned. The component of the combined action which stretches the muscle most will determine the action of the muscle. Therefore, in the example above, a muscle may act primarily as a flexor, secondarily as an adductor and lastly as an external rotator. For example, to achieve the greatest stretch on the psoas, the leg is positioned in extension, abduction and medial rotation, and con-

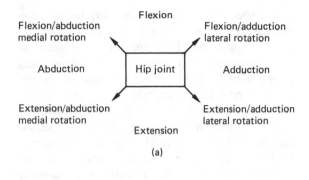

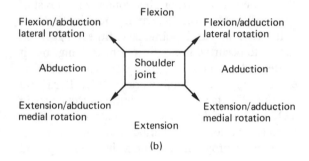

**Figure 6.5** PNF patterns. (a) Hip joint. (b) Shoulder joint. After Hollis (1977).

tracted to its shortest position by the opposing action (flexion-adduction-lateral rotation).

In addition to the position of the muscle, the timing of the muscle contraction is important. Normal timing aims to achieve smooth maximum contraction throughout the range, using accommodating manual resistance. Rotation begins the action, and the movement continues initially with the distal joints and then the proximal. Instead of normal timing, 'timing for emphasis' may be used. This technique employs the principle of irradiation or overflow to allow the athlete's stronger muscles to facilitate the weaker ones. This may be achieved by using manual resistance to prevent the strongest muscles in a group from moving the limb on their own. As the movement is performed, a greater resistance is offered to the stronger muscles in the hope that some stimulus will overflow to the weaker muscles encouraging them to contract more forcefully.

The third method is that of slow reversals. This uses the principle of successive induction, which demonstrates that immediately following a flexor withdrawal reflex the extensor thrust is stronger. Carrying this over to volitional movement, the motion required is immediately preceded by an action exactly opposite, with the result that the final pattern is produced more strongly (Atkinson, 1986).

These techniques, although originally designed for use with patients suffering from neurological conditions, adapt well to the rehabilitation of sports injuries. For example, with lower limb re-strengthening a flexion-adduction-lateral rotation movement may be combined with knee extension. This movement is far more functional than a simple leg extension action using a multistation weight training machine. Where quadriceps weakness is the major problem, the 'timing for emphasis' procedure may be used to focus on the knee extensors. Similarly, extension-abduction-medial rotation, combined with knee flexion may be used to precede the movement in a 'slow reversal' technique. Initially, manual resistance is used, but as rehabilitation progresses, a weight and pulley system may be used attaching a strap around the foot and ankle.

The use of muscle reflexes to facilitate stretching with PNF techniques such as contract-relax (CR) and contract-relax-agonist-contract (CRAC) is described on pp. 95–96.

### Implications for rehabilitation

The evidence from mixtures of sets, repetitions and types of muscle work indicates that no single combination yields optimum gains for everyone. In early rehabilitation, where the range of motion is severely limited, isometric exercise is useful. Performing this type of exercise in the inner range will contribute to joint stability, and it is important that this be obtained before resisted movement is begun.

Because isometric gains are joint angle specific, resistance training should progress rapidly to involve all types of muscle work. At the beginning of a weight training programme neurogenic changes predominate. Practising the skilled movement involved in the exercise is therefore important at this stage, so multiset regimes are likely to be more successful. As rehabilitation progresses, all the fitness components must be worked. Power and speed are important and should be combined with rapid eccentric contractions in plyometric routines. Cardiopulmonary fitness may be maintained using circuit weight training where lower limb injury prevents activities such as running, cycling or swimming.

For pure strength gains, high intensity programmes are more suitable for well-motivated individuals. Those who are poorly motivated may not be able to perform maximally in one set and so would be better to stay on more traditional multiset programmes.

For the effects of a weight training exercise to be maximal throughout the range of motion, the resistance offered to the muscle must change. Some form of accommodating resistance provided by an asymmetric cam or electronic braking system may be useful. Alternatively, free weights using body-building techniques such as 'forced repetitions' and 'cheating repetitions' can be used. In this, a training partner or body swing, respectively, is used to take the weight through the point of maximal leverage traditionally called the 'sticking point'.

Specificity of training makes it of paramount importance that exercise mimics as closely as possible the function which will be required of the athlete. At this stage sports specific skills should be practised in preference to pure strength work.

## Muscle pain

Muscle pain occurs under normal circumstances with exercise, and does not necessarily indicate injury. Two types of pain are generally recognized. First, pain which occurs during exercise, but disappears when the activity stops (ischaemic pain). Secondly, with unaccustomed exercise, discomfort may not occur immediately afterwards, but pain comes on a number of days later (delayed onset muscle soreness).

### Ischaemic muscle pain

Pain of this type begins in the working muscle and increases in intensity as exercise continues. It disappears when exercise stops and generally leaves no after-effects. The rise in intramuscular pressure during exercise can compress the blood vessels running through a muscle, producing ischaemic pain.

The accumulation of metabolites is generally accepted to be the cause of the pain. Lactic acid is often cited as the cause, but patients who are unable to produce lactic acid (McArdle's syndrome) still suffer ischaemic pain. Histamine, acetylcholine, serotonin (5-HT), potassium and bradykinin are the most likely agents to cause the pain of ischaemia (Newham, 1991).

## Delayed onset muscle soreness

Delayed onset muscle soreness (DOMS) is residual muscle pain which occurs 24–48 hours after unaccustomed bouts of intense exercise. Eccentric muscle work, and exercise with a long muscle length have been shown to increase the intensity of the delayed onset soreness (Talag, 1973; Clarkson and Byrnes, 1986; Newman et al., 1983; Jones, Newman and Torgan, 1989). A number of possibilities exist for the cause of this pain, and it is probable that a combination of factors occur, the contribution of each being related to activity type and individual differences.

Mechanical trauma can develop as a result of the high tensions developed during eccentric contractions (Newman et al., 1983). More trauma is likely with eccentric work than with other muscle actions, because the tensions created during eccentric contraction is usually greater. In a study of downhill running, increases in creatine kinase and myoglobin were seen, suggesting that structural damage was occurring within the muscle (Byrnes and Clarkson, 1985).

Disruption seems to be to the connective tissue elements, rather than the contractile tissue within the active muscles. McArdle, Katch and Katch, (1986) cited an example in which hydroxyproline, a product of connective tissue breakdown, was detected in the urine of subjects suffering from DOMS. They suggested that this is indicative of damage around the muscle or an imbalance of collagen metabolism. This disruption, and similar damage to tendons within the musculotendinous unit can give rise to pain (Abraham, 1979; McArdle, Katch and Katch, 1986). The connective tissue

surrounding the muscle becomes more permeable when damaged, allowing excess leakage of muscle enzymes and an increased uptake of injected radio-isotopes (Newham, 1991).

Unaccustomed exercise can also produce a build-up of metabolites within the working muscle. This, in turn, will give rise to osmotic changes in the cellular environment of the muscle, resulting in fluid retention and subsequent pressure on sensory nerves. Similarly, ischaemia of the working muscle can occur, leading to an accumulation of pain (p) substance, bringing on reflex muscle spasm (Abraham, 1977; DeVries, 1961).

Metabolite build-up or ischaemia is thought to be partially responsible for the pain of DOMS, but is unlikely to be the sole cause of the condition (McArdle, Katch and Katch, 1986; Byrnes and Clarkson, 1985).

A number of methods have been suggested to relieve DOMs. Stretching has been shown to reduce pain in the anterior tibial muscles (DeVries, 1961). Increasing the blood flow to the muscle during the warm down period is also helpful. This can be achieved by gentle exercise, hot showers, or massage. In each case, a possible mechanism of relief is that of flushing fresh blood through the muscle to remove metabolic wastes, and pumping the lymphatic vessels to remove local oedema and reduce interstitial pressure.

## Muscle fatigue

Muscular fatigue has been defined by Edwards (1981) as 'a failure to maintain the required or expected force', during muscular contraction. Changes in muscle function associated with fatigue include loss of force or power output, slowing of relaxation, changes in contractile characteristics, and alterations in electrical properties (Gibson and Edwards, 1985).

Two basic mechanisms of fatigue have been described, central and peripheral. Central fatigue refers to changes that occur proximally to the motor neurone, and involve neural and psychological changes such as motivation, and recruitment. Peripheral fatigue involves the motor unit itself, and occurs chiefly through exhaustion of the muscle energy supplies. The type and intensity of activity being performed will decide whether central and peripheral fatigue occur separately or in combination.

If a subject is told to push as hard as he or she can for as long as possible, without feedback, his or her force output will fall due to fatigue. If central fatigue occurs, more force can be generated only when the muscle is stimulated electrically.

Traditionally, fatigue types have been studied by comparing forces generated by maximum stimulated contraction (MStC), with those of maximal voluntary contractions (MVC). In unfatigued muscle, the MVC is the same as the MStC. With central fatigue, the force produced during MVC is less than that from a MStC, while in peripheral fatigue there is no difference between force of MVC and MStC (Bigland-Ritchie, 1981).

Peripheral fatigue can be further categorized into high and low frequency types. The natural firing frequencies of normal voluntary contractions are approximately 5–30 Hz. High frequency fatigue occurs when a muscle is stimulated at high frequencies between 50–100 Hz, while low frequency fatigue is the loss of force at low stimulation frequencies between l0 and 40 Hz.

# References

Abraham, W.M. (1977) Factors in delayed onset muscle soreness. *Medicine and Science in Sports*, **9**,(1) 11–20

Abraham, W.M. (1979) Exercise induced muscle soreness. *Physican and Sports Medicine*, **7**,(10) 57–60

Adams, J.A. (1961) The second facet of forgetting. A review of warmup decrement. *Psychological Bulletin*, **58**, 257–273

Albert, M. (1991) *Eccentric Muscle Training in Sports and Orthopaedics*, Churchill Livingstone, London

Allen, T.E., Byrd, R.J. and Smith, D.P. (1976) Hemodynamic consequences of circuit weight training. *Research Quarterly*, **47**, 299–306

American College of Sports Medicine (1978) The recommended quantity and quality of exercise for developing and maintaining fitness in healthy adults. *Medicine and Science in Sports and Exercise*, **10**, VII-X

American College of Sports Medicine (1990) The recommended quantity and quality of exercise for developing and maintaining cardiorespiratory and muscular fitness in healthy adults. *Medicine and Science in Sports and Exercise*, **22**, 265–274

Andzel, W.D., and Gutin, B. (1976) Prior exercise and endurance performance: a test of the mobilisation hypothesis. *Research Quarterly*, **47**, (3) 269–276

Andzel, W.D. (1982) One mile run performance as a function of prior exercise. *Journal of Sports Medicine*, **22**, 80–84

Ashton, D. and Davies, B. (1986) *Why Exercise?* Basil Blackwell, London

Astrand, P-O. and Rodahl, K. (1986) *Textbook of Work Physiology*, McGraw-Hill, Maidenhead

Atkinson, H.W. (1986) Principles of treatment. In *Cash's Textbook of Neurology for Physiotherapists*, 4th edn (ed. P.A. Downie), Faber and Faber, London, pp. 147–219

Bandy, W.D., Lovelace-Chandler, V. and McKitrick-Bandy, B. (1990) Adaptation of skeletal muscle to resistance training. *Journal of Orthopaedic and Sports Physical Therapy*, **12**,(6) 248–255

Barcroft, H. and Ebholm, O.G. (1943) The effect of temperature on blood flow and deep temperature in the human forearm. *Journal of Physiology*, **102**, 5–20

Barnard, R.J., Gardner, G.W., Diaco, N.V., MacAlpin, R.N. and Kattus, A.A. (1973) Cardiovascular responses to sudden strenuous exercise: heart rate, blood pressure, and ECG. *Journal of Applied Physiology*, **34**, 883

Berger, R A. (1962) Effect of varied weight training programmes of strength. *Research Quarterly*, **33**, 168–181

Bergh, U. (1980) Human power at subnormal body temperatures. *Acta Physiologica Scandinavica*, **478**, (Suppl.) 1–39

Bergh, U. and Ekblom, B. (1979) Physical performance and peak aerobic power at different body temperatures. *Journal of Applied Physiology*, **46**, 885–889

Bigland-Ritchie, B. (1981) EMG and fatigue of human voluntary and stimulated contractions. In *Human Muscle Fatigue: Physiological Mechanisms* (ed. R. Porter amd J. Whelan), Ciba Foundation Symposium 82, Pitman Medical, London

Bonner, H.W. (1974) Preliminary exercise: a two-factor theory. *Research Quarterly*, **45**, 138–147

Borms, J. (1984) Importance of flexibility in overall physical fitness. *International Journal of Physical Education*, **11**, 2

Borms, J., Van Roy, P., Santens, J-P. and Haentjens, A. (1987) Optimal duration of static exercises for improvement of coxofemoral flexibility. *Journal of Sports Science*, **5**, 39–47

Bosco, C. and Komi, P.V. (1979) Potentiation of the mechanical behaviour of the human skeletal muscle through pre-stretching. *Acta Physiologica Scandinavica*, **106**, 467

Braith, R.W., Graves, J.E., Pollock, M.L., Leggett, S.L., Carpenter, D.M. and Colvin, A.B. (1989) Comparison of 2 vs 3 days/week of variable resistance training during 10 and 18 week programs. *Interna-*

*tional Journal of Sports Medicine*, **10**, (6) 450–454

Bray, J.J., Cragg, P.A., Macknight, A.D.C., Mills, R.G., and Taylor, D.W. (1986) *Lecture Notes on Human Physiology*, Blackwell Scientific, Oxford

Byrnes, W.C. and Clarkson, M.C. (1985) Delayed onset muscle soreness following repeated bouts of downhill running. *Journal of Applied Physiology*, **59**, 283

Carlisle, F. (1956) Effect of preliminary passive warming on swimming performance. *Research Quarterly*, **27** (2) 143–151

Cavagna, G.A. (1977) Storage and utilisation of elastic energy in skeletal muscle. *Exercise and Sports Sciences Reviews*, **5**, 89–129

Clarke, D. H. and Stull, G. A. (1970) Endurance training as a determinant of strength and fatigability. *Research Quarterly*, **41**, 19–26

Clarkson, P.M. and Byrnes, K.M. (1986) Muscle soreness and serum creatine kinase activity following isometric, eccentric, and concentric exercise. *International Journal of Sports Medicine*, **7**, 152–155

Cornelius, W.L. and Hinson, M.M. (1980) The relationship between isometric contraction of hip extensors and subsequent flexibility in males. *Journal of Sports Medicine and Physical Fitness*, **20**, 75–80

Costill, D.L., Fink, W.J., Getchell, L.H., Ivy, J.L., and Witzmann, F.A. (1979) Lipid metabolism in muscle of endurance trained males and females. *Journal of Applied Physiology: Respiratory, Environmental and Exercise Physiology*, **47**, 787

Cureton, T.K. (1941) Flexibility as an aspect of physical fitness. *Research Quarterly*, **12**, (Suppl.) 381–390

Darden, E. (1975) Positive and negative work. *Scholastic Coach*, **45**, 6–12 and 85–86

Davies, C.T.M. and Young, K. (1983) Effect of temperature on contractile properties and muscle power of triceps surae in humans. *Journal of Applied Physiology*, **55**, 191–195

DeLorme, T. and Watkins, A. (1948) Techniques of progressive resistance exercise. *Archives of Physical Medicine and Rehabilitation*, **29**, 263–273

DeVries, H.A. (1959) Effects of various warm-up procedures on 100 yard times of competitive swimmers. *Research Quarterly*, **30**, 11–20

DeVries, H.A. (1961) Prevention of muscular distress after exercise. *Research Quarterly*, **32**, 177

DeVries, H.A. (1962) Evaluation of static stretching procedures for improvement of flexibility. *Research Quarterly*, **33**, 222–229

DeVries, H.A. (1980) *Physiology of Exercise for Physical Education and Athletics*, William C. Brown, Dubuque

Edwards, R.H.T. (1981) Human muscle function and fatigue. In *Human Muscle Fatigue: Physiological Mechanisms*. (ed. R. Porter and J. Whelan), Ciba Foundation Symposium 82, Pitman Medical, London, pp. 1–18

Ekstrand, J. and Gillquist, J. (1982) The frequency of muscle tightness and injuries in soccer players. *Ameri-can Journal of Sports Medicine*, **10**, (March–April) 75–78

Ekstrand, J., Gillquist, J., Moller, M. et al. (1983) Incidence of soccer injuries and their relation to training and team success. *American Journal of Sports Medicine*, **11** (March–April) 63–67

Etnyre, B.R. and Lee, E.J. (1987) Comments on proprioceptive neuromuscular facilitation stretching. *Research Quarterly for Exercise and Sport*, **58**, (2) 184–188

Etnyre, B.R. and Abraham, L.D. (1986) H-reflex changes during static stretching and two variations of proprioceptive neuromuscular facilitation techniques. *Electroencephalography and Clinical Neurophysiology*, **63**, 174–179

Fleck, S.J. and Schutt, R.C. (1985) Types of strength training. *Clinics in Sports Medicine*, **4**,(1), pp. 159–169

Gardner, G. (1963) Specificity of strength changes of the exercised and non exercised limb following isometric training. *Research Quarterly*, **34**, 98–101

Gettman, L.R. and Ayres, J.J. (1978) Aerobic changes through 10 weeks of slow and fast speed isokinetic training (abstract). *Medicine and Science in Sports and Exercise*, **10**, 47

Gettman, L.R. and Pollock, M.L. (1981) Circuit weight training: A critical review of its physiological benefits. *The Physician and Sports Medicine*, **9**, (1), 44–60

Gettman, L.R., Ayres, J.J. and Pollock, M.L. (1978) The effect of circuit weight training on strength, cardio-respiratory function, and body composition of adult men. *Medicine and Science in Sports and Exercise*, **10**, 171–176

Gettman, L.R., Ayres, J.J. and Pollock, M.L. (1979) Physiological effects on adult men of circuit strength training and jogging. *Archives of Physical Medicine and Rehabilitation*, **60**, 115–120

Gibson, H. and Edwards, R.H.T. (1985) Muscular exercise and fatigue *Sports Medicine*, **2**, 120–132

Goldberg, B., Saranitia, A., Witman, P. (1980) Preparticipation sports assessment – an objective evaluation. *Paediatrics*, **66**, 736–745

Gutin, B., and Stewart, K. (1971) Prior exercise and endurance. Physiology meeting. Springfield, Mass. Cited in Gutin et al. (1976)

Gutin, B., Stewart, K., Lewis, S. and Kruper, J (1976) Oxygen consumption in the first stages of strenuous work as a function of prior exercise. *Journal of Sports Medicine*, 60–65

Hardy, L. and Jones, D. (1986) Dynamic flexibility and proprioceptive neuromuscular facilitation. *Research Quarterly for Exercise and Sport*, **57**, 150–153

Harris, M.L. (1969) Flexibility: A review of the literature. *Physical Therapy*, **49**, (6) 591–601

Hogberg, P. and Ljunggren, O. (1947) Uppvarmningens inverkan pa lopprestationerna, *Svensk Idrott*, **40**

Holland, G.L. (1968) The physiology of flexibility: a review of the literature. In *Kinesiology Review*, pp. 49–62

Hollis, M. (1977) *Practical Exercise Therapy*, Blackwell Scientific, Oxford, pp. 164–213

Holt, L.E. and Smith, R. (1983) The effect of selected stretching programs on active and passive flexibility. Del Mar, CA: Research Center for Sport

Holt, L.E., Travis, T.T. and Okita, T. (1970) Comparative study of three stretching techniques. *Perceptual and Motor Skills*, **31**, 611–616

Hurley, B.F., Seals, D.R., Ehsani, A.A., Cartier, L.J., Dalsky, G.P., Hagberg, J.M. and Holloszy, J.O. (1984a) Effects of high- intensity strength training on cardiovascular function. *Medicine and Science in Sports and Exercise*, **16**,(5) 483–488

Hurley, B.F., Hagberg, J.M., Allen, W.K., Seals, D.R., Young, J.C., Cuddihee, R.T. and Holloszy, J.O. (1984b) Effect of training on blood lactate levels during submaximal exercise. *Journal of Applied Physiology: Respiratory, Environment, and Exercise Physiology*, **56**, 1260

Johns, R. J. and Wright, V. (1982) Relative importance of various tissue on joint stiffness. *Journal of Applied Physiology*, **17**, 824–828

Johnson, B.L., Adamezyk, J.W. Tenmore, K.O. and Stromme, S.B. (1976) A comparison of concentric and eccentric muscle training. *Medicine and Science in Sports and Exercise*, **8**, 35–38

Jones, D.A., Newham, D.J. and Torgan, C. (1989) Mechanical influences on long standing human muscle fatigue and delayed onset muscle pain. *Journal of Physiology*, **224**, 173–186

Karvonen, J. (1978) Warming up and its physiological effects. Acta Universitatis Ouluensis. Series D, No. 31. *Pharmacologica et Physiologica*, No. 6

Kisner, C. and Colby, L.A. (1990) *Therapeutic Exercise. Foundations and Techniques*, Davis, Philadelphia

Knight, K.L. (1979) Knee rehabilitation by the daily adjustable progressive resistance exercise technique. *American Journal of Sports Medicine*, **7**, 336

LaBan, M.M. (1962) Collagen tissue: implications of its response to stress in vitro. *Archives of Physical Medicine and Rehabilitation*, **43**, 461–466

Lehmann, J.F., DeLateur, B.J. and Silverman, D.R. (1966) Selective heating effects of ultrasound in human beings

Lindh, M. (1979) Increase of muscle strength from isometric quadriceps exercises at different knee angles. *Scandinavian Journal of Rehabilitation*, **11**, 33–36

Luithi, J.M., Howald, H., Claasen, H., Rosler, K., Vock, P., and Hoppeler, H. (1986) Structural changes in skeletal muscle tissue with heavy resistance exercise. *International Journal of Sports Medicine*, **7**, 1399–1403

MacDougal, J. D. (1992) Hypertrophy or hyperplasia. In: *Strength and Power in Sport* (P. V. Komi, ed.), Blackwell Scientific, Oxford, pp. 230–238

MacDougall, J.D., Ward, G.R., Sale, D.G. and Sutton, J.R. (1977) Biochemical adaptation of human skeletal muscle in heavy resistance training and immobilisation. *Journal of Applied Physiology*, **43**, 700–703

McArdle, W.D., Katch, F.I. and Katch, V.L. (1986) *Exercise Physiology. Energy, Nutrition, and Human Performance*, Lea and Febiger, Philadelphia

McKenzie, R.A. (1981) *The Lumbar Spine. Mechanical Diagnosis and Therapy*, Spinal Publications, Lower Hutt, New Zealand

Messier, S.P. and Dill, M.E. (1985) Alteration in strength and maximal oxygen uptake consequent to Nautilus circuit weight training. *Research Quarterly*, **56**,(4) 345–351

Morgan, R.E. and Adamson, G.T. (1962) *Circuit Training*, G. Bell, London

Nacson, J. and Schmidt, R.A. (1971) The activity-set hypothesis for warmup decrement. *Journal of Motor Behaviour*, **3**, 1–15

Nelson, A.G., Chambers, R.S., McGowan, C.M. and Penrose, K.W. (1986) Proprioceptive neuromuscular facilitation versus weight training for enhancement of muscular strength and athletic performance. *Journal of Orthopaedic and Sports Physical Therapy*, **7**, 250–253

Newham, D.J. (1991) Skeletal muscle pain and exercise. *Physiotherapy*, **77**, (1) 66–70

Newman, D.J., Mills, K.R., Quigley, B.M. and Edwards, R.H.T. (1983). Pain and fatigue after concentric and eccentric muscle contractions. *Clinical Science*, **64**, 55–62

O'Shea, P. (1963) Effects of selected weight training programs on the development of strength and muscle hypertrophy. *Research Quarterly*, **37**, 95–102

Palmitier, R.A., An. K., Scott, S.G. and Chao, E.Y.S. (1991) Kinetic chain exercise in knee rehabilitation. *Sports Medicine*, **11**, (6) 402–413

Pollock, M.L., Cureton, T.K. and Greniger, L. (1969) Effects of frequency of training on working capacity, cardiovascular function and body composition of adult men. *Medicine and Science in Sports*, **1**, 70–74

Reilly, T. (1981) The concept, measurement and development of flexibility. In *Sports Fitness and Sports Injuries* (ed. T. Reilly), Faber and Faber, London

Renstrom, P. and Kannus, P. (1992) Prevention of injuries in endurance athletes. In: *Endurance in Sport* (R. J. Shephard and P. O. Astrand, eds), IOC Medical Commission Publication, Blackwell Scientific, Oxford, pp. 325–350

Richards, D.K. (1968) A two factor theory of the warmup in jumping performance. *Research Quarterly*, **39**, 668–673

Rigby, B. (1964) The effect of mechanical extension under the thermal stability of collagen. *Biochemica et Biophysica Acta*, **79**, 634–636

Rutherford, O.M. (1988) Muscular coordination and strength training. Implications for injury rehabilitation. *Sports Medicine*, **5**, 196–202

Safran, M.R., Garrett, W.E., Seaber, A.V., Glisson,

R.R. and Ribbecsk, B.M. (1988) The role of warmup in muscular injury prevention. *American Journal of Sports Medicine*, **16**, (2)

Safran, M. R., Seaber, A. V. and Garrett Jr, W. E. (1989) Warm-up and muscular injury prevention: an update. *Sports Medicine*, **8**, 239–249

Sale, D.G., Upton, A.R.M., McComas, A.J. and McDougall, J.D. (1983) Neuromuscular function in weight-trainers. *Experimental Neurology*, **82**, 521–531

Sale, D.G. (1988) Neural adaptation to resistance training. *Medicine and Science in Sports and Exercise*, **20**, (5) 135–145

Sapega A.A., Quedenfel, T.C., Moyer, R.A. and Butler, R.A. (1981) Biophysical factors in range of motion exercise. *Physician and Sportsmedicine*, **9**, (12) 57–65

Sargeant, A.J. and Dolan, P. (1987) Effect of prior exercise on maximal short term power output in humans. *Journal of Applied Physiology*, **63**, 1475–1480

Sargeant, A.J. (1987) Effect of muscle temperature on leg extension force and short term power output in humans. *European Journal of Applied Physiology*, **56**, 693–698

Schmidt, R.A. (1982) *Motor Control and Learning*. Human Kinetics Publishers, Champaign, Illinois

Seger, J.Y., Westing, S.H., Hanson, M., Karlson, E. and Ekblom, B. (1988) A new dynamometer measuring concentric and eccentric muscle strength in accelerated, decelerated, or isokinetic movements. *European Journal of Applied Physiology*, **57**, 526–530

Shellock, F.G. and Prentice, W.E. (1985) Warming up and stretching for improved physical performance and prevention of sports related injuries. *Sports Medicine*, **2**, 267–278

Silvester, L.J., Stiggins, C., McGown, C. and Bryce, G. (1982) The effect of variable resistance and free-weight training programs on strength. *National Strength and Conditioning Association Journal*, **3**, 30–33

Smith, M.J. and Melton, P. (1981) Isokinetic versus isotonic variable resistance training. *American Journal*

of *Sports Medicine*, **9**, (4) 275–279

Stanton, P. and Purdam, C. (1989). Hamstring injuries in sprinting – the role of eccentric exercise. *Journal of Orthopaedic and Sports Physical Therapy*, **10**, (9)

Stokes, M. and Young, A. (1984) The contribution of reflex inhibition to arthrogenous muscle weakness. *Clinical Science*, **67**, 7–14

Stull, G.A. and Clarke, D.H. (1970) High resistance low repetition training as a determiner of strength and fatigability. *Research Quarterly*, **41**, 189–193

Talag, T.S. (1973) Residual muscular soreness as influenced by concentric, eccentric, and static contractions. *Research Quarterly*, **44**, (4) 458–469

Verhoshanski, Y. and Chornonson, G. (1967) Jump exercises in sprint training. *Track and Field Quarterly*, **9**, 1909

Voight, M.L. and Draovitch, P. (1991) Plyometrics. In *Eccentric Muscle Training in Sports and Orthopaedics* (ed. M.A. Albert), Churchill Livingstone, London

Voss, D.E., Ionta, M.K. and Myers, B.J. (1985) *Proprioceptive Neuromuscular Facilitation: Patterns and Techniques*, Harper and Row, Philadelphia

Warren, C.G., Lehmann, J.F. and Koblanski, J.N. (1971) Elongation of rat tail tendon: effect of load and temperature. *Archives of Physical Medicine and Rehabilitation*, **51**, 465–474

Westing, S.H., Seger, J.Y. and Thorstensson, A. (1991) Isoacceleration: a new concept of resistive exercise. *Medicine and Science in Sports and Exercise*, **23**, (5) 631–635

Wilmore, J.H. (1981) *The Wilmore Fitness Program*, Wallaby books, New York

Wilmore, J.H., Parr, R.B. and Girandola, R.N. (1978) Physiological alterations consequent to circuit weight training. *Medicine and Science in Sports and Exercise*, **10**, 79–84

Zinovieff, A.N. (1951) Heavy resistance exercise, the Oxford technique. *British Journal of Physical Medicine*, **14**, 129

# 7 Treatment modalities

The aim of this chapter is briefly to review some of the therapeutic modalities currently used in sports physiotherapy. The chapter does not attempt to teach medical or physiotherapy practitioners how to use a particular modality; instead, its aim is to give practitioners an insight into a technique so that they may judge whether it would be appropriate to study the subject further. Much of the material will be familiar to practising sports physiotherapists, although some modalities have only recently been introduced to the undergraduate physiotherapy syllabus. Medical practitioners and other specialists should find the introduction to electrotherapy techniques useful.

The information in this chapter comes from two sources. First, from the clinical experience of both the author and others who have published clinical findings, and secondly, from research papers which assess the effectiveness of the various modalities.

Although much research has been done, some of it is of limited value. Studies have often not been rigorously controlled, and in many instances the treatment parameters have not been quoted by the authors, making the reproducibility of a particular treatment regime impossible. In clinical physiotherapy practice many treatment modalities are used more through force of habit than with objectivity in mind. This is unfortunate, because whilst some treatments currently used may not be as effective as at first thought, others may be dismissed when they are in fact clinically useful.

In this chapter greater emphasis is given to modalities which are more frequently used in the treatment of sports injuries, while particular techniques relevant to a specific injury are left to Part Two.

## Therapeutic heating

Heat is a treatment which is widely used by both physiotherapists and athletes themselves. A large variety of apparatus exists to heat the body superficially by irradiation or conduction. Radiation sources cause heating without touching the skin and include heat lamps of various designs, while conduction therapies heat in direct contact with the skin and include hot packs, bathing and wax treatments.

Deep heating is achieved only by modalities whose effects pass through the insulating subcutaneous fat barrier of the body. The main modalities to do this are shortwave diathermy and microwave diathermy (which is less used). Some practitioners maintain that ultrasound can cause significant deep heating (see below).

### Effects of heating

Therapeutic effects are only achieved if tissue is heated to 40–45°C for at least 5 minutes (Lehmann and de Lateur, 1982). The effects of heating include metabolic and circulatory changes, pain reduction, alteration of collagen extensibility, and a reduction in muscle spasm.

#### Metabolic and cellular effects

Van't Hoff's law states that if the rate of a chemical reaction can be increased, it will be increased by a temperature rise. As metabolic reactions are basically chemical in nature they will be enhanced by heating and diminished by cooling, hence the usefulness of these modalities in the treatment of sports injuries. For every 1°C rise in tissue temperature, there is a 13% increase in metabolic rate (Low and Reed, 1990). However, proteins are denatured by heating, so metabolic enzymes may be affected detrimentally if heating is too great. An optimum temperature exists which is high enough to increase the rate of the metabolic chemical reactions without interfering with the metabolic enzymes.

The optimum temperature will depend very much on which chemical reaction is affected, but there are general guidelines. Above 45°C protein damage and tissue destruction is apparent. If the temperature drops too low, tissue damage may again result as body fluids are frozen. For deep tissues, therapeutic temperatures ranging from 5–6°C above or below that of the body core are recommended, while for superficial tissues lower temperature ranges are appropriate (Low and Reed, 1990).

Prolonged exposure to infra-red radiation (15 minutes, three times per week for 45 weeks) has been shown to increase the number of elastic fibres and ground substance in the skin of rats (Kligman, 1982). Inhibition of RNA, DNA and protein synthesis in cancer cells, and alterations in the amino acid make-up of proteins in normal cells has also been noted (Westerhof et al., 1987).

### Collagen extensibility

Various authors (LaBan, 1962, Lehmann et al.; 1970, Warren et al., 1971) have demonstrated increases in the extensibility of tendons *in vitro* when heat is combined with stretching (see pp. 98–99). Joint stiffness has also been shown to reduce with deeper heating (Wright and Johns, 1961), and this would seem logical as joint fluid viscosity will be lower.

Although these changes are useful, and may occur during exercise or following deep heating, it is doubtful if superficial heating will significantly affect the extensibility of collagenous tissues *in vivo* (Kitchen and Partridge, 1991). The increased range of movement sometimes demonstrated clinically following superficial heating is more likely to be the result of a reduction in pain and muscle spasm, which is a useful clinical response in itself.

### Circulatory changes

When heat is applied to the skin, the skin reddens giving an erythema. This is a protective effect as the body attempts to carry the heat away from the area and guard the skin. The vasodilation is caused by a reduction in sympathetic tone which opens the arteriovenous anastomoses. The resulting cutaneous hyperaemia is limited to the skin by the insulating properties of the subcutaneous fat.

The vasodilation is brought about both by a direct effect of heat on the local blood vessels, and by the increase in metabolic products in the area. The increased rate of metabolic reactions produces more carbon dioxide and lactate, which in turn cause a greater acidity within the tissues. Any protein damage which occurs as a result of heating will cause histamine release which perpetuates the vasodilation.

There are generally no significant alterations in either blood pressure or blood flow to the deeper tissues (Kitchen and Partridge, 1991), and the superficial cutaneous effect is, on the whole, limited to the local area receiving exposure, although some heat spread will occur.

The pace of interstitial fluid drainage increases with temperature, and blood flow to active organs is increased. The release of histamine and prostaglandin seen with heating raises hydrostatic pressure within the blood capillaries, forcing fluid into the surrounding tissues as oedema. Severe heating consequently reinforces acute inflammation, promoting further oedema and pain (Goats, 1989), although mild heating may have a pain relieving effect particularly in chronic conditions.

### Neural effects

The fact that heat can be felt is testament to its effect on skin receptors. Clinical experience would suggest that it can produce some sort of analgesic effect, and Barbour, McGuire and Kirchoff (1986) found that heat was used for pain relief by 68% of cancer patients in their study. When heat is applied, afferent nerves from skin receptors may affect the pain gate and produce an analgesic effect, but evidence for this mechanism is sparse. Kanui (1985) showed inhibition of nociceptive impulses in rats, whereas Kumazawa, Mizumura and Sato (1987) demonstrated heat sensitization and hyperalgesia with similar temperature changes.

Its effect on muscle spindles and Golgi tendon organs has been suggested as a mechanism for muscle spasm reduction with deep heating, and superficial heating may cause similar changes through decreased gamma fibre activity (Lehmann and de Lateur, 1982).

## Infra-red radiation

Infra-red lamps heat the body tissues by radiation and are not in contact with the skin. Their effect is achieved through heating rather than by photochemical changes (Kitchen and Partridge, 1991). Infra-red radiation has a wavelength of 0.78–1000 μm and lies between microwaves and visible light in the electromagnetic spectrum. Infra-red modalities used in physiotherapy are either luminous with a peak wavelength of 1 μm, or non-luminous, with a peak of 4 μm. The wavelength of the infra-red radiation produced will be inversely proportional to the temperature of the heat source (Wien's law), thus a cooler source will produce infra-red radiation with a longer wavelength.

The non-luminous type of infra-red lamp consists of a wire wound around a ceramic material. This heating unit is placed at the focus point of a parabolic reflector. Luminous lamps (the type available over the counter in chemist's shops) are made up of a tungsten filament encapsulated in a glass bulb filled with a low pressure inert gas. Part of the bulb is silvered to provide a reflective surface behind the heating element.

The penetration depth (by definition the point at which 63% of the radiation energy has been absorbed, so reducing the intensity to 37% of its original value) will depend on the type of apparatus used, the technique of application and the properties of the tissues treated. Long wavelengths only penetrate to 0.1 mm, while shorter wavelengths may penetrate to a depth of 3 mm (Kitchen and Partridge, 1991). The most effective response occurs when the infra-red radiation is applied at a 90° angle to the skin.

## Conduction heating

Conduction heating encompasses modalities which are in contact with the skin surface and heat mostly by conduction rather than radiation. Conduction heating apparatus includes moist packs, paraffin wax, hot-water bottles and hot-water bathing (including whirlpools).

Moist packs usually consist of a silicate gel enclosed in a cotton fabric sleeve. The pack is heated in water at 75–80°C and the gel will absorb some of the hot water. The gel pack is then wrapped in a number of layers of towelling to intervene between it and the patient's skin, preventing the skin temperature from rising above 42°C (Low and Reed, 1990). The pack is left in position for 20–30 minutes, and gradually reduces in temperature, thus providing a safe method of therapeutic heating.

Paraffin wax is used in particular on the hands and feet. The wax is kept in a stainless steel or enamelled container and maintained in a molten state at a temperature of 42–52°C. The body part to be treated is washed, immersed in the liquid wax are then withdrawn and allowed to dry for 2–3 seconds before being reimmersed. Using this method a thick layer of wax is gradually built up and the body part is covered with a plastic bag and towelling to maintain the heat.

Hot-water bathing is a simple form of heat application, with the advantage that exercise may be carried out at the same time. Whirlpool baths combine the benefits of hot water with mechanical agitation to stimulate the skin surface. Various types and sizes of baths are available. The water jet may be varied and the water changed with each treatment. The agitation of the water may be used for wound debridement, in which case an antibacterial agent is added to the water.

Heat is a widely used and useful treatment modality in sports medicine, but there is a tendency for athletes to apply heat too intensely, in the belief that 'more is better', and therapists must emphasize safety precautions. Heat should not be applied when the skin has any ointment or 'rub' on it, as this can severely impair skin sensation. Gentle heating is all that is required, and athletes must be warned that heat which is too intense can cause severe burning. Heat should obviously never be applied if skin sensation is impaired.

## Microwave diathermy

Microwave radiation lies between radiowaves and infra-red radiation in the electromagnetic spectrum. The normal frequency used therapeutically is 2450 MHz, at a wavelength of 12.245 cm, although 915 MHz is available and is probably more suitable for use in sport (see below). The maximum safe output is usually limited to about 25 W, which contrasts markedly with values of up to 1000 W used in commercial microwave ovens.

Microwaves are produced by the oscillation of an electric current at high frequency. However, it is not possible for electrons in a current to oscillate fast enough to produce microwaves if they have to pass through a valve or transistor. Instead, a device called a magnetron is used. This is similar in many respects to a large thermionic valve and consists of a centrally heated cathode surrounded by a positively charged metal block through which a strong magnetic field is passed. The electrodes emitted by the cathode are spun at high speed by the magnetic field. As these electrodes pass over small cavities

cut into the metal block of the magnetron, they oscillate and are then fed through a coaxial cable to an emitter which radiates the microwaves (Low and Reed, 1990). The output is varied by an intensity control on the machine.

As the microwaves enter the tissues they are reflected at the air–skin and skin–fat boundaries; the amount of reflection is as much as 50–75%, depending on the skin and fat thickness of the patient (Scowcroft, Mason and Hayne, 1977). Boundary reflection can result in an interaction between the incident and reflected beams of the microwaves, which may give rise to standing wave formation and intense heating. The rate of microwave absorption is lower in fat and higher in vascular tissue, and the reflection at the various tissue boundaries causes peaks of heating (Fig. 7.1). Lower frequency microwaves penetrate further, with less heat being lost to the fat layer, and more reaching the muscle tissue. Optimum therapeutic heating is achieved at 750 MHz (Lehmann et al., 1970), and for this reason commercial units which generate a frequency of 915 MHz give a more efficient absorption of energy, and are more suitable for use in sport, than the 2450 MHz frequency units usually used.

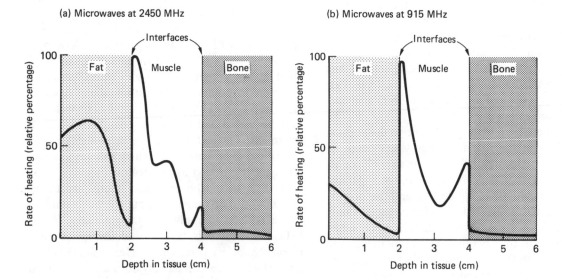

**Figure 7.1** Comparison of microwave heating effects at tissue boundaries. (a) 2450 MHz, (b) 915 MHz. From Low and Reed (1990), with permission.

The effective heating depth of microwaves is often given as 3 cm (Forster and Palastanga, 1981), but this will obviously vary depending on the thicknesses of the different tissue layers being heated. The penetration depth of a 2450 MHz machine has been given as 1.7 cm into muscle and skin and 11.2 cm into fat and bone, whilst for a 915 MHz unit the values are 3.04 cm and 17.7 cm, respectively (Goats, 1990a).

The main results of microwave diathermy have traditionally been thought to be due to heating. Blood flow has been shown to increase following microwave treatment (Gersten et al., 1949; Sekins et al., 1984), and superficial contractures have been effectively treated with microwave and stretching (Delateur, Stonebridge and Lehmann, 1978). However, it now appears that non-thermal effects may also be important. Biological effects at exposure levels as low as 10 mW/cm$^2$ have been reported (McRee, 1980). Changes in endocrine function, bodyweight, fertility, electrolyte balance, electroencephalogram, phagocytosis and neurone membrane function have been described in Soviet and Eastern bloc literature (Goats, 1990a).

## Short-wave diathermy

Short-wave diathermy (SWD) units generate radio frequency electromagnetic energy at 27.12 MHz. Continuous output is used primarily for heating, while pulsed output (which allows heat dissipation) is used at higher intensities for non-thermal effects.

Application of SWD is either by the capacitor field method, or by inductance. In the capacitor field method, electrodes are placed on either side of a body part, separated from it by insulating material. The electrodes act as capacitor plates, with the body tissues and insulating material forming a dielectric. In the inductance method, an insulated cable is wound into a flat spiral and placed inside a casing. This applicator is placed adjacent to the body tissues, which in turn behave as an electromagnetic conductor.

The oscillating electric and magnetic fields produced in the body tissues by SWD create heat through rapid ionic vibration and rotation of dipolar molecules. Highly vascular tissues are rich in electrolytes and therefore heat easily, while fibrous tissue in contrast heats only moderately (Goats, 1989b). By far the most significant effect of SWD is deep heating, which causes the physiological changes described above.

## Pulsed short-wave

Pulsed short-wave, or pulsed electromagnetic energy (PEME) operates at the same frequency as SWD, but as the output is pulsed, any heat formed is dispersed during the resting periods between the pulses. Consequently, a greater peak power output can be used than with SWD, without the risk of burning, giving non-thermal biophysical effects. Both electric (E) and magnetic (H) fields are produced, usually in combination.

A number of processes have been postulated for the effects of PEME therapy. Cell oscillation is thought to occur, and asymmetrical bodies within the blood, may be 'pushed along' through an electromotive effect. In addition, changes in cell potentials occur, and ionic interchange is altered (Hayne, 1984).

Ions within the cell membrane are thought to be redistributed, and metabolic processes active during inflammation modified. Neurones and ATP-ases may be affected, and blood vessels could act as conductors and have weak electric currents induced in them. These currents in turn may affect repair processes, brain activity and vascular muscle tone (Goats, 1989a).

Pain relief and reduction of swelling in ankle sprains has been reported as a result of PEME therapy applied daily for 60 minutes over a 3 day period at 38 W mean power output (Wilson, 1972). Haematoma induced in rabbits showed significant improvement when treated with PEME twice daily for 30 minutes at a mean power output of 25 W (Fenn, 1969). Golden et al. (1981) showed significant improvements in healing of the donor site of a split skin graft, using a mean power output of 25.3 W for 30 minutes (pulse duration 65 ms), given 6-hourly, over a 12 day period. Barclay et al. (1983) claimed 'definite biological and healing effects' following treatment of hand injuries (including lacerations and contusions). They used a pulse duration of 65 ms and treated within 36 hours of injury. Of their initial treatment group of 30 matched patients, all but 2 showed complete resolution of swelling 3 days after injury, compared with 7 days for the control group.

The effects of PEME on soft tissue injury are listed below (Golden et al., 1981; Hayne, 1984; Goats, 1989a).

1 Increased number of white cells, histocytes and fibroblasts in wound.
2 Electromotive effect on asymmetrical blood products.
3 Cell oscillation.
4 Oedema dispersion and haematoma absorption improved.
5 Inflammation modified/reduced.
6 Effects on fibrin and collagen.
7 Osteogenesis encouraged.
8 Peripheral and CNS healing improved.
9 Ionic effect on cell membrane.
10 Weak electric currents induced in blood vessels.
11 ATPases affected.

## Laser

### Production of laser light

The term laser is an acronym for 'light amplification by stimulated emission of radiation'. Some basic principles of atomic theory are needed to explain how a laser works. The nucleus of an atom contains neutrons and positively charged protons, and is itself surrounded by negative electrons. Overall, the atom will have a neutral charge unless an electron is lost or gained, in which case a charged atom or 'ion' will be produced. The electrons are contained within orbits or shells each at a specific energy level. If an electron absorbs enough energy, in the form of heat or electricity for example, it will jump to a higher energy shell. It cannot exist between two shells. When an amount (quantum) of energy collides with an electron, it will cause the electron to move energy levels and the atom becomes 'excited'. The atom will stay in this state only momentarily, and as the electron falls back into its previous orbit it will emit energy in the form of electromagnetic pulses or 'photons'. This process is called spontaneous emission.

In a laser, stimulated emission occurs. In this case, the photon of energy released from the first atom stimulates a similarly excited neighbouring atom to release an identical photon, setting up a chain reaction.

An electrical power source is used for therapeutic low-powered lasers (LPL). This is applied to a lasing medium which, in the case of LPLs, is usually either helium neon (HeNe) gas, or the solids gallium arsenide (GaAs) or gallium arsenide aluminium (GaAsAl). The lasing medium is positioned in a chamber between two mirrors, one of which is semipermeable. Gradually, the amount of energy created by stimulated emission builds up, until the chamber can no longer contain the power and photons are ejected through the semipermeable mirror.

### Properties of laser light

The light emitted by the laser is in an organized pattern, unlike the haphazard light from a fluorescent tube for example. Laser light has three distinct properties, known as coherence, monochromaticity and collimation. All the photons of light emitted by the laser are of the same wavelength and the waves are in step with each other (in phase). The light is therefore termed coherent. The light is also monochromatic, that is, of the same wavelength. If the light is in the visible spectrum it will be only one pure colour. Finally, the laser beam is said to be well collimated, meaning that there is little divergence of the photons even over a great distance.

LPLs have wavelengths of 630–1300 nm, and these will include both visible light and near infrared (NIR). Goldman et al. (1989) claimed that 99% of radiation within the range 300–1000 nm will be absorbed by the epidermis. However, Parrish (1981) claimed that an optical window exists in the range 600–1300 nm, allowing penetration through the entire skin layer and into the subcutaneous fat. A direct response appears to occur through absorption of laser light in the superficial tissues, and an indirect effect is thought to occur in deeper tissues (Saliba and Foreman, 1990).

The question of whether laser light actually penetrates the dermis is obviously an important one. Walker (1988) argued that skin contains optically active molecules (chromophores) which are also found within myelin, neuronal membranes and intraneuronally. In addition, the same author claimed that the central nervous system possesses a photosensitive enzyme. These factors could enable laser light to have effects below the dermis and stimulate underlying nerves.

### Effects of laser therapy

LPL has been shown to stimulate cell proliferation compared with incandescent light (Abergel, Lyons and Castel, 1987). Increases in fibroblastic proliferation have been shown for ruby lasers with a wavelength of 694.3 nm and HeNe lasers with a wavelength of 632.8 nm (Mester, Mester and Mester, 1985). HeNe and GaAs lasers with a wavelength of 904 nm have been shown to give a three-fold increase in procollagen production (Abergel, Lyons and Castel, 1987).

Increases in tensile strength of lased wounds have been reported (Lyons et al., 1987). A decrease in prostaglandin E has been shown, and this is thought to accelerate the resolution of acute inflammation (Mester, Mester and Mester, 1985). Wound healing is thought to be improved following LPL therapy. Faster healing, less scarring, and more regular alignment of collagen have been demonstrated following burn wounds in mice (Trelles and Mayayo, 1987). Dyson and Young (1986) showed accelerated wound contraction and an increase in the cellularity of the wound bed in mice. Interestingly, the level of improvement was linked to the pulsing frequency of the LPL. Increases in angiogenesis (Hickman and Dyson, 1988) and total collagen (Glassberg, Lask and Uitto, 1988) have also been shown.

### Application

Safe application of LPL therapy requires adequate annual maintenance of equipment, which should include a check of the unit's output using a radiometer. The main hazard represented by physiotherapy lasers is ocular damage. An LPL may produce a spot as small as 1 mm in diameter. A 20 mW beam concentrated over this area would give a power density of 2.4 $W/cm^2$. Radiation within the visible and near-infra-red range can be focused onto the retina, causing retinal damage, while near-infra-red radiation itself may also damage the anterior eye (CSP, 1991). As with any light source, phototoxic and photo-sensitizing chemicals may dangerously increase a laser's effect on the skin.

To protect the eye, suitable goggles should be worn to attenuate the wavelength of the device being used to non-hazardous levels. Goggles suitable for one wavelength may not necessarily be suitable for another.

A number of application methods are currently used. The first, point application, involves locating the most painful point of the lesion and treating this as a trigger spot. The technique has been compared to accupuncture (Saliba and Foreman, 1990). When point application is used, the tip of the LPL applicator is held in contact with the patient's skin, perpendicular to the skin surface. When an area is to be treated, it may be divided into a grid of 1 cm squares for guidance. Each square is radiated for a specific time.

The dosage given must be recorded accurately if treatment is to be standardized. The output of the laser in mW, the time exposure in seconds, the beam surface area, the distance the applicator is held from the skin and the pulsing frequency and wavelength of the unit are all variables to be considered.

Saliba and Foreman (1990) suggested that the periphery of a laceration wound should be treated, as the heavy exudate in the central portion will diminish the laser's penetration. They recommended a 'scanning' technique in which there is no contact between the laser tip and the skin. They argued that the laser tip should be 5–10 mm from the wound and, because some divergence may occur, the beam will cover a greater area. The same authors recommend a gridding technique over oedematous tissue, claiming that treatment will reduce inflammation and swelling.

Gordon (1990) claimed to have reviewed 20 000 LPL treatments for soft tissue injuries over a 9-year period. He maintained that 75–80% of patients were discharged showing 'marked improvement in function and symptoms'. Four treatments were given for an average of 30 minutes daily in most cases. His treatment involved a GaAs laser with a peak power output of 1 W and a wavelength of 904 nm, pulsed at a frequency of 72 Hz. The pulse width was 200 ns. The same author argued that patients who were heavy smokers or who had an excessive intake of caffeine responded poorly.

## Cold

Cold or ice is probably the most convenient modality available for the treatment of sports injuries. Ice is a low cost, effective treatment often recommended by practitioners for use by a patient at home. As with heat, however, the ready availability of the modality can lead to misuse with the potential for injury.

### Effects of cold

Cryotherapy may be used both in the immediate treatment of sports injuries, and in later rehabilitation. During immediate treatment, the aim is to limit the body's response to injury, in particular hypoxic tissue damage, swelling, pain and muscle spasm. Later, during the rehabilitation phase, the aims change. The goal then is to restore function and, at that stage, the effects of other techniques, such as exercise and manual therapy, are augmented by ice application.

Ice is often used in combination with rest, compression and elevation (RICE) as an effective initial treatment for sports injuries. Ice alone has been shown to be effective in the treatment of ankle injuries (Hocutt et al., 1983), but it is usually more effective when used to treat soft tissue injuries in conjunction with compression (Santiensteban, 1990). The main physiological effects of cryotherapy are listed below (Knight, 1989).

1  Decreased metabolism.
2  Decreased circulation.
3  Transiently increased, followed by decreased, pain.
4  Decreased muscle spasm.
5  Decreased inflammation.
6  Increased stiffness.

During immediate treatment, the most important effect is often claimed to be a reduction in blood flow through the local capillary network. However, blood clotting will usually seal these damaged vessels within 3–5 minutes of injury (Knight, 1989), about the same time as it takes to remove an athlete from the sports field and get him or her into the treatment room. Consequently, by the time an athlete is first seen, local bleeding may have stopped. For this reason decreased tissue metabolism is now thought to be a more important effect of cryotherapy during the immediate treatment of sports injuries (Knight, 1989; McLean, 1989). After injury, further tissue damage occurs through local hypoxia secondary to a disruption in blood flow. A reduction in metabolic rate and oxygen requirement is seen with ice treatment (Abramson et al., 1957), and this gives the body cells a better chance of survival for the period they are without oxygen, almost in a state of 'temporary hibernation' (Knight, 1989).

Circulatory changes occur during ice application, and are the subject of some debate. Blood flow has been shown to decrease during cold application and remain reduced for up to 45 minutes after treatment (Knight, Byrant and Halvorsen, 1981). Cold applications produce an easily observed reactive hyperaemia of the skin, but deeper vasodilation may not occur during therapeutic cooling (Knight, 1989). Certainly, the cyclical skin changes (the hunting response) originally described by Lewis (1930), including tissue temperature increases above pre-immersion levels, have been shown to occur only in fingers which have been cooled to 20°C prior to ice-water immersion (Knight et al., 1980).

The immediate response to ice application is a short-lived (5–60 s) dull pain, which is more intense in some individuals than others. Following this, pain reduction occurs through a reduction in nerve conductivity (Tepperman and Devlin, 1983), and stimulation of pain receptors (Halvorson, 1990). Cold-induced analgesia will allow an athlete to perform therapeutic exercise, but unlike some pain-killing injections, will not abolish the protective function of pain sensitivity (McLean, 1989).

Local cooling depresses muscle spindle activity (Halvorson, 1990; Mense, 1978) and so muscle spasm initiated through gamma nerve stimulation can be reduced. Inflammation is thought to be reduced by ice application (Schmidt et al., 1979), and joint viscosity and, with it, joint stiffness has been shown to increase (Knight, 1989).

## Cryotherapy techniques

Common cold applications include the use of flaked ice in towelling or plastic bags, cold compression, ice massage, cold sprays, ice baths, and cryogel or chemical packs.

The choice between the various methods often depends on cost and convenience. Ice soaks are better for uneven and small body parts, such as the hand and foot. With this technique some ice should be left floating on the surface of the water throughout the treatment to ensure that a low enough temperature is maintained.

Ice packs are better for larger tissue areas, such as the knee, hip and shoulder. Flaked ice in a plastic bag will give a lower tissue temperature than ice in a towelling bag, as the towelling provides insulation. Although mild frostbite is unusual (Knight, 1989) the body part should be inspected regularly. Wet towelling provides less insulation, but will still not give tissue temperatures as low as ice in a plastic bag. Knight (1989) claimed that two layers of dry wrap placed below an ice pack resulted in ankle temperatures which were 16°C higher after a 30 minute application than when ice was applied directly to the skin. Using wet wraps gave temperatures which were 5.7°C higher than with direct application. These temperature differences may, however, be of use if a patient demonstrates ice sensitivity.

Cryogel bags usually give a lower temperature than flaked ice, depending on the freezer setting used. This type of pack should not be placed directly on the skin, as mild frostbite has been observed repeatedly (Knight, 1989). Chemical packs have the advantage of convenience, and are easily carried by athletes themselves. However, they rarely produce temperatures which are low enough, and the temperature reduction which does occur is usually too short lived. Some packs also have the potential to cause chemical burns if punctured.

Similarly, temperature changes produced by cold sprays are slight and short term. The place of cold sprays is really as a stimulant for use with spray stretch techniques. Here, the vapocoolant spray (usually fluoromethane) is applied as a jet, either to overcome guarding muscle spasm or to treat irritable trigger points (Travell and Simons, 1983).

Ice or cold can be combined with compression to good effect. Several methods exist, including the use of elasticated bandage around a layer of ice, or a similar ice layer below a compression (IPC) boot. Machines which produce continuous cold air, or iced water and compression are also available.

Ice massage is particularly useful for pain relief in smaller tissue areas. Massage is carried out until cold anaesthesia ensues. The usual sensations are of cold, then burning, deep aching, and, finally, numbness (Halvorson, 1990). Once numbness has occurred, no additional skin sensation follows with more prolonged treatment, but underlying tissue temperature will continue to fall.

During the immediate treatment of sports injuries ice should be applied preferably within 5–10 minutes of injury, but certainly as soon as possible, and kept on for 20–30 minutes. Continuous application is not recommended, as its effectiveness is not increased, and frostbite has been reported (Proulx, 1976). Reapplication is made every 2 hours, it taking 2–4 hours for the ankle, knee, forearm and thigh to return to preapplication temperature (Knight, 1989). Ice may have no effect on joint swelling once intra-articular effusion has occurred (McLean, 1989).

## Cryokinetics

The use of ice in rehabilitation includes cryokinetics, the combination of cold therapy with active exercise. Cold is used to reduce pain and allow active exercise to be performed earlier than would otherwise be possible. The benefits of the therapy are from the exercise itself and not the ice application. By allowing exercise to be performed earlier, cryokinetics reduces muscle atrophy and mobility loss. The muscle pump is restored sooner, reducing swelling and consequent adhesions.

The time after which cold anaesthesia occurs will depend on the depth of the injury and the amount of insulating tissue covering it, as well as the psychological profile of the patient. Numbness of the ankle may occur 20 minutes after ice water soaking and remain for 3 minutes. While the numbness lasts, exercise is used. Further anaesthesia will occur if the ankle is then resoaked for 5 minutes. Exercise is increased progressively throughout the treatment for mobility, strength and function.

## Cryostretch

Cryostretch is the combination of cold application to relieve pain (Kowal, 1983) and reduce muscle spasm, and stretching to increase mobility. Ice is applied until cold anaesthesia is present, or for 20 minutes, whichever occurs sooner. Stretching is carried out for as long as numbness lasts, and then ice may be reapplied and stretching recommenced. Static or PNF stretching can be used, with both contract release (CR) and contract-release–agonist-contract (CRAC) methods being suitable.

This type of stretching is only of use where muscle spasm is the limiting factor in mobility. When connective tissue contracture has occurred, heat would be the treatment of choice as it will aid tissue elongation, and is less likely to cause tissue damage (Warren et al., 1976; Halvorson, 1990).

## Ultrasound

Ultrasound has a frequency greater than 20 kHz and is consequently above the limit of human hearing. It is a mechanical vibration created (transduced) by passing an alternating current through a transducer displaying piezo-electric properties. The frequency of the current used must match the resonance of the piezo-electric material, and so ultrasound units should only be used with transducers which have been matched to them.

The most common frequencies used in sport are 1.0 and 3.0 MHz, differing considerably from the diagnostic frequency in the range of 10 MHz. Higher frequency ultrasound is more readily absorbed and is therefore used to treat superficial structures.

The intensity of the ultrasound beam is expressed as average or point values over time or space. Space-averaged intensity is usually taken over the area of the transducer head, while time-averaged intensity is more important when pulsed modes are used (ter Haar, 1987). Space-averaged, time-averaged (SATA) is the space-averaged intensity over a specified time. Clearly, when quoting frequencies in research studies, it is not enough simply to give the intensity of ultrasound used in $W/cm^2$. The authors should always state which measure of intensity was used. The output of machines may alter, so calibration should be carried out annually (Docker, 1987).

### Physical effects

Both thermal and biological (non-thermal) effects have been described for ultrasound. Higher intensities may cause heating, more so in tissue with a high protein content, such as muscle and tendon. However, ultrasound of 1 $W/cm^2$ at 1 Mz will only raise the tissue temperature by 0.86°C per minute (Williams, 1987). Additional heating will occur if standing wave formation is allowed by not moving the treatment head (ter Haar, 1987) a condition particularly important when treating over bone.

The higher intensities required to achieve heating may in addition cause potentially dangerous biophysical effects. Dyson (1987) claimed that the high intensities once popular in physiotherapy treatment could have caused transient cavitation and may have been responsible for petechial haemorrhaging.

Non-thermal effects of ultrasound include both micro-streaming and cavitation. Within a fluid, micro-steaming is circulation induced by the ultrasound beam, and cavitation is the formation of pulsating gas-filled bubbles. These effects can lead to changes in the cell membrane, causing an influx of calcium. Such changes may cause secretion, synthesis or motility changes, depending on the type of cell affected (Dyson, 1987).

### Effects on soft tissue injury

The inflammatory phase of healing appears to be accelerated by ultrasound (Dyson, 1987). Histamine release from mast cells has been demonstrated as a result of insonation (Fyfe and Chahl, 1984; Hashish, Harvey and Harris, 1986), and chemotactic agents responsible for pulling polymorphonuclear leucocytes into an injured area may also be increased (Dyson, 1987). Insonated fibroblasts have been shown to produce more collagen, and the rate of scar contraction can be accelerated. This process may be brought on by contraction of myofibroblasts when insonated (Dyson, 1987).

Ultrasound treatment which commences during the inflammatory phase of healing can give stronger and more elastic scar tissue, due to increased deposition of collagen and a change in its fibre pattern (Dyson, 1989). During the proliferative phase, regeneration of blood vessels (angiogenesis) occurs following insonation, possibly due to an acceleration in the release of angiogenic factors from mast cells. Blood flow improves gradually as new vessels develop, and ultrasound itself has little direct effect on blood flow in normal muscle.

Low levels (0.5 W/cm$^2$) of ultrasound have been shown to be anti-inflammatory, while higher levels stimulate inflammation by increasing mast cell activity (Hashish, 1986; quoted in Dyson, 1989). These higher levels could be of use where inflammation is short term, and its resolution can be speeded up. However, where the stimulus to inflammation is still present, such as with an overuse syndrome, the cause of the inflammation must obviously be removed first.

Bone healing has been shown to occur following ultrasound treatment (Dyson and Brookes, 1983) possibly by stimulating the release of growth factors from macrophages. Stress fractures have been shown to be present by using ultrasound assessment (Lowden, 1986).

The effects of ultrasound are summarized in the following list (Dyson, 1987; Kitchen and Partridge, 1990).

1 Increased mast cell activity
2 Increased histamine
3 Increased chemotactic agents?
4 Altered cell membrane function
5 Increased calcium transport
6 Stimulation of fibroblast activity
7 Increased protein synthesis
8 Increased vascular permeability
9 Increased angiogenesis
10 Stronger and more elastic collagen
11 Altered smooth muscle function
12 Placebo effect (increased endorphins, decreased pain perception)
13 Heating

### Application

Accurate location of the injured tissue requiring treatment is essential, especially when pain is referred. Tissue depth measurement is important to calculate the dosage required allowing for attenuation. Three techniques are generally used, surface contact, water bag and water bath. With surface contact a coupling medium is required to exclude air from the region between the skin and the transducer head. Various preparations are available, some as creams and others as gels. All coupling media should be chemically inert and not absorbed too rapidly by the skin. They should have high viscosity, low attenuation and a low susceptibility to bubble formation. Their acoustic impedance should be similar to, or higher than, that of the tissue to be treated (Williams, 1987). The transducer head is kept moving slowly a rate of 4 cm/s being sufficient. The direction of motion will depend on the underlying anatomy. Circular movement is appropriate within a fossa and longitudinal movement is better along a tendon, for example.

The coupling medium may contain a medication, usually hydrocortisone, which is pushed through the skin by the ultrasound beam, a process known as phonophoresis. Griffen and Touchstone (1963) drove hydrocortisone through pig's skin, and Griffen et al. (1967) used the technique with 102 patients suffering from chronic joint inflammation. Of these, 68% were pain free and able to move through a full range of motion following treatment, compared with only 28% of the placebo group. Kleinkort and Wood (1975) reported good results using phonophoresis with conditions including tennis elbow and sub-deltoid bursitis. A total of 63% were relieved when 1% hydrocortisone was used, and 95% when 10% ointment was used. These authors also suggested that the increased permeability of the insonated cell may make it more susceptible to hydrocortisone. Cyriax (1982) quoted Searle (1981) as achieving good results with supraspinatus tendinitis and bursitis using 10%

hydrocortisone at a setting of 0.75 W/cm$^2$ for 4 minutes pulsed at 1:1 with a 1.5 MHz transducer.

If the body surface is irregular, a water bag may be used, although with the advent of smaller (1 cm diameter) treatment heads this process is used less often. A thin-walled rubber bag or balloon is used. Both it and the skin beneath are coated with coupling medium.

An alternative is to use a water bath, again less frequently used nowadays. Degassed water is used, and the ultrasound head is held 1–2 cm from the skin. Any bubbles forming on the transducer head should be wiped off. Multiple reflections within the water reduce the effectiveness of the ultrasound beam, and may mean that the therapist's hand will also receive exposure (Williams, 1987).

## Electrical stimulation

### Body electricity

When an electrical current is applied to the body therapeutically the intention is to bring about certain physiological changes. Some of these effects will be due to the interaction between the electrical current applied, and electrical charges created by the body as a result of normal physiological processes.

Body cells are bathed in fluid, so much so that two thirds of the bodyweight is water and half of this amount is found within the cells themselves. A great variety of ions are dissolved in the body fluids, and the water molecules themselves are dipolar and therefore capable of adhering to ionic compounds and being affected by electrical charges.

The extracellular fluid is held apart from the intracellular fluid by the cell membrane. Water and solutes may pass through the membrane by diffusion or active transport, thus altering the ionic balance inside and outside the cell and creating a potential difference between the two sides.

The main ions involved are sodium ($Na^+$) and potassium ($K^+$). Within the cell there is a high concentration of $K^+$ and a low concentration of $Na^+$. Conversely, the extracelluar fluid contains a higher concentration of $Na^+$ than $K^+$. An active transport system (the sodium/potassium pump) exists to bring $K^+$ ions into the cell and expel $Na^+$. The difference between the ionic charge of the intracellular and extracelluar fluid is called the resting potential and is negative ($-60$ to $-90$ mV) in normal circumstances. Others ions, such as hydrogen ($H^+$) and calcium ($Ca^{++}$) are also of importance to acid–base balance and muscle cell contraction, respectively.

An alteration in the cell membrane potential is an important factor in a number of physiological mechanisms. The passage of nervous impulses and muscle contraction are the two most widely accepted processes, and electrical currents have traditionally been used therapeutically to affect nerve and muscle. However, membrane changes are also important in inflammation and tissue repair/adaptation, and recent developments in electrotherapy have focused more closely on these mechanisms.

### Types of current

Various electric currents are used therapeutically in physiotherapy, and each type has its own particular name. The names sometimes refer to the shape or duration of the pulse, or the current frequency, and sometimes the name is taken from the person or company who first marketed a machine producing a certain current. When there is no change in current direction (or only a very slow change), the current is referred to as direct (d.c.). This type of current will cause chemical changes by ionic movement in non-excitable tissue at the electrode–tissue junction. If the current is interrupted to give a series of unidirectional pulses, it is referred to as an interrupted direct current (i.d.c.). However, by custom only those currents with long duration pulses (1 ms or more) are actually termed interrupted direct currents. Short duration interrupted direct currents (1 ms or less) are categorized as faradic, transcutaneous electrical nerve stimulation (TENS), or high voltage galvanic (see below).

When any interrupted direct current is used, the ionic balance of excitable membranes will be altered, stimulating either nerve or muscle tissue to produce sensory (tingling) or motor (twitching) effects. This type of current at low intensity is used in TENS, and at higher intensity in faradism. The greater the intensity of current, the more nerve fibres are stimulated. If the current intensity is increased and reduced gradually, a more comfortable impulse is produced — a process known as surging or ramping.

If the current alternates (a.c.), any chemical changes due to ions moving in one direction will be immediately cancelled out by the ions moving back again. Such currents include sinusoidal, diadynamic, Russian and interferential modalities. If an alternating current varies in the fashion of a sine wave it is termed sinusoidal. When pulses of 10 ms duration at 100 or 50 Hz are used the current is termed diadynamic, and alternating sine waves of 2500 Hz applied in bursts constitute Russian currents (Low and Reed, 1990). Two alternating sine waves, with frequencies of about 4000 Hz are used in interferential therapy.

## Application of electric current

Electric current is passed to the body through two electrodes to complete a circuit. In the wires of the modality the current moves via electrons, but in the body tissues this same current movement occurs between ions, the interface between the two systems is the point of application of the current. The electrochemical effect of the current is lessened as it passes from the modality to the body tissues with an evenly alternating current and one of low intensity. However, as the skin surface is irregular, simply placing a metal electrode directly on the skin would cause peaks of current at the contact points. In addition, the epidermis of the skin has a high electrical resistance. To create a smooth surface and to lower the skin resistance, a layer of ion-containing fluid is interspaced between the metal electrodes and the skin surface. This fluid may be either water or an electroconductive gel.

Water may be used in a water bath. Here, the limb is immersed in water (usually salinated) and the two electrodes are placed in the water at a distance from the skin surface. Alternatively, the metal electrode may be wrapped in a pad of water-retaining material (usually wet lint). The thickness of the pad is normally about 0.5–1.25 cm,

made up of a number of lint layers (Low and Reed, 1990).

More convenient are carbon impregnated silicone rubber electrodes which conform to the body surface. These are normally used with wet sponge pads or conducting gel and held in place with straps or tape. Self-adhesive electrodes using karaya gum or synthetic polymers are better still and more suitable for patient self-use or long-term application of modalities such as TENS.

### Direct current

With d.c. the main effect is one of electrolysis, with the formation of acids at the positive electrode (anode) and alkalis at the negative electrode (cathode). In addition to these effects, the anode may produce sclerosis (tissue hardening) and the cathode sclerolysis (tissue softening) (Santiesteban, 1990).

The electrolysis effect of d.c. may be used to move ions across biological membranes, a process known as iontophoresis or ion transfer. This technique was used extensively in the past, but went out of favour because a number of unsubstantiated claims were made for its benefit. However, the process is now becoming more widely used and has the advantage that it is sterile and non-invasive, and therefore causes no tissue damage if used correctly.

Various medications may be moved with iontophoresis and, although some studies have shown this treatment capable of placing drugs into deeply placed tissues (Glass, Stephan and Jacobsen, 1980), the effect is mainly on the subcutaneous tissues to a depth of about 1 cm. If the drug disseminates into the tissue fluids and away from the immediate treatment site, a minor systemic effect may be produced.

Any substance which dissociates easily into ions may be introduced into the body by iontophoresis, but current interest in sports physiotherapy has concentrated on anti-inflammatory and pain relieving drugs (Russo, Lipman and Comstock, 1980; Bertolucci, 1982; Antich and Brewster, 1985). Positive ions must be placed under the anode and negative ions beneath the cathode. To avoid the possibility of burns (especially caustic burns beneath the cathode) the lint pad covering the electrode must extend significantly further than the area of the metal electrode itself. Santiesteban (1990) recommended maintaining a 2:1 ratio of cathode-to-anode electrode surface area to disperse the current further and reduce its density.

The concentration of the drug entering the body is proportional to the current density and the treatment time. The current density is limited to 0.1–0.3 mA/cm² by skin tolerance, and solutions of 1 or 2% have been found to be the most satisfactory concentrations (Low and Reed, 1990).

### Faradic stimulation

Electrical stimulation of innervated muscle using a faradic current (50-100 Hz) has been used extensively in the past, but is now passing out of favour. The main reason for this is probably its overuse in the past, and unproven claims for its effectiveness. It does, however, have its place in the management of the injured athlete. First, it may be used to maintain muscle broadening to prevent adhesions when voluntary contraction is not possible, secondly, for muscle re-education, and thirdly, to assist in maximal muscle contraction.

Faradism has been used extensively in the past in an attempt to strengthen muscle, although Lloyd, De Domenico and Strauss (1986) concluded that this modality was not a satisfactory substitute for voluntary exercise. Its use with damaged muscle is more promising. Electrical stimulation has been shown to reduce atrophy of the quadriceps when given for one hour daily over a 6 week period (Gibson, Smith and Rennie, 1988), and stimulation of chronically weakened quadriceps (Singer, 1986) showed increased muscle force output.

Matching the stimulation frequency to that of the motor unit action potential (eutrophic stimulation) has been used successfully in the rehabilitation of hand injuries to improve both muscle force and endurance (Kidd, Oldham and Stanley, 1989).

### High-voltage stimulation

High-voltage pulsed galvanic stimulation (HVPGS) consists of a twin electrical pulse lasting for only 0.1 ms, with each separate pulse remaining for microseconds only. The frequency varies from 2–100 Hz and very high voltages (2–2.5 A) are used. The current passes easily through the body tissues, and is usually quite comfortable for the patient.

This modality has been used in the treatment of oedema. Reed (1988) demonstrated reduced capillary permeability to plasma proteins following HVPGS in hamsters. Bettany, Fish and Mendel (1990) showed significant reductions in oedema formation following HVPGS to frog limbs, and Griffin et al. (1990) demonstrated clinically significant oedema reduction when treating chronic hand conditions using HVPGS. Stimulation of wound healing has also been described (Ross and Segal, 1981).

Low frequencies (20–50 Hz) will stimulate a muscle pumping action, and fluids may be drawn to, or repelled from, the HVPGS current. Plasma proteins and blood cells have a negative polarity at normal blood pH, and have been shown to clump together when stimulated with a positive current, a situation which is reversed by stimulation with a negative polarity (Williams and Carey, 1959).

The use of electrical stimulation (d.c.) to retard micro-organism growth has been described (Rowley 1972; Rowley, McKenna and Chase, 1974; Barranco, Spadero and Berger, 1974), as has cell migration within a wound (Carey and Lepley, 1955; Harrington, Meyer and Klein, 1974). It has been suggested (Newton, 1987) that in using HVPGS the negative pole may retard bacterial activity, while the positive pole promotes cell migration in the proliferative phase of wound healing. However, the clinical usage of HVPGS in the treatment of sports injuries has yet to be fully investigated.

### Interferential

An interferential current is produced by combining two medium frequency currents which interfere with each other to produce a third current (the resultant) which is of low frequency. The two original currents oscillate, rising and falling at regular intervals. If these currents rise and fall at the same time, they are said to be in phase, but when the rising segment of one coincides with the fall of the other, the currents are out of phase. When waves are in phase, the resultant has an amplitude which is greater than that of the originals. When out of phase, the rising segment of one wave has an equal and opposite amplitude to the falling segment of the other and so the currents cancel each other out (Fig. 7.2). The result of this interference is the production of an alternating current in the tissues with an intensity (amplitude) which rises and falls regularly. This process is described as 'beating', the beat frequency is the difference between the frequencies of the two original currents. In practice, the first current has a fixed frequency of 4000 Hz and the other has a variable frequency of between 4000 and 4250 Hz. The resultant low frequency current has a beat frequency of 0–250 Hz.

*Physiological effects*
The current from each electrode is unable to stimulate nerve or muscle directly. However, the resultant interference current, produced within the body, has a greater amplitude through summation and can produce these effects. Discomfort through stimulation of cutaneous nerves is reduced, while effects are promoted in deeper tissues.

Traditional low frequency stimulation (faradic) will recruit only large fibre motor nerves which have a lower threshold than smaller fibred types. The pattern of discharge with this sort of stimulus is synchronous and unlike a normal muscle contraction. With interferential current, the amplitude of the majority of cycles is too low to reach the threshold stimulus required for a peripheral nerve. As the peak amplitude of the beat frequency is approached, the nerve fibre is depolarized by summation of the various current cycles, resulting in a more natural asynchronous muscle contraction. The optimum frequency for voluntary muscle stimulation is 40–80 Hz (Goats, 1990b).

Pain relief can be brought about both through the pain gate effect and the stimulation of opioid production. Large diameter fibres are stimulated optimally at 100 Hz (Low and Reed, 1990) and this frequency is often applied to acupuncture points. Increased activity in fibres descending from the raphe nucleus is caused by interferential currents of 15 Hz (De Domenico, 1982), and these fibres are thought to be important for descending pain suppression (see pp. 23–27). Stimulation of A delta and C fibres to give enkephalin and endorphin release may be produced with frequencies of 10–25 Hz (Low and Reed, 1990). The stimulation of sympathetic and parasympathetic nerves at frequencies of 0–5 Hz and 10–150 Hz, respectively, has also been described (Savage, 1984). An enhanced parasympathetic activity may increase blood flow through an area, thus assisting healing.

Vasodilation can be achieved with frequencies of 100 Hz, and 10 Hz will activate the muscle pump, the two applied in sequence are effective at reducing oedema (Goats, 1990b). The intracellular concentration of various metabolic substances is affected by interferential therapy. Concentrations of adenosine monophosphate, acetylcholine esterase, alkaline phosphatase and lysosomal enzymes have all been shown to alter (Goats, 1990b).

Acceleration of tissue repair, including that of bone, nerve, tendon and ligament has been reported. Interferential therapy at a frequency of 20 Hz has been used successfully in the treatment of mandibular fracture (Ganne, Speculand and Mayne, 1979). The rate of callus formation resulting from osteotomy of the radius and ulna of the foreleg of sheep was shown to be more rapid following interferential current treatment (Laabs et al. 1982; quoted in Nelson and Currier, 1987).

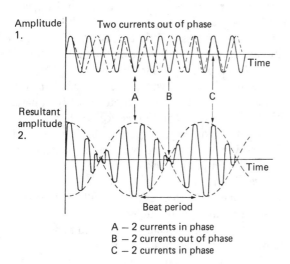

**Figure 7.2** Production of interferential current from two medium frequency currents. From Low and Reed (1990), with permission.

## Transcutaneous electrical nerve stimulation

Transcutaneous electrical nerve stimulation (TENS or TNS) also uses a current passed through surface electrodes. Low frequency (2 Hz) stimulation is applied to acupuncture points, and stimulates high-threshold A delta and C fibres, causing endorphin and enkephalin release. More conventional high frequency (50–100 Hz) currents are used to produce paraesthesia and effect low-threshold A beta fibres to give pain relief through the pain gate mechanism (Low and Reed, 1990).

As the pulse width is increased, the frequency will reduce and the current will be able to affect the body tissues for a longer period. In addition, longer pulse widths will enable smaller diameter afferent fibres to depolarize, a width of 200 ms being required to depolarize C and delta nociceptors fibres. Generally, TENS pulse widths are between 40 and 250 ms.

Output intensity will effect the depth of penetration of the current, and at least 50 mA is required to produce minimal muscle contraction in most subjects, a process thought to be beneficial in TENS stimulation (Santiesteban, 1990). The body will tend to accommodate to any electrical stimulation, and so the TENS impulse must regularly be changed slightly or modulated to prevent this.

Electrode placement is usually in one of three sites, over acupuncture points, over the pain area, or along the dermatome in which the pain is referred. Acupuncture points are often the most tender areas to palpation around the injury site.

Treatment of chronic conditions generally involves TENS of longer duration than the acute injury. Acute conditions are often treated for about 30 minutes, while chronic conditions may require long-term management with the patient operating the TENS unit themselves.

TENS has been used successfully for pain relief in the treatment of sports injuries (Roeser et al., 1976), and to treat torticollis (Ersek, 1977). Both osteoarthritis (Taylor, Hallett and Flaherty, 1981) and intra-articular haemorrhage (Roche et al., 1985) have been shown to respond to TENS treatment, as has postoperative pain (Vander Ark and McGrath, 1975; Cooperman et al., 1977; Solomon, Viernstein and Long, 1980; Smith et, al. 1986).

## Intermittent pneumatic compression

Intermittent pneumatic compression (IPC) devices have been used extensively since the l950s in the treatment of circulatory disorders of the legs (Pflug, 1974). Increasingly, they are used to reduce oedema and increase circulation in sports injuries, particularly to the ankle.

Various units are available. The usual type produces positive pressure and consists of a compression pump linked to a double-walled airtight bag. This is generally cylinder shaped, pliable and opened by a slide fastener. The compression time and pressure may be variable. An extension to this basic system uses a multicompartment garment. Here, a number of overlapping but separate air compartments are used, which are sequentially inflated starting distally and progressing proximally, to produce a 'milking effect'.

### Clinical uses of IPC

IPC is used in the treatment of sports injuries mainly to reduce oedema and improve circulation. When treating oedema, one of the aims is to enhance the transfer of fluid from the interstitial spaces into the vascular and lymphatic compartments (hydrodynamic flow). Formation and absorption of tissue fluid depends on the balance between the various pressures inside and outside the blood capillaries due to blood pressure, osmosis, and interstitial fluid pressure. The imposition of an external pressure on the limb with IPC will alter the fluid pressure balance.

IPC has been shown to be effective in the treatment of oedema of venous and lymphatic origin (Pflug, 1975), and to reduce swelling following both hand surgery (Hazarika, Knight and Frazer-Moodie, 1979) and post-traumatic hand oedema (Griffin et al., 1990).

Several manufacturers combine compression with temperature reduction by filling the IPC pressure garment with chilled water or Freon gas. Alternatively, flaked ice may be placed beneath the garment, or an electrical current may be incorporated within the unit to passively activate the muscle pump at the same time as compression is applied.

Both increases and reductions in circulatory volume have been reported with IPC, depending on the pressure cycle time (Allenby et al., 1973). The effects of IPC on blood flow will depend on a number of factors including haemodynamics, blood vessel structure, machine design and pressure variables. Sayegh (1987) claimed that slow inflation/deflation cycles cause a reduction in blood flow, while faster cycles may cause an increase.

Pflug (1975) argued that IPC exerts its haemodynamic action at the micro-circulatory level by increasing the osmotic attraction of blood and lymph, and later by increasing lymph production. He suggested affects were achieved on lipoprotein transfer through interstitial spaces, and protein and fibrinogen content in peripheral lymph.

# References

Abergel, R.P., Lyons, R.F. and Castel, J.C. (1987) Biostimulation of wound healing by lasers: experimental approaches in animal models and fibroblast cultures. *Journal of Dermatology and Surgical Oncology*, **13**, 127–133

Abramson, D.L., Kahn, A., Tuck, S., Turman, G.A., Rejal, H. and Fleisher, C.J. (1957) Relationship between a range of tissue temperature and local oxygen consumption in the resting forearm. *Laboratory Clinical Medicine*, **59**, 789–793

Allenby, F., Boardman, L., Pflug, J.J. and Calnan, J.S. (1973) Effects of external pneumatic intermittent compression on fibrinolysis in man. *Lancet*, **2**, 1412–14

Antich, T.J. and Brewster, C.E. (1985) Osgood–Schlatter disease: Review of literature and physical therapy management. *Journal of Orthopaedic and Sports Physical Therapy*, **7**, 1

Barbour, L.A., McGuire, D.B. and Kirchhoff, K.T. (1986). Nonanalgesic methods of pain control used by cancer patients. *Oncology Nursing Forum*, **13**, (6) 56–60

Barclay, V., Collier, R.J. and Jones, A. (1983) Treatment of various hand injuries by pulsed electromagnetic energy (Diapulse). *Physiotherapy*, **69**,(6) 186–188

Barcroft, H. and Ebholm, O.G. (1943) The effect of temperature on blood flow and deep temperature in the human forearm. *Journal of Physiology*, **102**, 5–20

Barranco, S.D., Spadero, J.A. and Berger, T.J. (1974) In vitro effect of weak direct current on staphylococcus aureus. *Clinical Orthopaedics and Related Research*, **100**, 250

Bertolucci, L.E. (1982). Introduction of antiinflammatory drugs by iontophoresis. Double blind study. *Journal of Orthopaedic and Sports Physical Therapy*, **4**, 103–108

Bettany, J.A., Fish, D.R. and Mendel, F.C. (1990) Influence of high voltage pulsed direct current on edema formation following impact injury. *Physical Therapy*, **70**, (4) 219–224

Carey, I.C. and Lepley, D. (1955) Effect of continuous direct electric current on healing wounds. *Surgical Forum*, **13**, 33

Cooperman, A.M., Hall, B., Mikalacki, K., Hardy, R. and Sader, E. (1977) Use of transcutaneous electrical stimulation in control of postoperative pain – results of a prospective, randomized, controlled study. *American Journal of Surgery*, **133**, 185–187

CSP (1991) Safety of electrotherapy equipment working group. Guidelines for the safe use of lasers in physiotherapy. *Physiotherapy*, **77**,(3) 169–170

Cyriax, J. (1982) *Textbook of Orthopaedic Medicine*, Vol. 1, 8th edn, Baillière Tindall, London

De Domenico, G. (1982) Pain relief with interferential therapy. *Australian Journal of Physiotherapy*, **28**,(3) 14–18

DeLateur, B.J., Stonebridge, J.B. and Lehmann, J.F. (1978) Fibrous muscular contractures: treatment with a new direct contact microwave applicator operating at 915 MHz. *Archives of Physical Medicine and Rehabilitation*, **59**, 488–490

Docker, M.F. (1987) A review of instrumentation available for therapeutic ultrasound. *Physiotherapy*, **73**,(4) 154–155

Donley, P.B. and Denegar, C. (1990) Pain and mechanisms of pain relief. In *Therapeutic Modalities in Sports Medicine* (ed. W.E. Prentice), Times Mirror/Mosby College Publishing, St Louis, pp. 1–18

Dyson, M. (1987) Mechanisms involved in therapeutic ultrasound. *Physiotherapy*, **73**, 116–120

Dyson, M. (1989) The use of ultrasound in sports physiotherapy In *Sports Injuries (International Perspectives in Physiotherapy*, 4) (ed. V. Grisogno), Churchill Livingstone, Edinburgh, pp. 213–232

Dyson, M. and Brookes, M. (1983) Stimulation of bone repair by ultrasound. In *Proceedings of the Third Meeting of the World Federation of Ultrasound in Medicine and Biology*, (ed. R.A. Lerski and P. Morley), Pergamon, Oxford, pp. 61–66

Dyson, M. and Young, S (1986) Effects of laser therapy on wound contraction and cellularity in mice. *Lasers in Medicine and Science*, **1**, 125–130

Ersek, R.A. (1977a) Transcutaneous electrical neurostimulation – new therapeutic modality for controlling pain. *Clinical Orthopaedics and Related Research*, 314–324

Ersek, R.A. (1977b) Relief of acute musculoskeletal pain using transcutaneous electrical neurostimulation. *Journal of the American College of Emergency Physicians*, **6**, 300

Fenn, J.E. (1969) Effect of pulsed electromagnetic energy (Diapluse) on experimental haematoma. *Journal of the Canadian Medical Association*, **100**, 251–254

Forster, A. and Palastanga, N. (1981) *Clayton's Electrotherapy: Theory and Practice*, Baillière Tindall, London

Fyfe, M.C. and Chahl, L.A. (1984) Mast cell degranulation and increased vascular permeability induced by therapeutic ultrasound in the rat ankle joint. *British Journal of Experimental Pathology*, **65**, 671–676

Ganne, J.M., Speculand, B. and Mayne, L.H. (1979) Interferential therapy to promote union of mandibular fractures. *Australian and N.Z. Journal of Surgery*, **49**, 81

Gersten, J.W., Wakim, K.G., Herrick, J.F. and Krusen, F.H. (1949) The effect of microwave diathermy on the peripheral circulation and on tissue temperature in man. *Archives of Physical Medicine*, **30**, 7–25

Gibson, J.N.A., Smith, K. and Rennie, M.J. (1988) Prevention of disuse muscle atrophy by means of electrical stimulation: maintenance of protein synthesis. *Lancet*, **ii**, 767–769

Glass, J.M., Stephan, R.L. and Jacobsen, S.C. (1980) The quantity and distribution of radiolabeled depamethasone delivered to tissues by iontophoresis. *International Journal of Dermatology*, **19**, 519–522

Glassberg, E., Lask, G.P. and Uitto, J. (1988) Biological effects of low energy laser irradiation. *American Society for Laser Medicine and Surgery Abstracts, Lasers in Surgery and Medicine*, **8**, 186

Goats, G.C. (1989a) Pulsed electromagnetic (short-wave) energy therapy. *British Journal of Sports Medicine*, **23**, (4), 213–216

Goats, G.C. (1989b) Continuous short-wave (radiofrequency) diathermy. *British Journal of Sports Medicine*, **23**, (2) 123–127

Goats, G.C. (1990a) Microwave diathermy. *British Journal of Sports Medicine*, **24**, (4) 212–218

Goats, G.C. (1990b) Interferential current therapy. *British Journal of Sports Medicine*, **24**, (2) 87–92

Golden, J.H., Broadbent, N.R.T., Nancarrow, J.D., and Marshall, T. (1981) The effects of Diapulse on the healing of wounds: a double-blind randomised controlled trial in man. *British Journal of Plastic Surgery*, **14**, 267–70

Goldman, L., Michaelson, S.M., Rockwell, R.J., Sliney, D.H., Tengroth, B.M. and Wolbarsht, M.L. (1989) Optical radiation with particular reference to lasers. In *Nonionising radiation protection*, 2nd edn (ed. M. Suess and D. Benwell-Morison), WHO Regional Publication, European Series, no 25

Gordon, G.A. (1990) The use of low power lasers in sports medicine. *Clinical Sports Medicine*, **2**, 53–61

Griffen, J.E. and Touchstone J.C. (1963) Ultrasonic movement of cortisol into pig tissues. I. Movement into skeletal muscle. *American Journal of Physical Medicine*, **43**, 77

Griffen, J.E., Echternach, J.L., Price, R.E. and Touchstone, J.C. (1967) Patients treated with ultrasound driven hydrocortisone and with ultrasound alone. *Physical Therapy*, **47**, 77–85

Griffin, J.W., Newsome, L.S., Stralka, S.W. and Wright, P.E. (1990) Reduction of chronic posttraumatic hand edema: A comparison of high voltage pulsed current, intermittent pneumatic compression, and placebo treatments. *Physical Therapy*, **70**, (5) 279–286

Halvorson, G.A. (1990) Therapeutic heat and cold for athletic injuries. *Physician and Sportsmedicine*, **18**, (5), 87–94

Harrington, D.B., Meyer, R. and Klein, R.M. (1974) Effects of small amounts of electric current at the cellular level. *Annals of the NY Academy of Science*, **238**, 300

Hashish, I.I. (1986) *The Effects of Ultrasound Therapy on Post-operative Inflammation. Ph.D. Thesis*, University of London

Hashish, I, Harvey, W. and Harris, M. (1986) Antiinflammatory effects of ultrasound therapy: evidence for a major placebo effect. *British Journal of Rheumatology*, **25**, 77–81

Hayne, C.R. (1984) Pulsed high frequency energy – its place in physiotherapy. *Physiotherapy*, **70**,(12) 459–466

Hazarika, E.Z., Knight, M.T.N. and Frazer-Moodie, A. (1979) The effect of intermittent pneumatic compression on the hand after fasciectomy. *The Hand*, **2**,(3) 309–314

Hickman, R.A. and Dyson, M. (1988) The effect of laser therapy on angiogenesis during dermal repair. American society for laser medicine and surgery abstracts. *Lasers in Surgery and Medicine*, **8**, 186

Hocutt, J.E., Jaffe, R., Rylander, C.R. and Bebbe, J.K. (1983) Cryotherapy in ankle sprains. *American Journal of Sports Medicine*, **10**, 316–319

Kanui, T.I. (1987) Thermal alleviation of capsaicin chemogenic pain. *Pain Supplement*, **1–4**, S50

Kidd, G.L., Oldham, J.A. and Stanley, J.K. (1989) A comparison of uniform and eutrophic electrotherapies in a procedure of clinical rehabilitation of some hand movements in arthritics. *Clinical Rehabilitation*, **3**, 27–39

Kitchen, S.S. and Partridge, C.J. (1990) A review of therapeutic ultrasound. *Physiotherapy*, **76**,(10) 593–600

Kitchen, S.S. and Partridge, C.J. (1991) Infra-red therapy *Physiotherapy*, **77**,(4) April

Kleinkort, J.B. and Wood, F. (1975) Phonophoresis with 1% versus 10% hydrocortisone. *Physical Therapy*, **55**, 1320

Kligman, L.H. (1982) Intensification of ultraviolet-induced dermal damage by infra-red radiation. *Archives of Dermatological Research*, **272**, 229–238

Knight, K.L. (1989) Cryotherapy in sports injury management. In *International Perspectives in Physical The-*

*rapy* 4, (ed. V. Grisogono), pp. 163–185

Knight, K.L., Aquino, J., Johannes, S.M. and Urban, C.D. (1980) A reexamination of Lewis' cold induced vasodilation in the finger and the ankle. *Athletic Training*, **15**, 24–27

Knight, K.L., Bryant, K.S. and Halvorsen, J. (1981) Circulatory changes in the forearm in 1, 5, 10 and 15°C water (Abs). *International Journal of Sports Medicine*, **4**, 231

Kowal, MA. (1983) Review of the physiological effects of cryotherapy. *Journal of Orthopaedic and Sports Physical Therapy*, **5**, 66–73

Kramer, F.L., Kurtz, A.B., Rubin, C. and Goldberg, B.B. (1979). Ultrasound appearance of myositis ossificans. *Skeletal Radiology*, **4**, 19–20

Kumazawa, T. Mizumura, K. and Sato, J. (1987) Thermally potentated responses to analgesic substances of visceral nocioceptors. *Pain*, **28**, 255–264

LaBan, M.M. (1962) Collagen tissue: Implications of its response to stress in vitro. *Archives of Physical Medicine and Rehabilitation*, **43**, 461–466

Lehmann, J.F., Guy, A.W., Warren, C.G., DeLateur, B.J., and Stonebridge, J.B. Evaluation of a microwave contact applicator. *Archives of Physical Medicine and Rehabilitation*, **51**, 143–147

Lehmann, J.F. and de Lateur, B.J. (1982) Therapeutic heat. In *Therapeutic Heat and Cold*, 3rd edn (ed. J.F. Lehmann) Williams and Wilkins, Baltimore

Lehmann, J.F., Mascock, A.J., Warren, C.G. and Koblanski, J. N. (1970). Effect of therapeutic temperatures on tendon extensibility. *Archives of Physical Medicine and Rehabilitation*, **51**, 481–487

Lehmann J.F., DeLateur B.J, and Silverman D.R. (1966) Selective heating effects of ultrasound in human beings. *Archives of Physical Medicine and Rehabilitation*, **47**, 331–339

Lewis, T.S. (1930) Observations upon the reactions of the vessels of the human skin to cold. *Heart*, **15**, 177–208

Lewis, T. and Grant, R.T. (1924) Vascular reactions of the skin to injury. *Heart*, **11**, 209–265

Lloyd, T., De Domenico, G. and Strauss, G.R. (1986) A review of the use of electro-motor stimulation in human muscle. *Australian Journal of Physiotherapy*, **32**, 18–30

Low, J. and Reed, A. (1990) *Electrotherapy Explained. Principles and Practice*, Butterworth-Heinemann, Oxford

Lowden, A. (1986) Application of ultrasound to assess stress fractures. *Physiotherapy*, **72**,(3) 160–161

Lyons, R.F., Abergel, R.P., White, R.A., Dwyer, R.M., Castel, J.C. and Uitto, J (1987) Biostimulation of wound healing in-vivo by a helium–neon laser. *Annals of Plastic Surgery*, **18**, 47

McLean, D.A. (1989) The use of cold and superficial heat in the treatment of soft tissue injuries. *British Journal of Sports Medicine*, **23**, (1), 53–54

McMaster, P.D. (1937) Changes in the cutaneous lymphatics of human beings and in the lymph flow under normal and pathological condiditions. *Journal of Experimental Medicine*, **65**, 347

McRee, D. (1980) Soviet and Eastern European research on biological effects of microwave radiation. *Proceedings of the IEEE*, **68**,(1) 84–91

Mense, S. (1978) Effects of temperature on the discharges of muscle spindles and tendon organs. *Pflugers Archives*, **374**, 159–166

Mester, E., Mester, A.F. and Mester, A. (1985) The biomedical effects of laser application. *Lasers in Surgery and Medicine*, **5**, 31–39

Nelson, R.M. and Currier, D.P. (1987) *Clinical Electrotherapy*, Appleton and Lange, Norwalk, Connecticut

Newton, R. (1987) High-voltage pulsed galvanic stimulation: Theoretical bases and clinical applications. In *Clinical Electrotherapy* (ed. R.M. Nelson and D.P. Currier), Appleton and Lange, Norwalk, Connecticut

Parrish, J.A. (1981) New concepts in therapeutic photomedicine: Photochemistry, optical targeting, and the therapeutic window. *Journal of Investigative Dermatology*, **77**, 45–50

Pflug, J.J. (1974) Intermittent compression: a new principle in treatment of wounds? *Lancet*, **2**, 355–356

Pflug, J.J. (1975) Intermittent compression in the management of swollen legs in general practice. *Practitioner*, **215**, 69–76

Proulx, R.P. (1976) Southern California frostbite. *Journal American College Emergency Physicians*, **5**, 618

Reed, B.V. (1988) Effect of high voltage pulsed electrical stimulation on microvascular permeability to plasma proteins: A possible mechanism in minimizing edema. *Physical Therapy*, **68**, 491–495

Roche, P.A., Gijsbers, K., Belch, J.J.F. and Forbes, C.D. (1985) Modification of haemophilia haemorrhage pain by transcutaneous electrical nerve stimulation. *Pain*, **21**, 43–48

Roeser, W., Meeks, L., Venis, R. and Strideland, G. (1976) The use of transcutaneous nerve stimulation for pain control in athletic medicine. A preliminary report. *American Journal of Sports Medicine*, **4**, (5) 210

Ross, C.R. and Segal, D. (1981) High voltage galvanic stimulation – an aid to post-operative healing. *Current Podiatry*, **30**, 19–25

Rowley, B.A.(1972) Electrical current effects on E. coli growth rates. *Proceedings of the Society for Experimental Biology and Medicine*, **139**, 929

Rowley, B.A., McKenna, J.M. and Chase, G.R. (1974) The influence of electrical current on an infecting microorganism in wounds. *Annals of the NY Academy of Science*, **238**, 543

Russo, J., Lipman, A.G. and Comstock, T.J. (1980) Lidocaine anaesthesia: comparison of iontophoresis, injection and swabbing. *American Journal of Hospital Pharmacology*, **37**, 843–847

Saliba, E.N. and Foreman, S.H. (1990) Low power lasers. In *Therapeutic Modalities in Sports Medicine* (ed. W.E. Prentice), Times Mirror/Mosby college publishing, St Louis

Santiesteban, A.J. (1990) Physical agents and musculoskeletal pain In *Orthopaedic and Sports Physical Therapy*, (2nd edn.) (ed. J.A. Gould), St. Louis, pp. 181–193

Savage, B. (1984) *Interferential Therapy*, Faber and Faber, London

Sayegh, A. (1987) Intermittent pneumatic compression: past, present and future. *Clinical Rehabilitation*, **1**, 59–64

Schmidt, K.L., Ott, V.R., Rocher, G. and Schaller, H. (1979) Heat cold and inflammation (a review). *Zeitschrift fur Rheumatologie*, **38**, 391–404

Scowcroft, A.T., Nason, A.H.L. and Hayne, C.R. (1977) Safety with microwave diathermy: preliminary report of the CSP working party. *Physiotherapy*, **63**, 359–361

Sekins, K.M., Lehmann, J.F., Esselman, P., Dundore, D., Emery, A.F. and DeLateur, B.J. (1984) Local muscle blood flow and temperature responses to 915 MHz diathermy as simultaneously measured and numerically predicted. *Archives of Physical Medicine and Rehabilitation*, **65**, 55–75

Shealy, N. and Mauer, D. (1974) Transcutaneous nerve stimulation for control of pain. *Surgical Neurology*, **2**, 45–47

Singer, K.P. (1986) The influence of unilateral electrical muscle stimulation on motor unit activity patterns in atrophic human quadriceps. *Australian Journal of Physiotherapy*, **32**, 31–37

Solomon, R.A., Viernstein, M.C. and Long, D.M. (1980) Reduction of postoperative pain and narcotic use by transcutaneous electrical nerve stimulation. *Surgery*, **87**, 142–146

Smith, C.M., Guralnick, N.S., Gelfund, M.N. and Jeans, M.E. (1986) The effects of transcutaneous nerve stimulation on post-cesarian pain. *Pain*, **27**, 181–194

Taylor, P., Hallett, M. and Flaherty, L. (1981) Treatment of osteoarthritis of the knee with transcutaneous electrical nerve stimulation. *Pain*, **II**, 233–246

Tepperman, P.S. and Devlin, M. (1983) Therapeutic heat and cold. *Postgraduate Medicine*, **73**, 69

Ter Haar, G. (1987) Basic physics of therapeutic ultrasound. *Physiotherapy*, **73**, (3) 110–113

Travell, J. G. and Simons, D.G. (1983) *Myofascial Pain and Dysfunction: the Trigger Point Manual*, Williams and Wilkins, Baltimore

Trelles, M.A. and Mayayo, E. (1987) Bone fracture consolidates faster with low-power laser. *Lasers in Surgery and Medicine*, **7**, 36–45

Vander Ark, G.D. and McGrath, K.A. (1975) Transcutaneous electrical stimulation in treatment of postoperative pain. *American Journal of Surgery*, **130**, 338–340

Walker, J. (1988) Low-level laser therapy for pain management: a review·of the literature and underlying mechanisms. In *Low Level Laser Therapy. A Practical Introduction*, (ed. T. Ohshiro and R.G. Calderhead), John Wiley, Chichester

Warren, C.G., Lehmann, J.F. and Koblanski, J.N. (1971) Elongation of rat tail tendon: effect of load and temperature. *Archives of Physical Medicine and Rehabilitation*, **52**, 465–475

Warren, G.C., Lehmann, J.F. and Koblanski, J.N. (1976) Heat and stretch procedures: an evaluation using rat tail tendon. *Archives of Physical Medicine and Rehabilitation*, **57**,(3) 122–125

Westerhof, W, Siddiqui, A.H., Corman, R.H. and Scholten, A. (1987) Infra-red hyperthermia and psoriasis. *Archives of Dermatological Research*, **279**, 209–210

Williams, R. and Carey, L. (1959) Studies in the production of standard venous thrombosis. *Annals of Surgery*, **149**, 381

Williams, R. (1987) Production and transmission of ultrasound. *Physiotherapy*, **73**, (3) 113–116

Wilson, D.H. (1972) Treatment of soft tissue injuries by pulsed electrical energy. *British Medical Journal*, **2**, 269–270

Wright, V. and Johns, R.J. (1961) Quantitative and qualitative analysis of joint stiffness in normal subjects and in patients with connective tissue disease. *Annals of Rheumatological Disease*, **20**, 26–36

# 8 Manual therapy

The terms massage, mobilization and manipulation encompass the main manual techniques used in sports physiotherapy. Within this book the teachings of Cyriax, Maitland and McKenzie predominate, with reference being made to the work of other specialists where appropriate. The aim here is to give an overview of the various techniques which are available, and, as for modalities, specific techniques are described, if applicable, in the individual sections covering each injury.

## Massage

Various massage procedures are used in sports physiotherapy, and most influence the tissues by stretching or compression, resulting in both reflex and mechanical effects. The classical massage techniques are outlined below (Hollis, 1987).

1  Effleurage — unidirectional stroking movement travelling proximally.
2  Petrissage — soft tissue compression, including kneading, picking up, wringing, rolling and shaking.
3  Frictions — small, deep, circular or transverse movements at specific anatomical sites.
4  Tapotement — percussive actions, including clapping, hacking, beating and tapping.

### Effleurage

Two types of effleurage are used, the first is a deep action, aimed at assisting lymphatic and venous drainage. The second is a superficial stroking movement, designed to produce a sensory reaction, either of relaxation (slow stroking) or of stimulation (fast stroking).

The tissue manipulation starts distally and proceeds proximally in the direction of the heart, for example 'toes to groin' or 'hand to axilla'. The therapist uses his or her hands either one at a time, or together with one supporting the other to create more force. Skin contact is maintained throughout the action, and as they move, the hands change shape to contour the limb. The whole of the hand, and not just the leading edge, should apply the pressure, to avoid sticking or jerking.

The force for the movement should come from overall body motion and not simply from arm strength. The therapist adopts a stance with one foot in front of the other (walk standing) and transfers his or her weight from the rear to the front foot. The arms and hands transmit, rather than create, the force. At the beginning of the action the elbows will be bent, and at the end full reach is achieved by straightening the arms. At this end point a slight overpressure is applied and the movement pauses before being repeated.

Some therapists prefer to maintain skin contact with a light stroking action as the hand is returned to the starting position. The advantage of this technique is that the movement is continuous, but the disadvantage is that sometimes the light pressure can be uncomfortable to a ticklish patient.

### Petrissage

Various petrissage movements are used. In each case the hands maintain contact with the skin and do not glide over the skin surface except when progressing from one area to another.

Kneading is a circular motion carried out by compressing the tissues against underlying structures. This may be performed with the flat of the hand or the pads of the fingers and thumbs, applying pressure on the upward part of the circle. Picking up is performed by compressing, then lifting and squeezing the tissues. The therapist's thumb and thenar eminence work against the medial two or three fingers to compress rather than pinch — a lumbrical rather than pinch grip being used.

In a wringing movement, both hands pick the tissues up, and then work against each other pulling and pushing the tissues before they are released. With rolling, the skin is lifted and rolled between the thumbs and fingers of both hands. The thumbs slide along the skin surface and the fingers flex to pull the skin back towards the thumbs. In so doing, an area of skin is lifted away from the underlying tissues. Shaking is generally only used with larger muscles. In this case the muscle is picked up, with the fingers and thumb only, and shaken transversely.

## Frictions

With frictions, only the therapist's fingers or thumbs are used to give an accurate, deep, soft tissue manipulation. The fingers should be held in a locked but not hyperextended position. With small areas, the first and second fingers are used overlapping as one unit. Larger areas may require the use of all of the fingertips of one hand reinforced by the other hand. The friction may either be circular or transverse.

Circular frictions are normally used to break up thickened oedema, particularly around a joint. Three or four circular actions are used, gradually increasing in depth depending on patient tolerance. Pressure is released and the hand moved to another position before the friction is resumed.

Transverse frictions are a specific manipulation technique pioneered by Cyriax (1941). The transverse friction is performed with the skin of the patient and the therapist's finger acting as a single unit. The action demands great anatomical accuracy and must be of sufficient depth and sweep to affect the desired tissues. Tendons are generally frictioned in a stretched position, while muscles are treated in relaxed inner range. The aim is to produce local hyperaemia, massage analgesia and

a reduction in adherent scar tissue particularly near the musculotendinous (MT) junction where broadening during normal muscle contraction is limited.

## Tapotement

Percussive movements may be used to stimulate, or for evacuation of a hollow cavity, as used in respiratory therapy.

For stimulating tapotement the hands are relaxed, and follow each other in a succession of alternating movements. With clapping, the wrists are flail and the cupped hand strikes the body creating a hollow (rather than slapping) sound. Hacking involves striking the skin with either the ulnar border of the hand (severe) or the back of the tips of the fingers using a pronation/supination movement of the forearm (mild). Beating is performed with the ulnar border of the semi-closed fist and tapping with the fingertips.

## Effects of massage

Effects are achieved through mechanical, physiological, and psychological processes. Compression and squeezing will improve venous and lymphatic drainage, visible when superficial vessels are massaged (Hollis, 1987). Interstitial pressure is increased and fluid absorption aided. Fresh blood will enter the area. The superficial skin response to vigorous massage is an axon reflex. Redness (flare) results through dilatation of skin arterioles and slight swelling (wheal) through increased permeability of the capillary wall, allowing tissue fluid to escape into the surrounding area. Deep stroking and kneading of the calf for a 10 minute period has been shown to increase blood volume for 40 minutes (Bell, 1964), and blood pressure has been shown to reduce following back massage (Barr and Taslitz, 1970). Intradermal dye injections have been used to show lymph flow improvements with massage (McMaster, 1937), and massage has been shown to be significantly better at improving lymph flow when compared with electrical stimulation and passive movements (Ladd, Kottke and Blanchard, 1952).

Short-term pain relief, particularly through friction massage may be brought about by closure of the pain gate and stimulation of endogenous opioids. Tissues are mobilized as they are moved over each other, and adhesions stretched with more forceful actions. Massage has been shown to aid recuperation from muscle fatigue (Balke, Anthony and Wyatt, 1989).

## Mobilization

Passive movements of a joint may be either physiological, having large ranges of movement measured in degrees, or accessory, with small ranges measured in millimetres (see p. 15). Passive physiological movements have traditionally been used in physiotherapy to increase a joint's range of motion. If flexion were limited, the joint would be pressed manually further into flexion by the therapist, or by mobility exercise.

However, when pain and protective spasm limit physiological movement, mobilizing the restricted accessory movements of a joint can provide freedom to the physiological range and reduce pain.

Mobilization as described by Maitland (1986, 1991) is a passive movement which the patient can prevent at any time. He described two types, oscillation and sustained stretch. Mobilization techniques aim to improve joint mobility or reduce pain originating in a joint by using accessory movements of specific grades. If pain is the dominant factor, this is treated first. When stiffness overshadows pain the aim is to increase the patient's range of motion even though some pain or soreness may be produced during and following treatment. Most patients will present with a combination of pain and stiffness, and when there is doubt as to which is the predominant feature, pain is treated first.

When joint movement is limited, the point of limitation falls short of the anatomical range (that which is available to a joint because of its structure). As the joint is mobilized the point of limitation moves closer to the anatomical range. Within a range of movement four grades of mobilization techniques are used as listed below (Maitland, 1986).

1 Grade I — small amplitude movement near the starting position of the range.
2 Grade II — large amplitude movement occupying any free part of the range.
3 Grade III — large amplitude movement moving into stiffness.
4 Grade IV — small amplitude movement at the end of the range.

Represented diagrammatically (Fig. 8.1) grades I and II do not reach the end range, and are used when pain is the predominant feature. It is thought that these grades affect pain by stimulating mechanoreceptors and pain receptors within the joint (Wyke, 1972). Grades III and IV are performed to end range movement and are used when stiffness is the main problem. The ratios between the movements remain the same, as the limitation point (L) moves to the right, and range of movement increases.

## Manipulation

A manipulation is a high velocity thrust of small amplitude, performed at the end range of motion. The thrust may be accompanied by a pop or click from alteration of gaseous pressure within the synovial fluid when the joint surfaces are tractioned (Unsworth, Doverson and Wright, 1971), or a tearing sensation as adhesions are ruptured. The process of replacing a subluxed joint may also be audible.

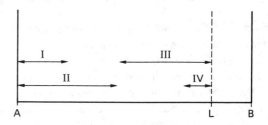

**Figure 8.1** Grades of joint mobilization.
A. Starting point of movement range. B. Anatomical limitation of range. L. Limitation point due to pain or resistance.

Cyriax and Cyriax (1983) claimed that three situations call for manipulation—capsular contraction, joint adhesions, and intra-articular displacement. They described manipulative stretching for capsular contraction as 'a slow steady movement carried out over a number of sessions' a definition more in line with a sustained stretch mobilization within the Maitland definition. Manipulative rupture of adhesions and manipulative reduction is achieved with a high velocity, low amplitude movement. Adhesion rupture of superficial ligaments is usually carried out after deep frictional massage, and reduction is achieved during traction using Cyriax methods.

Maitland (1986) used the term manipulation to describe a technique which is carried out at a speed too rapid for a patient to prevent. He stated that the technique is 'often gentle, always small in range, and rarely forceful'. He argued that manipulation is usually a progression of mobilization and is rarely used at the beginning of a treatment and never applied to a very painful joint or one which is protected by muscle spasm. The manipulation used within the Maitland concept is similar in amplitude and position in the range of motion to a grade IV mobilization, but performed at a greater velocity. This procedure is sometimes known as a grade V technique.

Massage, mobilization and manipulation are widely-used techniques of manual therapy, but the number of controlled trials undertaken to investigate their efficacy is quite low. Very few strictly controlled trials have been carried out on massage. Manipulation has received somewhat closer scrutiny, with most authors investigating the effects of rotatory manipulation on back pain of lumbar origin.

Evans et al. (1978) showed significant reductions in pain scores following three periods of rotational manipulation to the lower back carried out weekly. Spinal flexion increased during the period while manipulation was carried out, but decreased again when manipulation treatment had ceased. Farrell and Twomey (1982) compared mobilization and manipulation of the lumbar spine with microwave diathermy, isometric abdominal exercise and ergonomic instruction. The duration of the symptoms

of back pain was significantly shorter for the subjects treated by manipulation, and they were also symptom-free in a shorter period. Lewith and Turner (1982) used high velocity manipulation of the lumbar spine in 62 patients, and found the mean time for certificated sick leave to be 8.3 days for the manipulation group, compared with 16.3 days for the non-manipulation group. Buerger (1979) compared the effects of rotational manipulation of the lumbar spine with a control group who received soft-tissue massage to the area. The patients in the manipulation group showed improved musculoskeletal function (ability to bend, reach and sit) compared with the controls.

## Mechanical therapy

McKenzie (1981) claimed that the benefits of mobilization and manipulation have been exaggerated, and that this type of treatment provides only episodic relief, making the patient dependent on the therapy. He argued that the patient should be taught to become self-reliant.

McKenzie uses the terms posture, dysfunction and derangement with reference to the spine. Dysfunction represents, in its simplest form, adaptive shortening which hinders function. This may have occurred through previous injury or poor general back care, but in either case, the shortened tissue must be stretched, often giving short-term soreness for long-term gain. Derangement is a disturbance of the normal anatomic relationship within a disc. The purpose of treatment in this condition is to centralize and reduce or eliminate the patient's symptoms. The postural syndrome represents end range strain on otherwise normal tissues, through faulty posture. No pathology necessarily exists, and so no chemical treatment will give permanent relief. Once faulty posture is corrected, tissue strain is removed and pain disappears. In sport, the most common postural problems are loss of lumbar lordosis, coupled with excessive bending for the lower spine and exaggerated head protrusion for the cervical spine. Further details of mechanical therapy are given in Chapters 15, 16 and 17 on the spine.

# Autotherapy

Autotherapy consists of techniques which the patient applies to him or herself. These mostly combine elements of joint mobilization, soft tissue stretching, and traction, and although specific procedures are covered in Part Two, some illustrative examples are given below. Autotherapy mobilization procedures are used when there is painful limitation of joint movement due to capsular contraction. Some traditional joint mobility exercises use muscle force alone and so tend to compress the joint surfaces. Autotherapy techniques, however, emphasize the use of leverage and traction in an attempt to minimize muscle action and distract the joint surfaces. The pain-free joint position at end range is used as the starting point.

Autotherapy, if correctly applied, offers a number of definite advantages over more traditional techniques. First, as the patient is in the best position to assess his own pain, he or she can press a little further into the stiff range, while avoiding too much discomfort. Secondly, because the patient performs the techniques him or herself, the frequency of 'treatment' can be much greater with a 'little and often' programme generally being followed. Thirdly, because basic mechanical principles are used to advantage, the force required to mobilize a joint is far less than with traditional programmes, and so there is considerably less potential for tissue damage or pain following treatment. Finally, but perhaps most importantly, only a small amount of equipment is needed, and the techniques are quick and simple to apply, thus patient compliance is generally very good.

## Passive physiological movements with overpressure

Autotherapy mobilizations may be applied by stabilizing one part of a limb, and moving the other part against it. Either the proximal or distal limb segment may be stabilized, but movement is likely to be easier if the concave surface of a joint is the one being moved. In this situation both roll and glide (see p. 17) occur in the same direction, allowing a greater range of motion for substantially less pain (Hertling and Kessler, 1990).

Wrist mobility may be increased by using leverage with the hand fixed. The hand is stabilized on a table top and the patient moves the forearm to create the flexion/extension action, using the bodyweight as overpressure (Fig. 22.6, p. 314). Other examples include shoulder movements performed by fixing the hand on a high table and squatting down to place overpressure on shoulder elevation. Knee mobility may be increased using the crook sitting position to press into flexion. In most cases the movement occurs in closed chain fashion which is more functional than the open chain actions usually employed in traditional mobilization exercises.

## Traction

The same position used to mobilize the wrist above may be used to impart a traction force. Now, the forearm is fixed on the table top with the wrist crease at the edge of the table. The wrist is grasped with the ipsilateral hand, so that the forefinger and thumb surround the carpal bones. From this position, traction is applied by gently pulling on the wrist. In addition, an antero-posterior mobilization may be performed in traction by pressing towards the floor and then pulling up again.

Traction for the shoulder may be performed by fixing the axilla over the back of a chair. The contralateral hand, or a weight held in the hand, applies the traction force (Fig. 8.2).

## Accessory movements

Another method of applying autotherapy is to use a roll or pad as a fulcrum for the joint, and to perform a distraction mobilization by closing the joint against the roll. The roll is placed behind the flexor aspect of the joint in the case of the elbow and knee or in the axilla for the shoulder. Shoulder adduction or knee/elbow flexion is performed passively using overpressure from the contralateral limb (Fig. 8.3). The mobilization is performed with a rhythmical oscillation at a frequency of about two to four cycles per second.

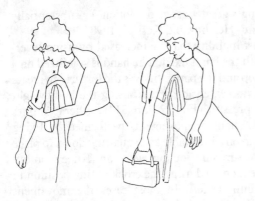

**Figure 8.2**    Inferior gliding of the glenohumeral joint.

## Stretching

Stretching procedures are also used, utilizing both static and PNF techniques. Again, stabilization and control are important factors. The patient must be made aware that the techniques applied differ considerably from normal stretching exercises used in sport, in application if not in design. Although any stretching procedure may be adapted to autotherapy use, a number are particularly important.

Postural deformity which results from tightness of soft tissue structures is a condition which responds well. A reduction in lateral flexion of the neck for example caused by prolonged sitting may be stretched in the sitting position. The patient laterally flexes the neck until tightness is felt. The ipsilateral hand is fixed by holding on to the chair seat, and the contralateral hand reaches over the top of the head to apply the overpressure (Fig. 17.2, p. 265). The contract-relax technique may be used to increase the range of movement. Many of the mechanical therapy techniques work equally well when used as part of an autotherapy programme. The controlling aim now is an increase in movement range, rather than centralization of pain.

### Uses of autotherapy

Autotherapy techniques are useful in any situation in which loss of movement range is the primary problem. Arthrosis, post-immobilization stiffness, and limitation of motion as a result of chronic swelling, are all examples. The stage of pathology with these conditions is clearly important. The general guideline is not to continue autotherapy through increasing pain. If pain is static or reducing the technique may proceed. But if a condition is acute or irritable it is not suitable for autotherapy until pain has been reduced using other therapeutic techniques.

The number of times the procedures are repeated each day is largely dependent on the amount of soreness which occurs in the hours after treatment. Generally, with chronic conditions the procedures are used twice daily to begin with and then increased to once every 2 hours through the working day. Sub-acute conditions require a more cautious approach, with treatment administered two or three times per week.

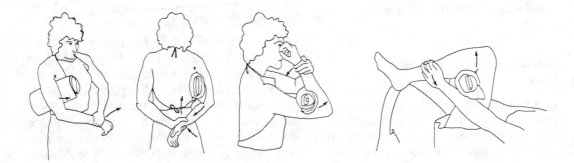

**Figure 8.3**    Various distraction mobilizations using a rolled towel. From Hertling and Kessler (1990), with permission.

Prior to treatment, superficial or deep heating may be used. Superficial heating may be applied by the patient, and may include the use of hot packs and hot-water soaking. This is used mainly for pain relief and to relax contractile structures. Deep heating is used by the therapist in the initial clinic session, to reduce pain and increase tissue pliability.

## Strapping

Strapping or taping is used extensively in the prevention and treatment of sports injuries, and this section seeks only to give a synopsis of the effects of strapping rather than the methods used. Where appropriate, specific strapping techniques are described in Part Two.

### Materials

A great variety of products are available, but these may be divided into strapping, padding, and splinting materials. Strappings may be either inelastic or elastic. The inelastic materials are usually zinc-oxide tapes. They may be air-permeable, and have a strong adhesive. They tear easily but are made from strong fabrics, giving good tensile strength. Elastic strappings can be either adhesive or adherent. Adhesive elastic tapes give some stretch longitudinally and have a strong adhesive backing, which may be hypoallergenic. Rather than tensile strength, they have good compression qualities. Adherent or cohesive tapes are normally impregnated with latex, enabling them to stick to themselves rather than to the patient's skin, and are to a certain extent reusable. Most tapes are water-repellent to some degree, but the latex-coated cohesive tapes may also be water-resistant, enabling the athlete to bathe with them on.

Padding materials are used under the tapes. These may be foam or fibre based. Foams of various thicknesses are used to prevent the tape adhering to the skin and to provide a more even compression. Fibre padding, such as orthopaedic felt or synthetic equivalents are used where thicker packing is required, and have the advantage that they may be cut and shaped.

Splinting or bracing materials vary from thermoplastic materials used to support unstable joints to anatomical braces used after surgery. In addition, a variety of elasticated stockinettes and purpose-designed braces are available for most major joints.

### Uses

Strapping in sport is normally used either to prevent injury or to promote the safe use of an injured body part, and may be used at any stage of healing. Its use in the acute phase of an injury must be treated with caution. Although its protective function is useful, accumulating swelling and the need for regular inspection of the body part usually make the use of compression bandages or inflatable splints more appropriate. The aim of taping in the sub-acute phase of injury is to support the injured structure, by reducing the range of motion of actions which place stress on the damaged tissues. The use of functional taping should allow near-normal movements in ranges other than those which stress the injury.

The great majority of publications describe strapping to the ankle, with particular reference to the lateral ligament, perhaps because this is one of the most commonly injured areas in sport. Reduction in the rate of ankle injuries following strapping application has been shown by a number of authors. In a study of 2562 college basketball players, Garrick and Requa (1973) showed an injury rate for non-strapped ankles of 32.8 sprains per 1000 players. This reduced dramatically to 14.7 per 1000 when a basketweave strapping with heel-lock was used. When the effect of strapping on players who had previous ankle sprains was studied, the injury rate reduced from 27.7 per 1000 to 16.4 per 1000. Ekstrand, Gillquist and Liljedahl (1983) taped half the previously injured or unstable ankles of Swedish football players. After a 6-month period, those taped had no lateral ligament injuries to the ankle, those without taping had suffered nine ligament injuries between them.

Some therapists believe that restricting movement at one joint by the use of taping may throw stress on other joints in the limb, although the evidence for this is inconclusive. Ankle taping has been shown to cause the heel to lift sooner in the stance phase of barefoot walking. In non-taped athletes, heel lift has been shown to occur at 71.5% of the stance phase, but at 67.1% in those athletes who wore ankle taping (Carmines, Nunley and McElhaney, 1988). This altered biomechanics may adversely affect the metatarsophalangeal joints (particularly the first), thereby increasing forefoot stress. This could make turf toe a contraindication to ankle taping. Neither Glick, Gordon and Nishimoto (1976), nor Garrick and Requa (1973) found an increase in knee injuries as a result of ankle taping in their subjects.

## Mechanisms

Two mechanisms of action have been proposed, mechanical stabilization and proprioceptive stimulation (Firer, 1990). During mechanical stabilization, the range of motion at the joint is reduced by the strapping, and the force required to displace the joint is therefore increased. Describing strapping to the normal ankle, Rarick et al. (1962) showed a significant resistance to an inversion and plantarflexion force, but this reduced by 40% after 10 minutes' exercise with the strapping in place. In ankles demonstrating chronic instability, Larsen (1984) showed that there was a significant reduction in both talar tilt and anterior displacement seen by radiographical assessment. In a study of ankle stability while walking on an inclined plane, Laughman et al. (1980) showed a 26.7% reduction in inversion-plantarflexion, and again there was a reduction in effectiveness following exercise.

In most cases, the mechanical effect of taping is a reduction in end-range motion and in abnormal movements of damaged joints, but in each case the effectiveness of taping is substantially reduced following exercise. As Firer (1990) points out, the force required to sprain the lateral ligament is far greater than that needed to passively displace the joint and, given that the strapping reduced its effectiveness following activity, it seems unlikely that the demonstrated effects of strapping are purely mechanical.

The second effect of strapping is one of proprioceptive stimulation through activation of the skin receptors, which in turn facilitate muscle contraction (McLean, 1989; Firer, 1990). Two methods seem to act here, first direct reflex stimulation, and, secondly, a learning process. Activation of a cutaneous reflex response is a familiar occurrence, and is demonstrated in both the abdominal reflex and the flexor withdrawal response. Cutaneous stimulation causes muscle contraction within the region of the stimulant, but with continual stimulation habituation will occur. It is possible that the stimulation of adhesive tape and particularly the drag caused by the tape on the skin with movement will initiate this response. Glick, Gordon and Nishimoto (1976) studied the effect of taping on the peroneus brevis in unstable ankles. This muscle contracted for a longer period at the end of the swing phase and start of the contact phase of the running cycle in the taped joint. The strapping seems to have had a beneficial effect by causing the peroneus to evert the ankle and may therefore have been instrumental in reducing the likelihood of lateral ligament injury.

The other way in which cutaneous stimulation seems to work is by reminding the athlete not to perform an unwanted action. Skin drag is uncomfortable, and can be used to great effect to correct faulty technique through feedback. A good example is the avoidance of repeated flexion of the lumbar spine. Strips of pre-stretched elastic adhesive tape placed either side of the spine will drag on the skin as the athlete flexes, reminding him or her to avoid this action.

This cutaneous stimulation of underlying protective mechanisms may be used in other regions. For example it is unlikely that a mechanical strapping could immobilize the hamstrings sufficiently to prevent tearing while still allowing unhindered function. However, elastic adhesive tape applied (pre-stretched) along the length of the muscle may remind the athlete not to overstretch and could therefore be useful in the sub-acute phase of injury.

## Application

The limb is generally positioned with the injured structure or part to be protected in a shortened position. For example, the lateral ligament of the ankle is strapped with the joint held everted and dorsiflexed. If a general limitation of all movements is required at a joint, the functional mid-range position is chosen.

The contact between the skin and the strapping should be as firm as possible to prevent excessive movement which may lead to skin abrasion. Anything that reduces this skin contact will result in a loss of adhesiveness. Substances which are secreted or excreted from the skin, such as the hydrolipid film, dead epidermal cells, and sweat, will stick to the tape and prevent direct skin contact. Clean and dry skin is therefore a requirement for good adhesion.

Some athletes will have hypersensitivity to components within the strapping and may show severe allergic reactions. Chemical skin reactions are more likely with strong zinc oxide adhesive than with hypoallergenic preparations based on polyacrylate. If this type of adhesive also causes irritation, cohesive strapping is chosen. Mechanical irritation can result if the drag of the strapping exceeds the elastic properties of the skin, or if the strapping starts to slip and 'burn' the skin. Frequent removal and re-application of adhesive tape is also irritating to the skin. Each time the tape is removed some of the protective corneum is stripped. To reduce mechanical irritation, the load taken by the strapping should be spread over a large area by using anchor strips and reins distant to the injured body part.

Small skin defects, such as minor cuts and scratches, should be protected by a sterile dressing or petroleum jelly. Larger wounds will require specific dressings rather than functional taping. If the part is not to be shaved or protected by underwrap, the hairs should be flattened down in their direction of growth and a skin preparation should be applied. Products such as tincture of benzoin or adhesive spray can be useful if strapping fixation is poor. The use of underwrap does allow the strapping to be applied onto non-shaved skin, but the cutaneous stimulation is likely to be less than with direct skin application. This may make underwrap better if mechanical rather than proprioceptive strapping is used.

In many circumstances the strapping is applied along the line of the tissue fibres, and thus knowledge of the underlying anatomy is important.

The aim is to reduce the movement which stresses the injured tissues, but allow a near-normal range of motion in other directions. If the strapping is applied in layers, the overlap between successive pieces is normally half the width of the tape. This ensures that the tape layers do not part during movement of the body (Adams, 1985). If the tape parts, then skin may be trapped between the tape layers, causing skin abrasion. The tape should be applied smoothly and moulded to the anatomical contours of the body part. Creases should be avoided as these will create pressure spots. The athlete must be observed for 2 or 3 minutes after the application of taping to check for possible circulatory complications. The fingernail or toenail of the treated limb should be pressed firmly and released to ensure that colour returns readily, demonstrating that an adequate circulation is reaching the nailbed. However, even with correctly applied strapping, complications may occur later, so the athlete must be told to remove the strapping immediately in the presence of skin discoloration in the fingers or toes, increasing swelling, increasing pain, or numbness/tingling.

When strapping adhered to non-shaven skin is removed, the strapping should be pulled in the direction of the hair growth, thus avoiding excessive epilation (Montag and Asmussen, 1990). Any remaining adhesive should be cleaned from the skin, and if the strapping is not to be reapplied, a moisturising cream should be used to form a protective cover to the treated area.

## References

Adams, I. (1985) *Strapping in Sport. Johnson and Johnson Wound Care*, Baillière Tindall, London

Balke, B., Anthony, J. and Wyatt, F. (1989) The effects of massage treatment on exercise fatigue. *Clinical Sports Medicine*, **1**, 189–196

Barr, J.S. and Taslitz, N. (1970) Influence of back massage on autonomic functions. *Physical Therapy*, **50**, 1679–1691

Bell, A.J. (1964) Massage and the physiotherapist. *Physiotherapy*, **50**, 406–408

Buerger, A.A. (1979) A clinical trial of spinal manipulation. *Pain Federation Proceedings*, **38**

Carmines, D.V., Nunley, J.A. and McElhaney, J.H.

(1988) Effects of ankle taping on the motion and loading pattern of the foot for walking subjects. *Journal of Orthopaedic Research*, **6**, 223–229

Cyriax, J. (1941). *Massage, Manipulation and Local Anaesthesia*, Hamilton, London

Cyriax, J.H. and Cyriax, P.J. (1983) *Illustrated Manual of Orthopaedic Medicine*, Butterworth, London

Ekstrand, J., Gillquist, J. and Liljedahl, S. (1983) Prevention of soccer injuries. *American Journal of Sports Medicine*, **11**, 116–120

Evans, D.P., Burke, M.S., Lloyd, K.N., Roberts, E.E. and Roberts, G.M. (1978) Lumbar spinal manipulation on trial. Part 1– clinical assessment. *Rheumatology and Rehabilitation*, **17**, 46

Farrell, J.P., and Twomey, L.T. (1982) Acute low back pain. Comparison of two conservative treatment approaches. *Medical Journal of Australia*, **1**, 160–164

Firer, P. (1990) Effectiveness of taping for the prevention of ankle ligament sprains. *British Journal of Sports Medicine*, **24**,(1) 47–50

Garrick, J.G. and Requa, R.K. (1973) Role of external support in the prevention of ankle sprains. *Medicine and Science in Sports and Exercise*, **5**, 200–203

Glick, J.M., Gordon, R.B. and Nishimoto, D. (1976) The prevention and treatment of ankle injuries. *American Journal of Sports Medicine*, **4**, 13–14

Gould, J.A. (1990) *Orthopaedic and Sports Physical Therapy*, (2nd edn), C.V. Mosby, St. Louis

Hertling, D. and Kessler, R.M. (1990) *Management of Common Musculoskeletal Disorders*, J.B. Lippincott, Philadelphia

Hollis, M. (1987) *Massage for Therapists*, Blackwell Scientific, Oxford

Ladd, M.P., Kottke, F.J. and Blanchard, R.S. (1952) Studies of the effect of massage on the flow of lymph from the foreleg of the dog. *Archives of Physical Medicine and Rehabilitation*, **33**, (8) 971–973

Larsen, E. (1984) Taping the ankle for chronic instability. *Acta Orthopaedica Scandinavica*, **55**, 551–553

Laughman, R.K., Carr, T.A., Chao, E.Y., Youdas, J.W. and Sim, F. (1980) Three-dimensional kinematics of the taped ankle before and after exercise. *American Journal of Sports Medicine*, **66**, 425–431

Lewith, G.T. and Turner, G.M.T. (1982) Retrospective analysis of the management of acute low back pain. *Practitioner*, **226**, 1614–1618

Maitland, G.D. (1986) *Vertebral Manipulation*, 5th edn., Butterworth, London

Maitland, G.D. (1991) *Peripheral Manipulation*, 3rd edn., Butterworth-Heinemann, Oxford

McKenzie, R.A. (1981) *The Lumbar Spine. Mechanical Diagnosis and Therapy*, Spinal Publications, Lower Hutt, New Zealand

McLean, D.A. (1989) Use of adhesive strapping in sport. *British Journal of Sports Medicine*, **23**, (3) 147–149

McMaster, P.D. (1937) Changes in the cutaneous lymphatics of human beings and in the lymph flow under normal and pathological condidtions. *Journal of Experimental Medicine*, **65**, 347

Montag, H. J. and Asmussen, P.D. (1990) *Taping Seminar*, Beiersdorf medical bibliothek, Hamburg

Rarick, G.L., Bigley, G., Karst, R. and Malina, R.M. (1962) The measurable support of the ankle joint by conventional methods of taping. *Journal of Bone and Joint Surgery*, **44A**, 1183–1190

Unsworth, A., Doverson, D. and Wright, V. (1971) Cracking joints. *Annals of the Rheumatic Diseases*, **30**, 348

Wyke, B. (1972) Articular neurology: a review. *Physiotherapy*, **58**, 94

# Part Two

Part Two

# 9 Biomechanics of the lower limb

Most sporting activities involve movement of the human body over distance. An understanding of the biomechanical factors which affect gait is therefore fundamental to the prevention and management of sports injuries. Abnormal forces placed on the body through alterations in normal running or walking can cause injury. In addition, rehabilitation of lower limb injuries, if it is to be successful, must involve the restoration of correct gait. Failure to do so may impair performance and leave the athlete open to further problems.

## Closed and open chain motion

Motion at a joint is often described anatomically as though it occurred in isolation, yet functionally, isolated joint movements rarely occur. The limbs or trunk may be considered as moveable chains, the links of which are the joints themselves. Movement of one of the joints causes an effect on the other links in the chain, and so other joints respond.

Open chain motion occurs when the proximal bone segment in a limb is fixed but the distal segment remains free. Closed chain motion is the reverse; both the proximal and distal bone segments are fixed, and movement occurs between the two. When we evaluate a joint within a limb in open chain motion, the movement of the bony segment occurs distal to the joint being studied. Movement within a closed chain will occur both proximally and distally to the joint being studied.

Muscle function is also different in open and closed chain motion. Take, as an example, dorsi-flexion of the foot. Open chain dorsiflexion, for example sitting in a chair and pulling the foot upwards, results from concentric action of the anterior tibial muscles. Closed chain dorsiflexion, such as occurs in walking as the body weight moves forward over the foot, involves eccentric action of the calf muscles.

## Joint movements

### Hip joint

The hip joint is the articulation between the head of the femur and the acetabulum. In standing, the femoral head is not completely covered by the acetabulum. This occurs in a position which mimics a quadruped stance, hip flexion to 90°, abduction to 5°, and lateral rotation to 10°. Hip flexion is free, being limited by soft tissue contact, but extension is usually limited to about 30°. Common values for abduction and adduction are 45° each. The total range of rotation is about 90° with medial rotation being more limited than lateral.

In single leg standing, forces of 1.8–3 times body weight have been recorded at the hip, while in the stance phase of walking, forces between 3.3 and 5.5 times body weight have been measured. With running, higher forces would be expected (Palastanga, Field and Soames, 1989).

### Knee joint

The knee joint articulation is between the condyles of the femur and tibia. The posterior surface of the patella and the patellar surface of the femur is usually considered in the knee complex. The neutral position of the knee is full extension. From this position, approximately 140° of flexion is possible in the average subject. In full extension, no transverse plane motion is possible, but as the knee flexes rotation can occur.

During the last 15° of extension, the femur medially rotates on a fixed tibia, or if the tibia is free it will laterally rotate to bring the bones into close pack formation and lock the knee (the screw home mechanism). Flexion progresses as a combination of rolling and gliding movements of the femoral condyles. At the beginning of flexion, rolling occurs alone, and as flexion increases the amount of gliding increases, until at the end of range, gliding is the only movement present.

The medial condyle rolls only for the first 10–15° of flexion, while the lateral condyle continues until 20° flexion, and at the same time the two menisci deform. This range of motion is the amount required during normal gait, and means that the knee is more stable (with no gliding movement) during this functional range. Beyond 20° flexion, the knee becomes looser as the part of the femoral condyles now involved in the articulation is smaller. As a result the knee ligaments relax, and a wider range of rotation is available.

During walking, forces between two and four times bodyweight are taken by the knee. Peak forces correspond to hamstring, quadriceps and gastrocnemius contraction, and occur at heel strike and during propulsion. In jumping, forces may approach 24 times bodyweight (Palastanga, Field and Soames, 1989).

**Ankle joint**

The ankle, or talocrural, joint consists of the trochlea surface of the talus and the distal ends of the tibia and fibula. The talar trochlea is wider anteriorly, and so plantarflexion is more free than dorsiflexion, average values being 30–50° and 20–30° respectively (Palastanga, Field and Soames, 1989). Marked variations occur both between individuals and following injury, and normal foot function can be achieved with as little as 20° of plantarflexion and 10° of dorsiflexion (McPoil and Brocato, 1990). Greater amounts of dorsiflexion are required as running speed or stride length increase.

The ankle is essentially a hinge, externally rotated to 20–25° with the malleoli (Fig. 9.1). In

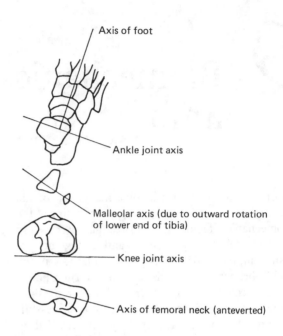

**Figure 9.1** Relationship between the ankle, knee and hip joint axes. From Pallastanga, Field and Soames (1989), with permission.

the neutral position, with the foot perpendicular to the lower leg, there is very little frontal or transverse plane motion. With dorsiflexion, abduction of the foot is possible, and during plantarflexion, adduction can occur. In dorsiflexion the broad anterior part of the talus is forced into the narrower mortice between the tibia and fibula. The interosseous and transverse tibiofibular ligaments are stressed, as the bones part slightly, and the joint moves into close pack position (Table 1.1).

Plantarflexion sees the narrow posterior part of the trochlear surface of the talus moving into the broader tibio-fibular mortice. Recoil of the above ligaments causes the malleoli to approximate and maintain contact with the talus.

**Sub-talar joint**

The sub-talar joint (STJ) lies between the concave undersurface of the talus and the convex posterior portion of the upper surface of the calcaneum. The STJ is in neutral position when the posterior aspect of the heel lies vertical to the supporting surface of the foot, and parallel to the lower one-third of the leg (Subotnick, 1989). An essential feature of the STJ is its ability to perform tri-plane motion. This occurs when movement of one joint is in all three body planes, because the joint axis is oblique.

Pronation of the foot is a tri-plane movement of the calcaneum and foot consisting of calcaneal eversion (frontal plane), abduction (transverse plane) and dorsiflexion (sagittal plane). Supination is an opposing movement of calcaneal inversion, adduction and plantarflexion in the same planes. These are both open chain movements in their pure forms. Functionally, the movements occur in closed chain formation with the foot on the ground. Abduction and adduction, and dorsiflexion and plantarflexion will not therefore occur in their pure form. Instead, the talus takes over these movements with supination consisting of calcaneal inversion with adduction and dorsiflexion of the talus, while pronation combines calcaneal eversion with adduction and plantarflexion of the talus (Fig. 9.2).

The foot has two important functions during the gait cycle. The first is to act as a mobile adaptor, adjusting to alterations in the ground surface and reducing the shock travelling up to the other lower limb joints. Secondly, the foot must efficiently transmit force from the muscles of the lower leg to provide propulsion to push off. For this, the foot must change into a rigid lever. These two diame-trically opposed functions of mobile adaptor and rigid lever are achieved by changing the bony alignment of the foot joints, and 'locking' or 'unlocking' the foot.

### Mid-tarsal joint

The movement of the STJ alters the alignment of the two components of the mid (transverse) tarsal joint (MTJ). These are laterally the calcaneal cuboid joint, and medially the talocalcaneonavicular joint. The mid-tarsal joint has two axes of motion, one oblique and one longitudinal. The longitudinal axis primarily allows inversion and eversion of the forefoot, while the oblique axis permits adduction/abduction and plantarflexion/dorsiflexion. The direction of the motions at the mid-tarsal joint causes the dorsiflexion force created by weight bearing to lock the forefoot against the rearfoot.

The position of the STJ alters the neutral alignment of the mid-tarsal joint axes (Fig. 9.3b). Supination of the STJ causes the axes to become more oblique (Fig. 9.3c), and less motion can take place. The foot is said to be locked, and acts as a rigid lever ideal for propulsion. Pronation of the STJ causes the mid-tarsal joint axes to become more parallel (Fig. 9.3a), and therefore more mo-

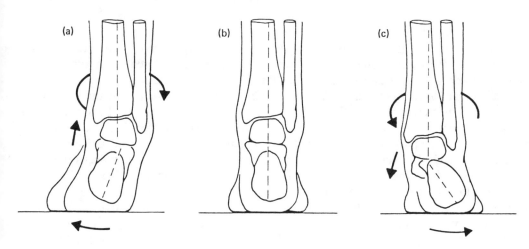

**Figure 9.2** Weightbearing motion of the sub-taloid joint. (a) Supination. (b) neutral position. (c) Pronation. From Gould (1990), with permission.

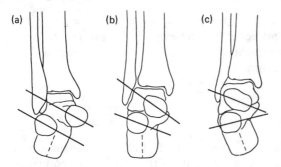

**Figure 9.3** Position of mid-tarsal joint axes. (a) Pronation, axes parallel increasing mobility. (b) Neutral. (c) Supination, axes oblique reducing mobility. From Gould (1990), with permission

bile. Now the foot is unlocked, and acts as a mobile adaptor capable of accommodating to changes in the ground surface.

### First ray complex

The first ray is a functional unit consisting of the 1st metatarsal and the 1st cuneiform. Its axis is at 45° to the sagittal and frontal planes. The joint does have tri-plane motion, but little abduction and adduction occur functionally. Dorsiflexion of the first ray is accompanied by inversion, and plantarflexion is combined with eversion.

### The gait cycle

The gait cycle can be divided conveniently into two phases. The stance phase occurs when the foot is on the floor, supporting the body weight. Closed chain motion occurs in the lower limb, as it decelerates. The swing phase takes place as the foot comes off the ground and open chain motion follows. This time the limb is accelerating.

The foot moves through four positions in three phases during stance. Initially, the heel strikes the ground (contact phase) and as the bodyweight moves forwards, the foot flattens (mid-stance). Forward movement continues and the heel lifts off the ground, finally the toes push off (propulsion) and the leg moves into the swing phase.

At the start of the swing phase the limb is accelerating. In the mid-swing position the speed is constant, and finally the leg decelerates, and is lowered to the ground where heel strike again occurs and the cycle is repeated (Fig. 9.4).

The stance phase in walking is approximately 60% of the total gait cycle, while the swing phase is 40%. Walking at a normal rate of 120 steps/min the total cycle takes 1 s, so stance occurs for 0.6 s while swing takes only 0.4 s. With running, the movements occur more rapidly, and the stance phase occupies less of the total cycle time. A runner with a pace of 6 min/mile has a total cycle time of only 0.6 s. The stance phase would last for 0.2 s, and so events occurring within this phase are performed three times faster.

During the walking gait cycle, overlap of the stance phases of both legs occurs so that for a short period both feet are on the ground at the same time (double leg support). As walking speed increases, the double leg support period reduces. When the stance leg 'toes off' before the swinging leg contacts the ground, double leg support is eliminated and an airborne period is created. Walking has now progressed to running.

### Stance phase

#### Contact

With the contact phase, the lateral aspect of the calcaneum strikes the ground. The ankle joint is close to its neutral (90°) position, and the sub-talar joint is slightly supinated. The hip is flexed to about 30°. The pelvis and the body's centre of gravity are moving laterally over the weight-bearing leg, producing closed chain adduction of the hip.

The STJ starts to pronate, and the mobility of the mid-tarsal joint is increased. The ankle begins to plantarflex to bring the foot flat onto the ground for mid-stance. Pronation causes the tibia to internally rotate, and this in turn unlocks the knee, allowing it to flex to about 20°, in a movement opposite to the screw home effect. The hip begins to extend and internally rotate and this continues until heel raise occurs.

The anterior tibials contract eccentrically to stop the foot slapping at heel strike, and the posterior tibials decelerate pronation. The quadriceps work

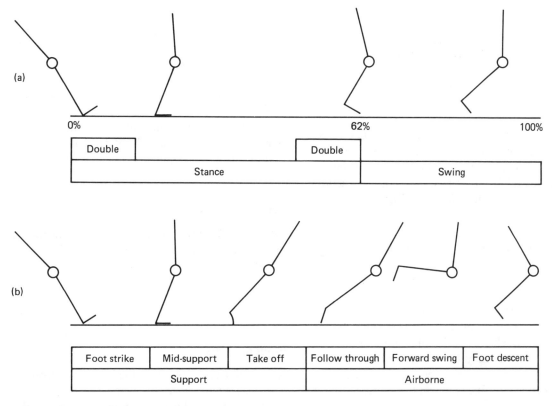

**Figure 9.4** (a) The walk cycle, and (b) the run cycle. Subotnick (1989).

eccentrically to allow the knee to bend, and the hamstrings prevent forward tilting of the pelvis on the hip. Later, the hamstrings work concentrically to extend the hip (closed chain extension). The hamstrings are used in favour of the gluteals here possibly because they have been prestretched. When the knee bends, the hamstrings can no longer produce hip extension, and the gluteals take over.

The hip abductors work eccentrically to control lateral movement over the supporting leg and then concentrically to pull the bodyweight back again in preparation for the next cycle.

### Mid-stance

In mid-stance, the transition of the foot from mobile adaptor to rigid lever occurs. The STJ starts to supinate, reducing mid-tarsal mobility and locking the foot. When hip abduction is completed,

closed chain abduction occurs for the rest of the stance phase.

The action of the calf is eccentric to control dorsiflexion and with it forward motion of the body, and the posterior tibials contract concentrically to supinate the foot.

### Propulsion

The heel rises with the plantarflexion at the ankle and the propulsion phase begins, the knee reaching its point of maximal extension. At toe off, dorsiflexion again occurs at the ankle to prevent toe drag, and the hip begins to flex. The calf now works concentrically to actively plantarflex the ankle, and the peroneus longus and brevis are eccentric to control supination. The peroneus longus also stabilizes the first ray. The quadriceps work eccentrically to control the knee.

## Swing phase

During the swing phase, the maximally supinated STJ moves back to its position of slight supination just before heel strike. The knee continues to flex during the acceleration position of the swing phase, and starts to extend again before heel strike. The hip continues to flex, until it has reached its 30° position to begin the cycle again. The quadriceps continue to contract eccentrically to stop the knee 'snapping' back, and the hip flexors are concentric to accelerate the leg forwards. Phasic muscle action during running is summarized in Fig. 9.5.

## Abnormal biomechanics of the foot

### Excessive pronation/supination

These conditions occur if the normal pronation and supination periods of the gait cycle are extended, or when there is a change in the angulation of the foot segments. Causes may be extrinsic, such as tight muscles or abnormal lower leg rotation, or intrinsic, as occurs with fixed deformities of the STJ and MTJ.

Severe pronation causes foot flattening. The range of motion at the STJ is increased, making the mid-tarsal joint axes more parallel and unlocking the foot. The foot can then remain pronated and mobile after the stance phase, hence the terms 'hypermobile' or 'weak' foot.

With excessive supination the MTJ is locked, the foot is more rigid, and the arch higher (cavus). In time the plantar fascia and intrinsic foot muscles become tight, reducing the capacity of the foot to dissipate shock.

### Rearfoot varus

With this condition, the calcaneus appears inverted when the foot is examined in the neutral position. Left uncompensated (Fig. 9.6) the forefoot would invert and leave the medial side of the foot off the ground. To compensate, the STJ pronates excessively on ground contact. This deformity has been associated with an increased number of lateral ankle sprains (Weil, 1979).

Rearfoot varus is usually a result of developmental abnormality. From the eighth to twelfth fetal week the calcaneum lies at the side of the talus. As the fetus develops the calcaneum rotates to a more plantar position, so that it lies below the talus. However the calcaneus may not be completely perpendicular to the ground until the child is 6 years of age, and in some cases the rotation is never complete. In addition to the subtalar deformity, the condition is also associated with tibial varum.

### Rearfoot valgus

This unusual condition can occur if the calcaneum rotates excessively in its development, or following a Pott's fracture. The posterior surface of the calcaneum will appear everted, and the foot will hyperpronate, giving a severe flatfoot.

### Forefoot varus

In this deformity (Fig. 9.7), the forefoot is inverted in respect to the rearfoot, when the STJ is in a neutral position. To compensate, and bring the forefoot to the ground, the STJ everts and the entire plantar surface of the foot becomes weight-bearing, flattening the medial longitudinal arch. The head of the talus bulges proximally to the tuberosity of navicular. Plantar calluses are apparent over the second and third metatarsal heads, and an associated hallux valgus deformity may be present.

If the STJ is unable to pronate sufficiently, the entire plantar surface of the foot will be unable to touch the ground. Weight bearing will therefore be lateral, with callus formation this time over the fourth and fifth metatarsal heads.

Abnormal pronation continues into the propulsive phases of the gait cycle, and the foot tries to push off without becoming a rigid lever. This instability causes shearing forces between the metatarsal heads giving rise to associated pathologies. Interdigital neuroma, postural fatigue, fasciitis, chondromalacia and shin pain have all been described as resultant to this deformity (McPoil and Brocato, 1990).

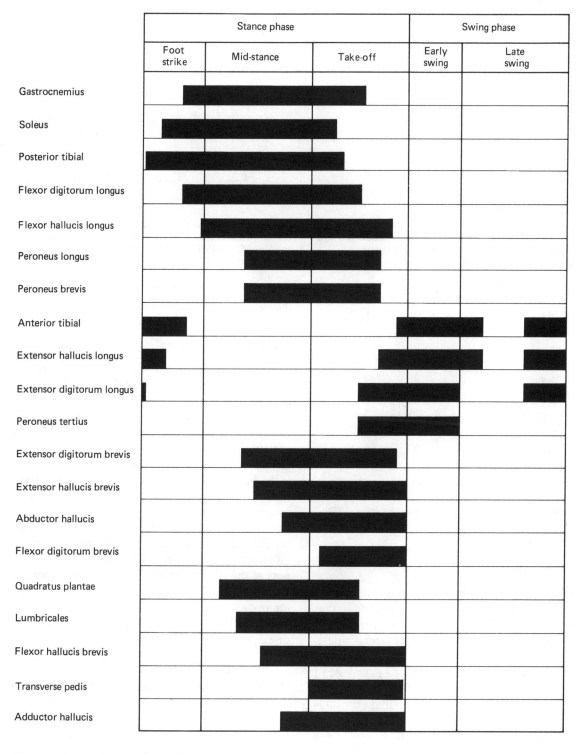

**Figure 9.5**  Phasic muscular activity during normal ambulation. From McGlamry (1987), with permission.

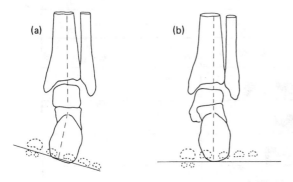

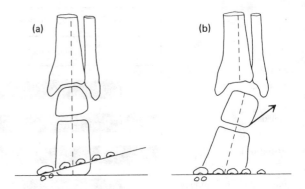

**Figure 9.6** Rearfoot varus (posterior view). (a) Uncompensated — both rearfoot and forefoot are inverted. (b) Compensated — the talus is abducted and plantarflexed to bring the calcaneus to a vertical position. From Gould (1990), with permission.

**Figure 9.8** Forefoot valgus (anterior view). (a) Uncompensated, (b) Compensated — the talus abducts and dorsiflexes (arrow). The calcaneus inverts. From Gould (1990), with permission.

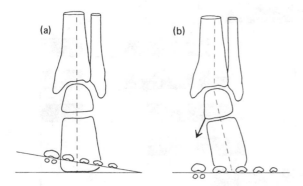

**Figure 9.7** Forefoot varus (anterior view). (a) Uncompensated. (b) Compensated — the talus adducts and plantarflexes (arrow). The calcaneus everts. From Gould (1990), with permission.

### Forefoot valgus

Here, there is an eversion of the forefoot in relation to the rearfoot, a situation exactly opposite to that above (Fig. 9.8). The medial foot structures are in contact with the ground, while the lateral side is suspended. Deformities greater than 6° (McPoil and Brocato, 1990) will require STJ and MTJ compensations. To place the foot flat on the ground, the calcaneus will invert, pulling the talus into an abducted-dorsiflexed position. During the contact phase of gait, the foot will pronate more than normal, and remain pronated and therefore mobile into the propulsive phase. Symptoms as-

sociated with hypermobility of the metatarso-phalangeal and interphalangeal joints occur.

### Plantarflexed first ray

This condition is present when the first metatarsal lies below the level of the other metatarsals in neutral position, causing the forefoot to appear slightly everted relative to the rearfoot. When forefoot eversion continues, a forefoot valgus is present.

Various conditions may give rise to this problem. If the first metatarsal phalangeal (MP) joint is rigid (hallux rigidus, see p. 212) the foot is forced rapidly into supination (a supinatory rock) to allow the lateral side of the foot to bear weight. In so doing, the fifth metatarsal head strikes the ground rapidly (Wernick and Langer, 1985). In addition, weakness of the tibialis anterior will allow the peroneus longus to pull the first ray into plantarflexion unopposed. Deformity occurs over time, and is particularly exaggerated in certain neuromuscular diseases.

### Biomechanical examination and treatment

Examination of the lower limb may reveal problems with the spine, pelvis, hip or knee. The aim of this section, however, is to deal with the examination of the limb in relation to foot problems, assessment procedures for the other body parts are covered in the chapters describing injuries to these areas. Equally, foot examination in isolation is not enough. Forces acting through the kinetic chain, and referral of pain from other structures, make holistic evaluation of lower limb function essential.

Subjective examination and inspection of the lower limb will act as pointers to further assessment, and give clues about any additional tests which may be required.

Objective examination is made both with the athlete weight-bearing and then non-weight-bearing. Positions include standing, sitting, walking and then running. With walking and running, video analysis is often used to slow the motion down and aid in the identification of faults. In each case the examination may be carried out with the athlete in shorts and bare feet, and then while wearing their normal training shoes.

In standing, the alignment of the various body segments is assessed. Starting from the top of the body and working downwards, viewed from behind, the head and shoulder positions are noted, as is the symmetry of the spine. Shoulder and pelvic levels are assessed. Buttock and knee creases are examined for equal level. Knee position gives a clue to the presence of coxa valga/vara and genu vara/valga (Fig. 9.9).

Tibial vara can be measured in a standing position, by comparing the line of the distal third of the leg with a line perpendicular to the supporting surface which passes through the posterior contact point of the calcaneus (Fig. 9.10).

From the front, similar comparisons of shoulder, pelvic, spinal and leg alignments are made. The position of the patella relative to the foot will suggest any tibial torsion. Tibial torsion can be further assessed with the patient in a sitting position with the knee flexed to 90° over the end of the couch. The examiner places his or her thumbs over the patient's malleoli and compares an imaginary line connecting these two points with the knee axis.

In supine lying, active and passive range of movement at the knee and hip are measured and any asymmetry or alteration in normal end feel is noted. Resisted strength is measured and limb girths measured. The distribution of any pain or alteration in sensation is mapped. The appearance of the foot is observed and any skin abnormalities are noted. In prone lying, the range of movement of the foot is measured and compared with normal values.

Calcaneal inversion and eversion are measured by marking a line bisecting the back of the calcaneus and comparing this with a line bisecting the calf and Achilles tendon. The forefoot position is assessed by placing the foot in its neutral position. This is achieved by inverting and everting the foot (with the ankle in neutral), palpating the head of the talus and placing the STJ in its mid-position

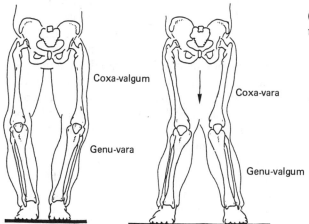

Figure 9.9   Femoral and tibial alignment. From Subotnick (1989), with permission.

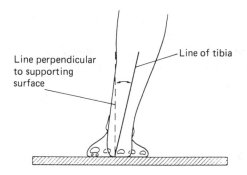

Figure 9.10   Tibia vara measurement made from standing position.

(see below). The neutral position of the foot is detailed in the following list (Subotnick, 1989).

1 Mid position (90°) at the ankle joint.
2 STJ aligned so that the posterior surface of the heel is vertical to the supporting surface and parallel to the lower leg.
3 Maximum pronation of the MTJ, so the line of the metatarsal heads is perpendicular to the line of bisection of the calcaneus, and on the same plane.
4 The first ray is in neutral position, neither plantarflexed nor dorsiflexed, and on the same plane as the other metatarsals.
5 The fifth ray is in mid position as above and on the same plane as the other metatarsals.
6 The second, third and fourth rays are dorsiflexed and the metatarsal heads are approximately at the same level as the other metatarsal heads.
7 The first metatarsal phalangeal joint is dorsiflexed to 20–25° relative to the long axis of the 1st metatarsal, in its neutral position.
8 The lesser metatarsal phalangeal joints are slightly dorsiflexed.

A goniometer is placed over the metatarsal heads, and its line compared with one perpendicular to the line of calcaneal bisection. Alternatively, a forefoot measuring device (FMD) may be used. This has a slit which is placed over the line of calcaneal bisection, the plateaux on the front of the FMD is placed over the plantar surface of the foot in line with the metatarsal heads, and a value for forefoot–rearfoot alignment read from the scale. Using both goniometry and the FMD the most common forefoot–rearfoot relationship is one of varus, with average values being 7.5° (Garbalosa, Donatelli and Wooden, 1989).

Significant biomechanical faults of the foot can be managed by using a functional orthotic device.

## Orthotics

An orthotic device is usually made after taking a plaster impression of the foot in the neutral position. This may be sent to an orthotic laboratory, where a device is fabricated according to the practitioner's prescription and laboratory assessment of the cast.

The orthotic device aims to alter the mechanical functioning of the foot, and so is more than a simple arch support. When worn, the device changes the foot's alignment to make the lower limb function more normally. There are generally few long-term benefits, and much as with a pair of eye glasses, once the orthotic is removed, the body returns to its previous state.

The most common casting technique is the neutral impression cast or slipper cast, and this will be described. Initially, the line of bisection of the calcaneus in marked on the skin in ink, so that the line will bleed into the cast and act as a reference point.

The patient lies supine on a couch with the lower third of the leg over the couch end. The foot should be vertical, and not allowed to fall to one side; a sand bag can be used to support the leg if necessary. Two or more strips of plaster of Paris are used, each about 13 x 75 cm, folded in half. Each splint is folded over by 1 cm on the upper border to strengthen the edge of the cast.

The first strip is placed over the calcaneus and along the medial and lateral border of the foot to the tips of the toes. The under edge is moulded over the sole of the foot. The second strip is again placed in a U fashion, this time starting over the toes and overlapping the first. The two strips are moulded using a wet finger, into the sole of the foot and together into one unit. When the cast is in place, the foot is placed into a neutral position and the cast kept moulded firmly into the foot until set. When tapped, the plaster should sound hollow.

The neutral position of the foot is obtained by firstly finding the STJ mid-position. This is done by palpating the head of the talus as it begins to emerge from behind the navicular. The point where it is just palpable is the mid-position. At this point the skin lines above and below the lateral malleolus should be equal. Taut skin indicates that the foot is supinated, and excessive skin folding shows a pronated foot position. In addition, the concavities above and below the lateral malleolus should appear equal.

The neutral position is maintained while the cast is setting by locking the MTJ. The practitioner dorsiflexes the foot until slight resistance is felt by pushing the sole of the foot up and slightly outwards (abduction). Pressure is over the fourth and fifth digits, while constantly palpating the head of the talus to ensure neutral STJ position is maintained.

When dry, the cast is removed by grasping it behind the calcaneus and removing the heel first, and then sliding the foot out as though the cast were a slipper. This cast can now act as mould for the foot model.

At the orthotic laboratory, the cast is lined with plaster parting agent and then filled with liquid plaster. Once hardened, the original slipper cast is removed, leaving a positive model of the athlete's foot, which is then trimmed and smoothed.

Various substances are used for orthotic fabrication, such as acrylics for rigid devices and plastics for semi-rigid orthotics. These materials are vacuum-formed over the positive cast. Forefoot and rearfoot posts are added and ground down so that the cast will align with the calcaneal bisection line perpendicular to the supporting surface.

Forefoot posts are needed to ensure that the MTJ will lock to provide a rigid lever during the propulsive gait phase. Rearfoot posts ensure proper STJ alignment at heel contact. As the foot rolls forward into mid-stance, the rearfoot post must allow adequate motion. This is achieved either by grinding down the distal medial aspect of the post, or by making this part of the post from a compressible material.

In some cases, a temporary orthotic device is all that is required. This may be to correct a temporary fault occurring as a result of injury, or to assess whether a permanent (and more expensive) orthotic device is justified. In this case, no cast is made, but the practitioner makes a temporary device using his or her own examination results as a reference. More malleable substances, such as cork or non-compressible foam materials, are used this time.

# References

Garbalosa, J.C., Donatelli, R. and Wooden, M.J. (1989). Dysfunction, evaluation and treatment of the foot and ankle. In *Orthopaedic Physical Therapy* (ed. R. Donatelli and M.J. Wooden), Churchill Livingstone, London, pp. 533–553

McGlamry, J.G. (1987) *Fundamentals of Foot Surgery*. Williams and Wilkins, Baltimore

McPoil, T.G. and Brocato, R.S. (1990) The foot and ankle: Biomechanical evaluation and treatment. In *Orthopaedic and Sports Physical Therapy*, 2nd edn. (ed. J.A. Gould), Mosby, St Louis, pp. 293–321

Palastanga, N., Field, D. and Soames, R. (1989) *Anatomy and Human Movement*, Butterworth-Heinemann, Oxford

Subotnick, S.I. (1989) *Sports Medicine of the Lower Extremity*, Churchill Livingstone, London

Weil, L.S. (1979) A biomechanical study of lateral ankle sprains in basketball. *Journal of the American Podiatry Association*, **69**, 687

Wernick, J. and Langer, S. (1985) *A Practical Manual for a Basic Approach to Biomechanics*, Langer Biomechanics Group, Stoke-on-Trent

# 10 The hip

## Screening examination

Hip conditions may refer pain anywhere within the L3 dermatome, over the front of the thigh and down to the knee. Initial observation includes resting position, muscle wasting, leg length and gait. Examination for range of motion may be carried out in a supine position for flexion, abduction and adduction and both rotations. Medial and lateral rotation are best compared between the affected and unaffected hip in a prone position with the knees flexed to 90°. Resisted abduction is better tested in a side-lying position with the affected joint uppermost.

Compression of the joint through the flexed knee and circumduction with compression to 'scour' the femoral head into the acetabulum is an important assessment for arthritic changes. Both the lumbar spine and sacroiliac joints must be examined to eliminate them as a potential cause of pain referral, and straight leg raising should be tested. Cyriax (1982) warned that serious pathology may be present if the sign of the buttock is positive. Here, hip flexion with the knee bent is more painful and more limited than straight leg raising. A non-capsular limitation is present, and pain may make the end feel empty. As straight leg raising is full the sciatica nerve is unimpinged, and the non-capsular limitation precludes the hip joint. Possibilities include an inflammatory disease state, neoplasm and fracture.

In addition to passive mobility checks, two procedures, the Thomas test and the Ober manoeuvre are of importance (see below).

## Muscle injuries

### Quadriceps

The majority of strains involve two-joint muscles, and so the rectus femoris is the most commonly injured of the quadriceps group. The other members of the quadriceps, the vasti, are usually injured by direct blunt trauma, as occurs in a collision with another player or sports implement. The quadriceps contusion so formed is often referred to colloquially as a 'dead leg' or 'charley horse'.

Initially, there is local swelling over the front of the thigh, with some superficial bruising appearing later and tracking down to the knee. The main danger with this injury is the development of myositis ossificans traumatica (MOT, see p. 43). Thigh contusions may be rated as grade one (mild), in which knee flexion beyond 90° is possible, grade two (moderate), in which motion is restricted to 45–90°, or grade three (severe), in which swelling and pain limit movement to less than 45°. This grading system can be an accurate predictor of the likelihood of MOT development. Jackson and Feagin (1973) assessed quadriceps contusions in 65 subjects, and found that none of the subjects with grade one injuries had developed MOT. However, 13 out of 18 subjects who had been graded two or three later went on to develop the condition. The amount of movement present in the initial stages is thus an important indicator of the severity of the lesion and the likely prognosis.

It is important to limit movement in grade one and grade two injuries, and to discourage the use of massage, vigorous stretching or exercise, and ultrasound, as these are contraindicated in the early post-injury stage. The RICE protocol is used to limit tissue damage, and an athlete resuming contact sports should wear padding over the damaged area. Calcification is slow, with fibroblasts beginning to differentiate into osteoblasts about 1 week after injury. Radiographic evidence of bone formation is usually visible after 3 weeks, and by 6–7 weeks after injury, the calcified mass generally stops growing. Total reabsorption may occur with minor lesions, but more major conditions may continue to show remnants of the mass. The mass rarely interferes with muscle contraction, so excision is not normally required (Estwanik and McAlister 1990).

### Rectus femoris

The rectus femoris is frequently injured by a mistimed kicking action. On examination, pain is usually apparent to resisted knee extension and hip flexion. Passive stretch into knee flexion coupled with hip extension and adduction is also painful. Injury is usually to either the upper insertion or the mid-belly. Upper insertion injuries are palpated with the patient half-lying to relax the muscle. The area of injury is usually the musculotendinous junction, approximately four finger widths below the anterior superior iliac spine.

Mid-belly tears are less common and usually occur within the middle third of the thigh. Here, the muscle is subcutaneous and any swelling is immediately apparent. The athlete should flex the hip and knee to 45° against resistance, and as the muscle stands out any abnormality will become apparent.

The rectus femoris can be worked concentrically by flexing the hip against a resistance supplied by a weight bag attached to the knee. Two-joint action of the muscle can be worked with the athlete in a supine position with the injured leg over the couch side, flexed at both the knee and hip. Manual resistance is applied to the foot of the athlete as he or she extends the knee and flexes the hip simultaneously.

Stretching must involve both knee flexion and hip extension and can be carried out in a side-lying position by the athlete him or herself, or by the therapist. Lunging actions are also useful. The athlete takes up a position of half kneeling, with the knee of the injured leg on the floor (Fig. 10.1). From this position, he or she lunges forwards, flexing the unaffected knee and forcing the affected hip into extension. Extra pressure may be applied by pressing the hand over the buttock of the affected side, and by resting the foot of the affected leg on a cushion and so increasing knee flexion.

### The hamstrings

The hamstrings may be injured either at their attachment to the ischial tuberosity or within their mid-bellies and, less commonly, at the knee (see below). The hamstring pull is the classic sprinting injury, with the athlete spectacularly pulling up in mid-flight with obvious pain.

Pain is apparent on straight leg raising and resisted knee flexion. Resisted flexion and tibial rotation will determine whether the biceps femoris or semi-membranosus and semi-tendinosus is affected.

To palpation, the structure of the muscles differentiates them. The semi-tendinosus and long head of the biceps have a combined attachment on the lower medial facet of the ischial tuberosity, and the two muscles travel together for a short distance until they form fusiform muscle bellies. The semi-tendinosus almost instantly forms into a long slender tendon, and travels around the medial condyle of the tibia to attach to the medial surface of the tibia below the gracilis. The biceps has two proximal attachments; the long head, as described,

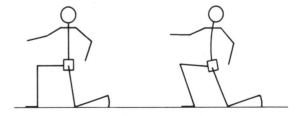

**Figure 10.1** Hip flexor stretch. The athlete half kneels, with the knee of the injured leg on the floor.

and the short head from the lower linea aspera. The muscle swings downwards and laterally across the posterior aspect of the thigh and around the lateral ligament to insert into the head of the fibula. The biceps has a dual innervation and asynchronous stimulation of the two heads has been described as a factor in injury (Burkett, 1975). The semi-membranosus comes from the lateral facet of the ischial tuberosity and travels down and medially, becoming flattened and broader as it does so. The semi-membranosus is deep to both the semi-tendinosus and the biceps, and divides into five components when it reaches the knee (Sutton, 1984). The principal insertion is to the posterior aspect of the medial tibial tubercle.

### Biomechanics and hamstring injury

During the running cycle (p. 154) the hamstrings contract eccentrically to decelerate the leg in late forward swing. This action also helps to stabilize the knee. During the support phase, the hamstrings act concentrically to extend the hip and continue to stabilize the knee by preventing knee extension. During push-off the hamstrings and gastrocnemius, both two-joint muscles, paradoxically extend the knee (see p. 14). This action is necessary because the mechanical efficiency of the quadriceps is reduced at this point (Sutton, 1984).

The ratio of the strength of the hamstrings to that of the quadriceps muscles (HQ ratio) is important. Normally, the quadriceps is the stronger of the two muscle groups, as demonstrated by its greater volume. However, any disturbance to this natural balance may leave the weaker muscle group vulnerable to injury. The optimum value of the HQ ratio varies from 50% to 80% (Kannus, 1989), with average values in the region of 60%. After knee injury, quadriceps wasting may result in the two muscle groups producing the same power, giving an HQ ration of 100% (Burnie and Brodie, 1986a).

Strength measures comparing the quadriceps with the hamstrings are traditionally carried out with an isometric dynamometer. However, the disadvantages of joint angle specificity and lack of movement make isokinetic testing more desirable. During isokinetic testing the speed of movement should match the speed of the sport as closely as possible. The speed must be quoted as the absolute value of the HQ ratio increases as velocity of movement increases (Burnie and Brodie, 1986b). Slow speeds (45°/s) have been shown to give ratios of 60% and high speeds (300°/s) ratios of 80% (Sutton, 1984). Isokinetic testing in the standard sitting position does not allow hip motion, and movement of the limb does not occur in a closed kinetic chain, so testing is not ideal.

## Aetiology of hamstring injury

Tears tend to occur when there is a breakdown in the reciprocal action of the quadriceps and hamstrings, and happen at one of two instances in the running cycle. First, during late forward swing as the hamstrings are decelerating the limb, and the athlete feels the muscle 'stretch', and secondly, during the take off phase as the athlete 'pushes'. Changes in muscle co-ordination as a result of an alteration in the sensitivity of muscle spindles have been cited as a contributory factor in injury. It has been suggested (Sutton, 1984) that when an athlete is fatigued he or she unconsciously increases the sensitivity of the muscle spindles, which respond to stretch with an exaggerated contraction, and this in turn causes injury.

Lack of flexibility may predispose to hamstring injury, and may be assessed with the athlete lying supine with one hip flexed to 90°. Maintaining this position by gripping the leg with the hands, the athlete attempts to straighten the leg using quadriceps power only. Adequate flexibility is indicated by an ability to lock the leg out while maintaining 90° hip flexion. Alterations in the normal 60% strength ratio between the hamstrings and quadriceps and a deficit greater than 10% between the two sets of hamstrings has also been cited as a predisposing factor (Burkett, 1970).

Many hamstring injuries tend to recur, and lack of full rehabilitation may be one cause. After injury, athletes are usually aware of lack of mobility in the hamstrings and are often conscientious about stretching exercises. However, muscle wasting is not so obvious in the hamstrings as it is in the quadriceps, and so many athletes forget to spend time regaining hamstring strength. In addition, the use of eccentric exercises as part of a general leg-conditioning programme may strengthen the series elastic components within the hamstrings, thus making them better equipped to withstand loading at heel strike (Stanton and Purdam, 1989). The inclusion of plyometric training in late stage rehabilitation of hamstring injury is therefore essential.

### Adductor strain

Variously called groin strain and rider's strain, a tear of the adductor muscles gives pain to resisted adduction, and abduction stretch. Damage is usually to the musculotendinous junction about 5 cm from the pubis, or more rarely the teno-osseous junction, giving pain directly over the pubic tubercle (adductor longus) or body of the pubis.

The condition is more common in sports requiring a rapid change of direction, and in which the adductors are used for propulsion. Pain is often experienced with sprinting, lunging, and twisting on the straight leg.

Ultrasound during the acute phase must be used with caution because of the proximity of this area to the genitalia. Isometric contractions may be carried out by gripping a foam pillow between the knees. During the sub-acute phase transverse frictions may be applied with the athlete in a supine position, with the affected leg abducted and the knee flexed and supported on a pillow.

The adductor muscles are often neglected with respect to strengthening and flexibility, particularly in the male athlete. Sagittal plane leg movements are common in weight training, and although frontal plane actions are possible, they are infrequently used.

Treatment for the condition must therefore involve stretching and strengthening the adductors.

Initially, strength exercises such as side-lying (injured limb down) (Fig. 10.2b), hip adduction with a weight bag over the knee (early) or ankle (more advanced) are useful. Later, adduction may be performed using a weight and pulley apparatus. Power training may be carried out by flicking a medicine ball with the foot with an adduction action. Swimming exercises, such as breast stroke, and hip adduction with a paddle secured to the lower leg are also of benefit. Closed kinetic chain actions using running, side stepping, jumping and hopping are included during late stage rehabilitation.

One complication of the disorder is the formation of myositis ossificans traumatica within the adductor origin. This is usually a consequence of inadequate rest during the acute stage of the condition. This condition is often described somewhat inaccurately under the general term 'osteitis pubis'.

### Osteitis pubis

True osteitis pubis is a condition affecting the pubic symphysis rather than the pubis itself, although the two conditions often coalesce. Shearing stress is placed on the pubic symphysis during mid-stance as the non-weight-bearing hip drops, tilting the pelvis. With distance runners, and particularly after pregnancy when the pubic symphysis is still mobile, this repetitive stress may inflame the pubic symphysis, a condition known as pubis stress symphysitis (Rold and Rold, 1986).

In osteitis pubis no instability of the pubic symphysis occurs, but there is tenderness over the area with rarefaction of the pubic bones and widening of the symphysis pubis apparent on X-ray. The athlete often has a waddling gait, and may describe occasional crepitus. Severe cases may progress to sclerosis and eventual narrowing of the symphysial joint space requiring wedge resection (Grace, Shires and Coventry, 1989). Differential diagnosis between the various persistent groin conditions calls for radiographic investigation and, possibly, bone scan.

# Bursitis

### Trochanteric bursitis

Any of the bursae around the hip may become inflamed and cause pain, but the one most likely to cause problems is the trochanteric bursa, which lies between gluteus maximus and the posterolateral surface of the greater trochanter. The condition may arise if flexibility of the ilio-tibial band (ITB) is reduced. Normally, the ITB moves forwards with flexion and backwards with extension of the hip. The bursa may be irritated if the movement of the ITB is limited, a cause of 'snapping hip syndrome' (see below). Biomechanical faults in running which tax the gluteus maximus or alter pelvic tilt in the frontal plane are also a causal factor. Running on a banked surface with one foot lower than the other, and excessive posterolateral heel wear, which increases supination at heel strike, will increase pressure on the bursa via the ITB. Muscle imbalance between the adductors and abductors, especially in an athlete with a wide pelvis, or, in young athletes with a tendency to run with the feet crossing, may also be a contributory factor.

Pain often comes on gradually over the lateral aspect of the hip, in some cases radiating down to the knee. It may be aggravated by crossing the legs, climbing stairs and getting into and out of a car. Pain may be elicited by passively flexing, adducting, and medially rotating the affected hip, and with resisted hip abduction allowing muscle tension to compress the bursa beneath the gluteus maximus. Palpation for tenderness is carried out in a side-lying position, with the injured limb uppermost and slightly flexed. The patient can often feel the injury while lying in this position because of the hip adduction involved. Pressure for palpation should be directed behind, rather than on top of, the trochanter. The Ober manoeuvre is often positive.

Treatment which aims to reduce pain and inflammation must be linked to a removal of the cause, be it training or biomechanically related. Phonophoresis with hydrocortisone gel is often useful as the bursa is fairly superficial. If the ITB is shortened (the Ober manoeuvre will confirm this) stretching is obviously called for.

In patients in whom pain is referred and point tenderness is not present, trochanteric bursitis may be differentiated from arthritis by the absence of a capsular pattern.

### Ischial and psoas bursitis

Less common causes of bursitis around the hip include psoas bursitis, giving pain to passive hip flexion and adduction, but also slight pain on contraction of the psoas in a position of maximal hip flexion. Ischial bursitis (Weavers' bottom) gives pain after prolonged sitting and to palpation of the bursa between the ischial tuberosity and the gluteus maximus. It can be mistaken for a hamstring pull, but is differentiated by the absence of pain to resisted knee flexion. The condition is aggravated by tight hamstrings, speed work and excessive hill running. The condition can also occur in cycling.

## Neural structures and posterior thigh pain

### Discal involvement

As already mentioned, the hip is an L3 structure and so can refer pain down the front of the thigh. However, posterior thigh pain frequently accompanies low back pain and may be a result of nerve entrapment in the absence of accompanying symptoms in the back. Distinguishing between sciatic impingement and hamstring injury is not always straightforward. A history of trauma is important, and if straight leg raising causes pain but resisted knee flexion does not, the spine should be examined further. Weakness on resisted knee flexion could be through intramuscular trauma, pain inhibition, or impaired neural conduction. Laseague's sign will cause pain from sciatic and hamstring stretch, but adding neck flexion will not affect the hamstrings but will stretch the dural covering of the cord and nerve roots. Pain of discal origin will therefore be worse and that of hamstring origin unchanged.

The slump test is helpful, both diagnostically and therapeutically. This test is used to assess tension in the pain-sensitive structures around the vertebral canal or intervertebral foramen. To perform the manoeuvre the patient sits unsupported over the couch side, with the knees flexed to 90° and the posterior thigh in contact with the couch. The patient is then instructed to relax the spine completely and 'slump' forward. The therapist places overpressure onto the patient's shoulders to increase the movement. From this position the patient is asked to flex the neck and then straighten the leg on the affected side (Maitland, 1986). A hamstring tear will give pain as the leg is straightened, but will not be made worse by slumping the spine, providing the pelvis does not tilt.

Kornberg and Lew (1989) assessed athletes with grade I hamstring tears using the slump test. Where the test was positive, they used the slump therapeutically as a stretching exercise, and found that the addition of the slump procedure to standard physiotherapy management of the injuries (which had included stretching exercises) was significantly more effective in returning a player to full function. They argued that abnormal neural tension had produced symptoms which mimicked hamstring injury. In addition, they made the point that increased tension in the neural structures could elevate the resting tone of the hamstrings predisposing them to intrinsic injury.

### Piriformis syndrome

The piriformis muscle attaches from the front of the second to fourth sacral segments, the gluteal surface of the ileum and the sacrotuberous ligament. It then travels through the greater sciatic notch to attach to the upper medial side of the greater trochanter. Its position is such that the sciatic nerve rests directly on the muscle, and in 15% of the population (Calliet, 1983) the muscle is divided into two, with the sciatic nerve passing between the two bellies.

Piriformis syndrome occurs in women more frequently than in men (ratio 6:1). If the muscle is inflamed, shortened, or in spasm it will impinge on the sciatic nerve giving pain in the posterior thigh. Pain is deep and localized and examination of the lumbar spine and sacro-iliac joints is unrevealing. Palpation of the muscle may be carried out with the

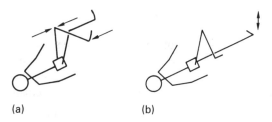

**Figure 10.2**  (a) Gluteal stretch. (b) Adductor strengthening.

patient prone in the frog position (hip flexed and abducted, bringing knee to chest), or rectally. Resisted lateral rotation of the affected hip gives pain, and passive stretch into internal rotation is painful and may be limited.

Management involves pain-relieving modalities and stretching the external rotators of the hip. A simple self-stretch can be taught to the patient. If the right hip is affected, the left hip is flexed to 90° and the right foot is placed on the left knee. The right hip is pushed gently into abduction and external rotation (Fig. 10.2).

### Hamstring syndrome

Puranen and Orava (1988) described athletes with gluteal pain radiating into the posterior thigh who had no history of trauma. Pain occurred most often in the sitting position, and when stretching the hamstrings. Local tenderness was evident to the ischial tuberosity, neurological examination was normal, and extensive physiotherapy, including electrical modalities, stretching and strengthening (no specific details given), failed to remove the symptoms.

At operation, tight fibrotic bands were found from the semi-tendinosus and biceps femoris, with the thickest actually within the bulk of the biceps. These were located close to the sciatic nerve and in some cases actually adhered to it.

Release of the tight bands gave symptomatic relief to 52 of the 59 patients treated. The authors proposed that excessive stretching may have led to hypercompensation within the muscles, particularly in sprinters and hurdlers.

# Hip pain and the young athlete

Pain and limitation of movement in the hip in children should always be treated with caution. The extreme forces placed on the hip by weight bearing, combined with osseous and vascular changes occurring about the joint during adolescence, can lead to a variety of serious orthopaedic conditions.

The blood supply to the femoral head may be compromised in the very young. From birth until the age of 4 years blood reaches the femoral head via the metaphysis. From the age of 8 years, vessels through the ligamentum teres supply the head. Between these two periods the lateral epiphyseal vessels are the only source of blood to the femoral head (Cyriax, 1982). In addition, the upper femoral epiphysis does not fuse with the shaft until about 20 years of age.

Persistent hip or groin pain and/or a limp in young males (4–12 years) may be the result of Perthes' disease, an avascular necrosis (osteochondrosis) of the femoral head. The bony nucleus of the epiphysis becomes necrosed. The upper surface of the femoral head flattens and the epiphyseal line widens, altering the biomechanical alignment of the joint. When the bone is revascularized it hardens again, leaving a permanent deformity. Objective examination often reveals slight limitation of all hip movements with protective spasm. The condition may be precipitated by joint effusion at the hip following trauma, or a non-specific synovitis (Apley and Solomon, 1989).

Trauma, or more usually simply weight bearing, in the young athlete (10–20 years) may result in slipping of the upper femoral epiphysis. Pain is usually felt in the hip or knee. The epiphyseal junction may soften and with weight bearing or trauma may cause the head of the femur to slip on the neck, usually downwards and backwards. If left, the epiphyses will fuse to the femoral neck in the abnormal position. Objective examination often reveals limitation of flexion, abduction and medial rotation with the limb often lying in lateral rotation. Leg shortening of up to 2 cm is common, and radiographs reveal widening and a 'woolly' appearance of the epiphyseal plate. On the X-ray, a line

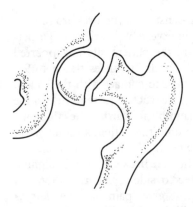

**Figure 10.3** Slipped upper femoral epiphysis. The step deformity is apparent on X-ray.

traced along the superior aspect of the femoral neck will reveal a step deformity (Fig. 10.3). The line remains superior to the head, rather than passing directly through it (Trethowan's sign).

# Capsular tightening

Inflammation within the hip joint leads to the characteristic capsular pattern of marked limitation of flexion and medial rotation with some limitation of abduction. Adduction and lateral rotation are generally full (Cyriax and Cyriax, 1983). Initially, the synovium becomes inflamed, causing synovitis. Pain is due to the chemical stimulation of sensory nerve endings within the synovium and is often dull and throbbing in nature, being worse at night and at rest. If the synovitis does not resolve, swelling causes capsular pain by mechanically stretching nerve endings between the collagen fibres of the capsule. Eventually, secondary capsular fibrosis occurs, leading to capsular tightening and deformity. When pain and inflammation abate, the capsular tightening and associated loss of muscle stretch and strength leave the patient with hip dysfunction.

Capsular tightening will respond to mobilization procedures and later to stretching exercises. Longitudinal mobilizations, followed by full hip traction, may be used, with a belt to prevent the patient from sliding on the couch. Accessory movements should be restored using joint mobilizations at grades I and II where pain is the predominant feature, and grades III and IV where stiffness is the main problem. Hip flexion may be stretched using the Thomas test as an exercise (see p. 172). The patient lies supine with the popliteal area of the knees over the couch end. The unaffected leg is straight and hangs below couch level, while the knee and hip of the affected side are flexed to chest level. Hip extension may be promoted with the modified lunge described above. (Fig. 10.1).

## Hip pointer

The relatively unprotected iliac crest is vulnerable to direct blows from any hard object, be it a hockey ball, boot or another player's head. Contusion is often persistent, especially if the periosteum is affected, and the condition is described as a 'hip pointer'. The pain from the injury is so severe that the trunk is flexed to the affected side. The athlete is often unable to take a breath and may panic.

Following reassurance, the iliac crest is examined and usually reveals dramatic pain but little bruising or swelling. The abdominal muscles are often rigid and the hips pulled into flexion. After 24–48 hours more extensive bruising appears and local tenderness may last for several weeks. A raised area may persist for many months. Ice may be used initially to relieve pain, and the area may be padded when the athlete resumes sport.

## Snapping hip syndrome

This is a condition in which an audible click or snap is heard when the hip is flexed and extended in certain positions. The condition is usually painless but of obvious concern to the athlete, as in some cases the sound is loud enough for others to hear. On examination, the snap may be reproduced by flexing and extending the hip in adduction,

revealing the cause to be the ilio-tibial tract moving over the greater trochanter.

The condition may be a result of inflexibility of the ITB and gluteal muscles as often the Ober manoeuvre is positive. If the condition is painful, treatment designed to reduce local inflammation may be required. In painless instances stretching of the ITB and hip adductors is required. One method is for the athlete to stand sideways on to a wall with the affected leg innermost and crossed over the unaffected limb. He or she then side flexes away from the pain and adducts the hips simultaneously.

## References

Apley, A.G., and Solomon, L. (1989) *Concise System of Orthopaedics and Fractures*, Butterworth–Heinemann, Oxford

Burkett, L.N., (1975) Investigation into hamstring strains: the case of the hybrid muscle. *American Journal of Sports Medicine*, **3**, 228–231

Burkett L.N. (1970) Causative factors in hamstring strains. *Medicine and Science in Sports and Exercise*, **2**, 39–42

Burnie, J. and Brodie, D.A. (1986a) Isokinetic measurement in preadolescent males. *International Journal of Sports Medine*, **7**, 205–209

Burnie, J. and Brodie, D.A. (1986b) Isokinetics in the assessment of rehabilitation: a case report. *Clinical Biomechanics*, **1**, 140–146

Cailliet, R. (1983) *Soft Tissue Pain and Disability*, F.A. Davis, Philadelphia

Cyriax, J.H. and Cyriax, P.J. (1983) *Illustrated Manual of Orthopaedic Medicine*, Butterworth, London

Cyriax, J. (1982) *Textbook of Orthopaedic Medicine*, Vol. 1, 8th edn, Baillière Tindall, London

Estwanik, J.J. and McAlister, J.A. (1990) Contusions and the formation of myositis ossificans. *Physician and Sportsmedicine*, **18**,(4) 52–64

Grace, J.N., Shives, T.C. and Coventry, M.B. (1989) Wedge resection of the symphysis pubis for the treatment of osteitis pubis. *Journal of Bone and Joint Surgery*, **71A**, 358–364

Jackson, D.W. and Feagin, J.A. (1973) Quadriceps contusions in young athletes. Relation of severity of injury to treatment and prognosis. *Journal of Bone and Joint Surgery (America)*, **55**,(1) 95–105

Kannus, P. (1989) Hamstring/quadriceps strength ratios in knees with medial collateral ligament insufficiency. *Journal of Sports Medicine and Physical Fitness*, **29**,(2)

194–198

Kornberg, C. and Lew, P. (1989) The effect of stretching neural structures on grade one hamstring injuries. *Journal of Orthopaedic and Sports Physical Therapy*, June, 481–487

Maitland, G.D. (1986) *Vertebral Manipulation*, 5th edn, Butterworth, London

Puranen, J. and Orava, S. (1988) The hamstring syndrome. A new diagnosis of gluteal sciatic pain. *American Journal of Sports Medicine*, **16**, (5) 517–521

Rold, J.F. and Rold, B.A. (1986) Pubis stress symphysitis in a female distance runner. *Physician and Sportsmedicine*, June, **14**, 61–65

Stanton, P. and Purdam, C. (1989) Hamstring injuries in sprinting – the role of eccentric exercise. *Journal of Orthopaedic and Sports Physical Therapy*, **10**, (9) 343–349

Sutton, G. (1984) Hamstrung by hamstring strains: a review of the literature. *Journal of Orthopaedic and Sports Physical Therapy*, **5**, (4) 184–195

# 11 The knee

## Biomechanics of the extensor mechanism

The patella is the largest sesamoid bone in the body. It is attached above to the quadriceps tendon, below to the patellar tendon, and medially and laterally to the patellar retinacula. The breadth of the pelvis and close proximity of the knee creates a valgus angulation to the femur. Coupled with this, the direction of pull of the quadriceps is along the shaft of the femur and that of the patellar tendon is almost vertical (Fig. 11.1). The difference between the two lines of pull is known as the Q angle and is an important determinant of knee health. Normal values for the Q angle are in the region of 15–20°,

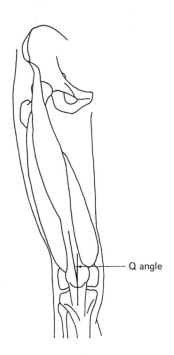

Q angle

**Figure 11.1** The Q angle.

and knees with an angle greater or less than this can be considered malaligned.

As the knee flexes and extends, the patella should travel in line with the long axis of the femur. However, the horizontal force vector created as a result of the Q angle tends to pull the patella laterally, a movement which is resisted by the horizontal pull of the lower fibres of vastus medialis. These lower fibres can be considered as a functionally separate muscle, the vastus medialis oblique (VMO) (Speakman and Weisberg, 1977). The quadriceps as a whole have been shown to undergo reflex inhibition as the knee swells (de Andrade et al., 1965; Stokes and Young, 1984). However, the VMO can be inhibited by as little as 10 ml effusion while the vastus lateralis and rectus femoris require as much as 60 ml (Arno, 1990). Minimal effusion occurs frequently with minor trauma and may go unnoticed by the athlete. However, this will be enough to weaken the VMO and alter the biomechanics of the patella.

In full extension the patella does not contact the femur, but lies in a lateral position. As flexion progresses, the patella should move medially. If it moves laterally it will butt against the prominent lateral femoral condyle, and the lateral edge of the patellar groove of the femur. As flexion progresses different areas of the patella's undersurface are compressed on to the femur. At 20° flexion the inferior pole of the patella is compressed and by 45° the middle section is affected. At 90° flexion, compression has moved to the superior aspect of the knee. In a full squatting position, with the knee reaching 135° flexion, only the medial and lateral areas of the patella are compressed (Fig. 11.2). Compression tests of the patella to examine its posterior surface must therefore be performed with the knee flexed to different angles.

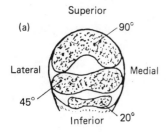

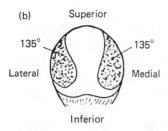

**Figure 11.2**   Contact areas of the patella at different angles of flexion.

Patello-femoral loads may be as high as three or four times body weight as the knee flexes in walking, and nine times body weight when descending stairs (Cox, 1990). While the posterior surface of the patella is compressed, the anterior aspect receives a tensile force when seen in the sagittal plane (Fig. 11.3b). The effect of the Q angle is to create both horizontal and vertical force vectors which tend to compress the lateral aspect of the patella but submit the medial aspect to tensile stress (Fig. 11.3a). Clearly, alterations in the Q angle will change the pattern of stress experienced by the patellar cartilage.

Knee angles in the stance phase of walking or running will be altered by foot and hip mechanics through the closed kinetic chain. Excessive foot pronation and hip internal rotation and adduction (causing a 'knock knee' posture) have been linked to anterior knee pain (see below).

# Anterior knee pain

## Pathology

Anterior knee pain is variously called chondromalacia patellae and patella malalignment syndrome. It

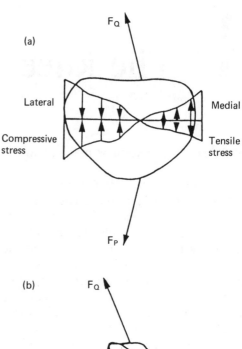

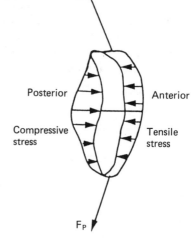

**Figure 11.3**   Patellar stress. (a) The Q angle causes the lateral edge of the patellar cartilage to be compressed, while the medial aspect is subjected to tensile stress. (b) The posterior surface of the patella is compressed. $F_Q$, quadriceps pull; $F_P$, patellar tendon. From Cox (1990), with permission.

is a condition affecting the posterior surface of the patella sometimes attributed to cartilage damage and on occasion incorrectly seen as a direct precursor to osteoarthritis. Since hyaline cartilage is aneural, changes in the patellar cartilage surface itself would not result in anterior knee pain. Furthermore, at arthroscopy cartilage changes are often seen in patients who have no anterior knee pain. If cartilage degeneration does occur with this condition, it is to the ground substance and collagen at deep levels on the lateral edge of the patella. This results in a blistering of the cartilage as it separates from the underlying bone, but the cartilage surface itself is still smooth (Gruber, 1979). In osteoarthritis (see pp. 39–40) the initial changes occur to the cartilage surface of the odd facet (medial) and are followed by fibrillation.

The retinacula supporting the patella may be a major source of pain (Fulkerson, 1982), as may be the subchondral bone of the odd facet (Hertling and Kessler, 1990). As we have seen, the odd facet is only occasionally compressed in a full squatting position, and so its sub-chondral bone is less dense and weaker. Lateral movement of the loaded patella could pull the odd facet into rapid contact with the patellar surface of the femur, causing pain.

The complex mechanical relations of the patella make biomechanical assessment of the lower limb a necessity in the treatment of anterior knee pain, and static and dynamic posture should be analysed.

## Muscle strength imbalances

Flexibility and strength of the knee tissues and muscles will often reveal asymmetry. The relationship between the hamstrings and quadriceps (HQ ratio) is particularly important and may require isokinetic assessment of peak torque values. In cases where genu recurvatum is present, strengthening the hamstrings may be necessary in attempting to correct the knee hyperextension. In addition to knee musculature, hip strength is particularly important. The hip abductors and lateral rotators warrant special attention, as weakness here has been associated with this condition (Beckman, Craig and Lehman, 1989). It is common for young athletes to allow the knee to adduct and medially rotate when descending stairs. This may be due to weakness in the hip abductors, particularly the gluteus medius, causing the ilio tibial band to overwork and tighten, pulling on the lateral retinaculum. Manual muscle testing of the gluteus medius in a side-lying position will often reveal weakness in the affected leg, and tightness in the ITB should be evaluated.

Weakness in the VMO will allow the patella to drift laterally as the quadriceps contract. Strengthening has traditionally been achieved by the use of short-range quadriceps exercises and straight leg raising exercises. However, these are both open chain movements and, as the knee is in closed chain motion during the stance phase of gait, closed chain actions are more likely to carry over into functional activities.

Closed chain VMO strengthening may be carried out by performing limited range squats or lunges moving the knee from 20–30° flexion to full extension. Step downs from a single stair are useful as they can retrain correct knee motion. The patient should be instructed to keep the knee over the centre of the foot (avoiding adduction and medial rotation) throughout the movement.

## Flexibility

Flexibility should be evaluated against accepted norms and against the contralateral limb. Normal values of flexibility are highly subjective, but comparisons with other athletes of a similar stature who are performing similar sports will give some guidance.

Tightness in the quadriceps will increase compression of the patello-femoral joint, while tight hamstrings (which tend to flex the knee passively) will place a demand on the quadriceps during knee extension. Quadriceps flexibility may be assessed by passively flexing the knee in a prone-lying position and flexing the knee and extending the hip in a side-lying position to test the rectus femoris. In the same position the ITB may be evaluated using the Ober manoeuvre. This is performed by adopting a side-lying position with the affected limb uppermost. The unaffected limb is flexed and the knee held by the patient to stabilize the pelvis. The therapist flexes the knee of the affected limb and then passively abducts and then extends the hip, to pull the knee behind the plane of the body. While maintaining knee and hip extension, the knee is passively pushed into adduction. Full movement occurs when the hip adducts far enough to allow the knee to touch the couch. Minimal ITB tightness is said to be present if the knee is unable to touch the couch but will adduct into the horizontal position. If the horizontal position cannot be reached, the tightness is moderate (Gose and Schweizer, 1989).

Hamstring flexibility may be assessed by actively extending the knee with the hip flexed to 90° in the sitting or lying position (see p. 69). Failure to extend the knee fully while maintaining 90° hip flexion constitutes inflexibility. The hip flexors are tested using the Thomas test. The patient lies supine with the popliteal area of the knee over the couch end. The unaffected limb is flexed and the knee gripped and pulled in towards the chest (Fig. 11.4a). Normal stretch of the hip flexors will allow the lower leg to remain in contact with the couch as the flexed limb contacts the patient's chest, but tightness is indicated if the lower leg starts to lift (Fig. 11.4b). Differentiation between the ilio-psoas and rectus femoris can be made by assessing the difference made to the movement by further flexing the knee of the lower leg. If the rectus is tight, the knee will not flex fully

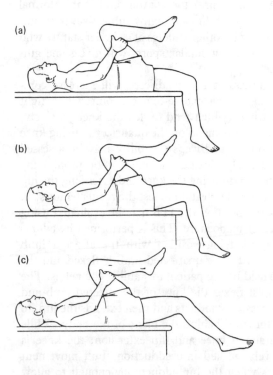

(a)

(b)

(c)

**Figure 11.4** The Thomas test. (a) Normal stretch. The lower leg remains on the couch as the upper hip is flexed to the chest. (b) Hip flexor tightness causes the lower leg to lift off the couch. (c) Rectus femoris tightness prevents the lower knee from flexing fully. From Saunders (1989), with permission.

(Fig. 11.4c). Satisfactory scores of knee flexion to 80° have been quoted for industrial workers, and if the lower hip flexes 10° or more off the table, and/or the lower knee does not flex to at least 70°, tightness is present (Saunders, 1989). If the lower leg drifts into abduction the ITB may be tight, and should be tested by pressing the leg into adduction. This position mimics the Ober manoeuvre.

A tight gastrocnemius will affect the sub-talar joint and can increase pronation, a condition which in turn will affect the patello-femoral joint. The gastrocnemius is assessed using a forward lunging position against the wall whilst maintaining full knee extension.

## Foot biomechanics

During normal running gait (pp. 152–154) the sub-taloid joint (STJ) is slightly supinated at heel strike. As the foot moves into ground contact, the joint pronates, pulling the lower limb into internal rotation and unlocking the knee. As the gait cycle progresses, the STJ moves into supination, externally rotating the leg as the knee extends (locks) to push the body forward. This biomechanical action combines mobility and shock absorbtion (STJ pronation and knee flexion) with rigidity and power transmission (STJ supination and knee extension), and shows the intricate link between foot and knee function.

If STJ pronation is excessive or prolonged, external rotation of the lower limb will be delayed. At the beginning of the stance phase, STJ pronation should have finished. But, if it continues, the tibia will remain externally rotated and prevent the knee from locking. The leg must compensate to prevent excessive strain on its structures, and so the femur rotates instead of the tibia, and the knee is able to lock once more. As the femur rotates internally in this manner, the patella is forced to track laterally.

In certain circumstances the patella can cope with this extra stress, but if additional malalignment factors exist, they are compounded. Anteversion of the femur (internal rotation), VMO weakness, and tightness of the lateral retinaculum may all increase the lateral patellar tracking causing symptoms (Tiberio, 1987). For anterior knee pain to be treated effectively therefore, a biomechanical

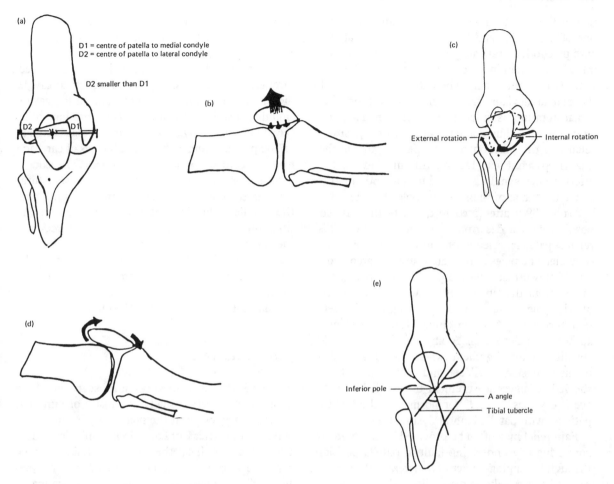

**Figure 11.5**  Assessment of patella position. (a) Patellar glide. (b) Patellar tilt. (c) Patellar rotation. (d) Anterior–posterior position. (e) The A angle. From Arno (1990), with permission.

assessment of the lower limb is mandatory. If hyperpronation is present, it must be corrected. This will involve assessment of sports footwear, patient education and orthotic prescription.

## Patella position

Quantifying the position of the patella is important because, as described above, excessive pressure on the odd facet may result if the patella position is at fault. McConnell (1986) described four different patellar position faults which could be assessed

with the patient in the supine position with the quadriceps relaxed. By using the patellar poles as landmarks and comparing their position with the planes of the femur any malalignment becomes evident. In addition, accessory patellar movements can be assessed with particular emphasis on medial and lateral gliding.

Patellar glide occurs when the patella moves from a neutral position. The distance from the centre of the patella to the medial and lateral femoral condyles is assessed (Fig. 11.5a). Tightness in the lateral retinaculum, a frequent occurrence in anterior knee pain sufferers, will cause lateralization of the patella. Patellar tilt evaluates the position of the medial and lateral facets of the patella, with patello-femoral pain patients frequently showing a more prominent medial facet (Fig. 11.5b). Patellar rotation occurs when the inferior pole of the patella deviates from a neutral position. Internal rotation is a change to the medial side (Fig. 11.5c). The anterior–posterior position relates to the position of the inferior pole as the quadriceps contract. During this movement, the inferior pole should remain inferior and not tilt above the plane of the superior pole (Fig. 11.5d).

Arno (1990) attempted to quantify the patellar position with a description of the A angle. This relates patellar orientation to that of the tibial tubercle. The poles of the patella are palpated and a line is drawn bisecting the patella. Another line is drawn from the tibial tubercle to the apex of the inferior pole of the patella and the angle of intersection forms the A angle (Fig. 11.5e). The same author argued that an A angle greater than 35° constituted malalignment when the Q angle remained constant. DiVeta and Vogelbach (1992) showed A angle measurement to be reliable, with average values of 12.3° for normals and 23.2° for patients with patellofemoral dysfunction.

Pain relief may often be provided by temporarily correcting any underlying fault in patella position through strapping. Excessive lateral tilt is corrected by passively medially tilting the patella and applying adhesive taping from the midpoint of the patella to the medial aspect of the knee. Decreased medial glide is corrected with a similar taping method, but this time extending from the lateral border of the patella to the medial knee. If the inferior pole of the patella lies posterior to the superior pole, taping is applied to the upper half of the patella to compress it. Patella rotations are corrected by placing the patella in a neutral position.

### Surgery

Before surgery is considered, conservative management must be attempted. Indeed, Insall (1979) stated that surgery was only indicated when continuous pain limited normal activities for at least six months and the condition had not responded to conservative management. The complex aetiology of the condition has led to a number of different approaches.

Release of tight lateral retinaculum is performed through a small incision or arthroscopy to divide the retinaculum from the lower fibres of the vastus lateralis. Patellar debridement/shaving has been carried out to remove degenerate articular cartilage on the patella undersurface. Small areas of cartilage may be removed *en bloc* or larger areas shaved.

Re-alignment procedures involve structural transfer to reduce or alter compression forces on the patella. The Maquet operation elevates the tibial tubercle to reduce patella reaction forces and the Hauser manoeuvre uses distal and medial transfer to reduce the valgus vector acting on the patello-femoral joint. Realignment of the attachment of the vastus medialis aims to increase the mechanical advantage of the VMO.

## Patellar fracture

Patellar fractures in sport occur most frequently in adolescent athletes, usually as a result of jumping. Fracture may occur at the pole of the patella, or as transverse, vertical, or comminuted injuries. Stress fracture at the distal third of the patella has been reported after sprinting (Jerosch, Castro and Jantea, 1989). Conservative treatment, consisting of immobilizing the limb in a cast for two to three weeks, is sufficient in 50–60% of cases (Exler, 1991). Surgical treatment involves internal fixation of the patellar fragments, and hemipatellectomy or total patellectomy in the case of comminuted injuries, combined with immobilization in a cast.

Following immobilization, mobility exercises and quadriceps strengthening are started. Strengthening begins with straight leg raising. An extension lag is common in these patients. The leg is locked from a long sitting position and, as it is raised, the tibia falls 2–3 cm as the patient is unable to maintain locking. Re-education of the knee-locking mechanism may be achieved in a side-lying (gravity eliminated) position. This is followed by knee bracing with a rolled towel under the knee, the patient being instructed to 'push down' on the towel with the back of the knee and at the same time to lift the heel from the couch surface. Short range movements over a knee block using a weight bag is the next progression. When 60–90° knee flexion is achieved, light weight training on a universal machine with a relaxation stop, or isokinetic training, is used before closed chain activities.

## Patellar dislocation

Patellar dislocation may occur traumatically with any athlete, but is more frequently seen in children between the ages of 8–15 years and middle-aged women who are overweight and have poor muscular development of the quadriceps. Biomechanically, the individual is more susceptible to this condition if they demonstrate genu valgum, excessive femoral anteversion or external rotation of the tibia, and if the VMO is weak.

The injury usually occurs when the knee is externally rotated and straightened at the same time, such as when the athlete turns to the left while pushing off from the right foot. In this position the tibial attachment of the quadriceps moves laterally in relation to the femur, increasing the lateral force component as the muscle group contracts. The patella almost always dislocates laterally and is accompanied by a ripping sensation and excruciating pain, causing the knee to give way. As the knee straightens, the patella may reduce spontaneously with an audible click.

Swelling is rapid due to the haemarthrosis, causing the skin to become taught and shiny. Bruising forms over the medial retinaculum, and the athlete is normally completely disabled by pain and quadriceps spasm.

Initial treatment is to immobilize the knee completely and apply the RICE protocol. Aspiration may be required if pain is intense, but swelling usually abates with non-invasive management. Quadriceps re-education plays an important part in the rehabilitation process, with VMO strengthening being particularly important. The medial retinaculum must be allowed to heal fully, and it is a mistake to allow these athletes to mobilize unprotected too soon. Only when 90° knee flexion is achieved and the patient is able to perform a straight leg lift with 30–50% of the power of the uninjured leg are they ready to walk without support.

## ITB friction syndrome

The ITB is a non-elastic collagen cord stretching from the pelvis to below the knee. At the top it is attached to the iliac crest, where it blends with the gluteus maximus and tensor fascia lata. As the tract descends down the lateral side of the thigh its deep fibres attach to the linea aspera of the femur. The superficial fibres continue downwards to attach to the lateral femoral condyle, lateral patellar retinaculum and anterolateral aspect of the tibial condyle (Gerdy's tubercle).

In standing, the ITB lies posterior to the hip axis and anterior to the knee axis and therefore helps to maintain hip and knee extension, reducing the muscle work required to sustain an upright stance. In running, during the swing phase the ITB lies anterior to the greater trochanter and hip flexion/extension axis, reducing the workload required for hip flexion.

### Aetiology

Tightness of the ITB can occur in a number of patient groups. The tall, lanky teenager who has recently undergone the adolescent growth spurt may experience pain if soft tissue elongation lags behind long bone development. Tightness in adolescent females is a frequent cause of anterior knee pain. The second major group of sufferers are adult athletes, particularly distance runners. A number of factors can contribute to problems within this group. Running on cambered roads and using shoes worn on their lateral edge will increase varus knee angulation and may overstretch a tight ITB. Rapid increases in speed or hill work can place excessive stress on the structure. In addition, imbalances of muscle strength and flexibility around the knee and hip may lead to the gradual onset of symptoms.

Pain normally occurs either over the trochanteric bursa or the lateral femoral condyle. Pain is experienced to palpation, but also to limited range squats or lunges on the affected leg. As the knee flexes to 30° and back, the ITB will pass over the lateral femoral condyle and may cause friction and pain which builds in intensity. Flexibility tests, particularly the Ober manoeuvre and Thomas test (p. 172) often reveal pain and a lack of flexibility.

## Management

The initial inflammation responds to anti-inflammatory modalities, but the underlying cause must be addressed. Modifications include alterations of running surface and footwear, and changes to training intensity, frequency, duration and content. Where limited-range motion is identified, stretching procedures are called for. Hip flexor and extensor flexibility is regained by using exercises previously described, and the ITB itself is stretched using an adaptation of the Ober manoeuvre.

The ITB insertion at the knee is first heated with hot packs or diathermy. The pelvis is stabilized by the patient flexing and holding the lower knee. The affected upper leg is initially abducted and extended at the hip and flexed at the knee. From this position, hip extension is maintained and the leg is pushed downwards into adduction, and held for 30–60 seconds, with the stretch being repeated four or five times. As adduction commences, the patient's pelvis will tend to tilt, and an assistant should press down on the rim of the ilium to stabilize the pelvis and increase the stretch.

Between treatment sessions the patient should attempt this procedure at home. The weight of the leg may be used to press it into adduction, and a weight bag on the knee will assist this. In addition, training partners or family members can be taught to help.

Weakness in the hip abductors may allow the pelvis to tilt or 'dip' during the stance phase of walking or running. This often gives the impression of a mild trendelenberg gait, and may be habitual following lower limb injury. Gait re-education and abductor strengthening are called for. The abductors may be strengthened from an open chain or more functional closed chain starting position. Open chain strengthening is performed using a weight bag in a side-lying hip abduction exercise. Closed chain strengthening is carried out

with the athlete standing on the affected leg, and keeping it locked. The unaffected leg is flexed at the knee. From this position the pelvis is allowed to drop towards the unsupported side and pulled back to the horizontal position by hip abductor action (Fig. 11.6).

## Collateral ligament injuries

The medial collateral ligament (MCL) is a broad flat band about 8 or 9 cm in length. It travels downwards and forwards from the medial epicondyle of the femur to the medial condyle and upper medial shaft of the tibia. The ligament has both deep and superficial fibres, with the deep fibres attaching to the medial meniscus, and the superficial fibres extending below the level of the tibial tuberosity. The superficial fibres have anterior, middle and posterior portions.

When the knee is in full extension, it is in close pack formation. The medial femoral condyle is pushed backwards, and the medial epicondyle lifts away from the tibial plateaux, tightening the posterior part of the MCL. As the knee is flexed, the posterior part of the ligament relaxes, but the anterior and middle parts remain tight. By 80–90° flexion, the middle of the ligament is still tight, but the anterior and posterior portions are lax. In this way, the strong middle section of the ligament remains tight for most of the range of movement. The changing distribution of tension strain in the ligament means that the section which is affected

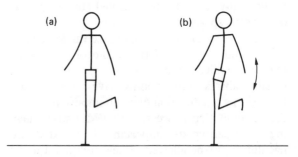

**Figure 11.6** Hip abductor strengthening. (a) Athlete stands on affected leg. (b) Allowing the opposite hip to drop and then pulling it up works the abductors of the weight-bearing limb.

through injury will depend on the knee angle when the injury occurred, so an accurate history is extremely helpful.

The lateral collateral ligament (LCL) is a round cord about 5 cm long, which stands clear of the joint capsule. It travels from the lateral epicondyle of the femur to the lateral surface of the head of the fibula. The ligament splits the tendon of biceps femoris, and is separated from the joint capsule by the popliteus muscle, and the lateral genicular vessels and nerve (Palastanga, Field and Soames, 1989). The lower end of the lateral ligament is pulled backwards in extension and forwards in flexion of the knee.

Damage to the MCL can result from excessive valgus angulation of the knee coupled with external rotation, while LCL damage is normally through varus strains coupled with internal rotation. MCL damage usually leads to pain over the medial epicondyle of the femur, the middle third of the joint line, or the tibial insertion of the ligament. With LCL damage, pain is normally over the head of the fibula or lateral femoral epicondyle. The integrity of the ligaments is tested by applying a varus and valgus stress to the knee flexed to 30°. It is ineffective to the same test with the knee locked, as this is the close pack position, and nearly 50% of medial and lateral stability is provided by the cruciate ligaments and joint capsule. The easiest way to perform the varus/ valgus test is with the patient's hip abducted, the thigh supported on the couch and the lower leg over the couch side.

First and second degree injuries are generally treated conservatively. Third degree injuries (complete rupture) have been treated surgically, but some authors argue that stability of the knee is not improved to a greater extent than with non-operative intervention (Keene, 1990). First degree injuries are generally treated partial or full weight bearing with the ligament supported by strapping. Second and third degree injuries are managed non-weight bearing.

Initially, the aim is pain relief, swelling reduction and the start of mobile scar formation. Isometric quadriceps drill is begun and modalities used to reduce pain and swelling. At night a knee brace may be used to protect the ligament. By the third or fourth day after injury (sometimes earlier with a first degree and later with a third degree injury) gentle mobility exercises are begun either in a side-lying starting position or in the pool. Gentle transverse frictions are used to encourage mobile scar formation. The sweep should be quite broad and a large section of the ligament treated. Free, or light resisted exercises are begun to the knee, hip and calf musculature within the pain-free range. Isokinetics may be used, with the aim of restoring the HQ ratio to that of the uninjured limb.

When 90° of pain free movement is obtained (usually 10–14 days after injury with a grade three sprain) the rehabilitation programme can be progressed further to include more vigorous activities, and increased mobility and strength training. An exercise cycle or light jogging may be used, and swimming (not breast stroke) started. Weight training is progressed to use leg machines, and some power training is added. Towards the end of this period, depending on pain levels, shallow jumping, bench stepping, circle running and zig-zagging in the gym are used to gradually introduce rotation, shear, and valgus stress to the knee. In addition to improving strength and power, these exercises build confidence and provide an assessment of knee stability.

## Cruciate ligaments

The cruciate ligaments are strong rounded cords within the knee joint capsule, but outside its synovial cavity. The ligament fibres are 90% collagen and 10% elastic tissue, arranged in two types of fasciculi. The first group travel directly between the femur and tibia as would be expected, but the second set spiral around the length of the ligament. This structure enables the ligament to increase its resistance to tension when loaded. Under light loads only a few of the fasciculi are under tension, but as the load increases, the spiral fibres unwind bringing more fasciculi into play and effectively increasing the ligament strength.

The anterior cruciate ligament (ACL) is attached from the tibia, anterior to the tibial spine. Here, it blends with the anterior horn of the lateral meniscus and passes beneath the transverse ligament. Its direction is posterior, lateral and proximal to attach to the posterior part of the medial surface of the lateral femoral condyle. As it travels from the tibia to the femur, the ligament twists in a medial spiral. The posterolateral part of the ACL is taut in extension and the anteromedial portion is lax. In flexion, all of the fibres except the anteriomedial portion are lax.

The posterior cruciate ligament (PCL) arises from the posterior intercondylar area of the tibia and travels anteriorly, medially and proximally, passing medial to the ACL to insert into the anterior portion of the lateral surface of the medial femoral condyle. The majority of the PCL fibres are taut in flexion, with only the posterior portion being lax, and in extension the posterior fibres are tight but the rest of the ligament is lax.

The ACL provides 86% of the resistance to anterior displacement and 30% to medial displacement, while the PCL provides 94% of the restraint to posterior displacement and 36% to lateral stresses (Palastanga, Field and Soames, 1989).

Of the two ligaments the ACL is far more commonly injured in sport. The athlete has usually participated in either a running/jumping activity or skiing. The history is usually of a non-contact movement such as rapid deceleration, a 'cutting' action in football, or a twisting fall. The combination is frequently one of rotation and abduction, a similar action to that which causes MCL or medial meniscus damage, and the three injuries often coalesce to form an 'unhappy triad'.

Swelling is usually immediate as a result of haemarthrosis, and instability may be noticed at this stage. A tense effusion is apparent within 24 hours of injury. The classic anterior drawer test is often negative early on, due to hamstring muscle spasm and effusion. The high strain rates encountered in sports cause the majority of injuries to occur to the ligament substance rather than the osseous junction and so X-ray is usually unrevealing.

Diagnosis relies heavily on clinical history and tests for instability, the latter being the subject of some debate. The two most common tests are the anterior drawer test and modifications on this, and the pivot shift.

The classic anterior drawer test (Fig. 11.7) involves flexing the patient's knee to 90° and stabiliz-

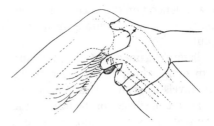

**Figure 11.7** Anterior drawer test for the cruciate ligament.

ing the foot with the examiner's body weight. The proximal tibia is pulled anteriorly and the amount of movement compared with the 'normal' value of the uninjured leg. Various grades of movement may be assessed, grade one being up to 5 mm of anterior glide, grade two 5–10 mm and grade three over 30 mm. The test can however give false negatives if haemarthrosis prevents the knee being flexed to 90°. Movement can also be limited by protective hamstring spasm or if the posterior horn of the medial meniscus wedges against the medial femoral condyle.

The Lachman test, a modification of the anterior drawer test, has been shown to be highly reliable (Donaldson, Warren and Wickiewicz, 1985). The test is performed with the patient lying supine. The examiner holds the patient's knee in 20° flexion, minimizing the effect of hamstring spasm and reducing the likelihood of meniscal wedging. One hand stabilizes the femur and the other applies an anterior shearing force to the proximal tibia, avoiding medial rotation (Fig. 11.8). If anterior translation of the tibia is felt, the test is positive. The movement is compared with that of the uninjured knee, both for range and end feel, an ACL tear giving a characteristically soft end feel. The same grading system is used as with the anterior drawer test.

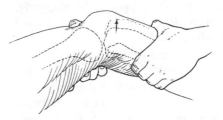

**Figure 11.8** Lachman test for the cruciate ligament.

Another frequently used test is the pivot shift, and its adaptations. These work on the basis that the ACL-deficient knee will allow the lateral tibial plateau to sublux anteriorly. By applying forces to enforce this and then moving the knee, the tibia can be made to reduce rapidly, causing a 'thud'. The pivot shift test starts with the affected leg in full extension. The examiner grasps the ankle of this leg with his or her distal hand and the outside of the ipsilateral knee with his or her proximal hand. The ankle and tibia are forced into maximum internal rotation, subluxing the lateral tibial plateau anteriorly. The knee is slowly flexed as the proximal hand applies a valgus stress. If the test is positive, tension in the ITB will reduce the tibia, causing a sudden backward 'shift'. The major disadvantage with this test is that the patient must be relaxed throughout the manoeuvre, a situation which often is not possible because of pain. Donaldson, Warren and Wickiewicz, (1985) tested more than 100 ACL-deficient knees preoperatively and found the pivot shift test to be positive in only 35% of cases. The same examination carried out under anaesthesia (with the muscles completely relaxed) gave 98% positive results.

This test is reversed in the jerk test (Table 11.1), while the flexion rotation drawer (FRD) test elim-inates the need for a valgus force by using gravity to sublux the tibia. A reliability of 62% has been reported for the FRD, rising to 89% with the anaesthetized patient (Jensen, 1990). The Slocum test uses a side lying position to perform a pivot shift and is particularly suitable for heavier patients.

Since the ACL has two functionally separate portions (see above), depending on the knee angle at the time of injury, only one portion may be damaged, thus resulting in a partial ligament tear. If the anteromedial band is damaged but the poste-rolateral portion is intact, the Lachman test may be negative, but the anterior drawer test positive. This is because the anteromedial portion is tightened as the knee flexes, and so will be tighter (and there-fore instability will be more apparent) with the 90° knee angle of the anterior drawer. Similarly, if the posterolateral band is disrupted (the more usual situation) the anterior drawer may be negative but the Lachman positive, as this portion of the liga-ment becomes tighter as the knee approaches extension.

Partial tears usually remain intact and show good long-term results. However Noyes et al. (1989) argued that progression to complete deficiency, although unlikely in knees which have sustained

**Table 11.1  Manual laxity tests of the knee**

| Test | Method |
| --- | --- |
| Anterior drawer | Knee flexed to 90°, foot stabilized, tibia drawn forwards. |
| Lachman | Knee flexed to 20° femur stabilized, tibia drawn forwards. |
| Pivot shift (MacIntosh) | Knee extended, foot/tibia internally rotated, valgus strain on knee as it is flexed. |
| Jerk (reverse pivot shift) | Knee flexed to 90° valgus stress on knee internally rotate tibia and extend knee. |
| Flexion/rotation drawer | Leg held by tibia only, knee in 20° flexion posterior force on tibia, then flex knee. |
| Slocum | Patient on uninjured side, pelvis rotated posteriorly. Ankle on couch. Knee flexed to 10°, apply valgus stress and push further into flexion. |
| Losee | Knee flexed to 45°, tibia externally rotated. Knee extended, and valgus force applied, allowing tibia to internally rotate. |

Adapted from Jensen (1990).

injury to one quarter of the ligament, may be expected in 50% of knees with half ligament tears and 86% of those with three-quarter tears.

## Management

First and second degree injuries may be immobilized initially and then subjected to intense rehabilitation to re-strengthen the supporting knee musculature. A derotation brace may be used to protect the knee until muscle strength is sufficient. Third degree injuries with marked instability may be treated surgically, although some authors argue that rehabilitation alone is the better solution (Garrick and Webb, 1990). Surgery involves repair and reconstruction, most authors agreeing that the latter is more appropriate. Reconstruction techniques may be extracapsular, intracapsular, or a combination of the two.

Extracapsular reconstruction has been described using the MacIntosh procedure (Wilson, Lewis and Scranton, 1990). A 10 x 1 cm strip of the ITB is passed beneath the fibular collateral ligament, under the lateral attachment of the gastrocnemius and then looped back on itself. The knee is flexed to 60° and the leg externally rotated before the ITB is pulled tight and secured with sutures.

Alternatively, a graft may be cut from the middle third of the patellar tendon, to include both non-articular patellar and tibial tubercle bone. This has the advantage that it leaves other structures around the knee intact. Tunnels are then drilled in the tibia and femur travelling through the attachments of the ACL. The graft is passed through the bone tunnel and attached to the lateral aspect of the lateral femoral condyle and the tibial tubercle. The graft is secured with cancellous screws and sutures. This procedure gives a very strong graft, but may have the complication of patellar pain following surgery. Flexion contraction of 5° or more may be present in almost one quarter of these patients (Sachs et al., 1989), and patello-femoral irritability can result. Where contracture is a likelihood, rehabilitation should place a greater emphasis on maintaining full knee extension. A similar technique has been described by Wilson, Lewis and Scranton (1990) using the semi-tendinosus tendon instead of the patellar tendon, to avoid patellar complications.

Several structures may be used for grafts, and Noyes, Butler and Grood (1984) showed the patellar tendon graft to have a strength of 168% of the ACL, while the semi-tendinosus had only 70%, gracilus 49% and the quadriceps/patellar retinaculum only 21%. Synthetic tissues, such as polytetrafluoroethylene (PTFE), are now used more frequently, and mobility may be attained more rapidly following surgery using these materials. However, synthetics are generally only used where intra-articular reconstructions have failed. Bovine substances have been used, but problems have been caused by reactive synovitis following these operations. Allogenic tendon grafts from cadavers and amputation specimens have been used to good effect in patients suffering chronic ACL insufficiency (Shino et al., 1986).

Rehabilitation will depend very much on the particular procedure which has been performed. The problem is that immobilization is thought to be desirable for healing of the graft, but early mobility is required to avoid cartilage degeneration, soft tissue contracture and muscle atrophy. The solution is to mobilize the patient early, providing the movement used does not overly stress the graft. The range of motion possible without placing undue tension on the graft must be established, and a protective brace may be used to limit undesirable movements. Sandberg, Nilsson and Westlin (1987) showed the time needed to return to sport to be five weeks shorter and range of motion significantly better following the use of a hinged cast allowing knee flexion from 20–70°. Noyes, Mangine and Barber (1987) mobilized patients on the second day after surgery and found no adverse effects on the ligament reconstruction.

The use of a leg extension regime using a sitting position has been criticized (Palmitier et al., 1991). Contraction of the quadriceps from this open chain position places considerable anterior shear on the knee and may stretch the ACL. Closed chain motions, such as the squat or leg press movement, reduce the shear. With these actions, a more functional co-contraction is used, with the hamstring contraction used primarily for hip extension now counteracting some of the shear created by the quadriceps.

## Posterior cruciate damage

The PCL is the strongest ligament in the knee (Baylis and Rzonca, 1988) and much less frequently damaged in sport than the ACL. When an injury does occur it may be the result of a force directed posteriorly onto a flexed knee, forced hyperextension, or forced flexion where the athlete falls into a kneeling position pressing the ankle into plantarflexion (Keene, 1990). Unlike ACL injury, the athlete with a damaged PCL can usually continue playing and may notice only minimal swelling, but there is marked pain on the posterior aspect of the knee. Posterior subluxation of the tibia may be seen from the side if the knee is flexed to 90°. This may be accentuated if the patient contracts their quadriceps against a resistance provided by the examiner. The patient is asked to 'slide the foot down the couch' (Daniel et al., 1988), as the examiner stabilizes the ankle. If not viewed from the side, the subluxation may be missed, and the injury wrongly diagnosed as an ACL tear, the tibia moving forwards to reduce and mimicking an anterior drawer sign.

As with ACL damage, conservative treatment involving intensive muscle strengthening is tried first. The PCL is contained within a synovial sheath which enhances its ability to heal in continuity (Fowler and Messieh, 1987). Reconstruction may be attempted, using a similar patellar tendon graft to that described above. This time, the graft is positioned lateral to the tibial attachment of the PCL and travels through the femur at the junction of the medial condyle and the intercondylar notch.

The knee with isolated PCL insufficiency producing unidirectional instability generally does well conservatively, but when PCL damage is associated with additional tissue damage which results in multidirectional instability, surgery should be considered (Torg, 1989). In a study investigating the long-term effects of non-operative management of PCL damage, Parolie and Bergfeld (1986) assessed 25 athletes on average 6.2 years after injury. Of these 84% had returned to their previous sport. Importantly, those who were not satisfied with their knee had less than 100% strength compared with the undamaged knee (measured as mean torque on an isokinetic dynamometer at varying angular velocities), and those who were satisfied had strength values greater than 100%. The importance of maintaining superior muscle strength following PCL injuries is therefore clear.

## The menisci → Intro

The menisci are fibrocartilage structures which rest on the tibial condyles. They are crescent-shaped when viewed from above, but triangular in cross-section. Their peripheral border is formed from fibrous tissue and attached to the deep surface of the joint capsule. These same fibres attach the menisci to the tibial surface forming the coronary ligaments. Anteriorly, the two menisci are joined by the transverse ligament, a posterior transverse ligament being present in 20% of the population (Palastanga, Field and Soames, 1989).

The medial meniscus is the larger of the two, semicircular in shape, and broader posteriorly. Its anterior horn is attached to the front of the intercondylar area of the tibia in front of the ACL. The posterior horn attaches to the posterior intercondylar area between the PCL and the lateral meniscus. It has an attachment to the MCL, and the oblique popliteal ligament coming from semimembranosus. The upper part of the meniscus is firmly attached to the MCL, the fibres here forming the medial menisco-femoral ligament. The lower part, attached to the coronary ligament, is more lax. This has important functional consequences because the medial meniscus is anchored more firmly to the femur than to the tibia. In flexion/extension the femur is thus able to glide on the tibia, while in rotation, the meniscus can slide over the tibial plateau (Evans, 1986).

The lateral meniscus is more circular, and has a uniform breadth. Its two horns are attached close together, the anterior horn blending with the attachment of the ACL. The posterior horn attaches just anterior to the posterior horn of the medial meniscus. The meniscus has a posterolateral groove which receives the popliteus tendon, and a few fibres from this muscle attach to the meniscus itself. In addition, the tendon of popliteus partially separates the lateral meniscus from the joint capsule, a configuration which makes the lateral meniscus more mobile than its medial counterpart. The posterior part of the lateral meniscus has two ligamentous attachments, the anterior and posterior meniscofemoral ligaments. These divide around the PCL, and in extreme flexion, as the PCL tightens, so do the anterior and posterior meniscofemoral ligaments. The lateral meniscus is thus pulled backwards and medially.

The menisci receive blood from the inferior genicular arteries which supply the perimeniscal plexus. Small penetrating branches from this plexus enter the meniscus via the coronary ligaments. Up until the age of about 11 years, the whole meniscus has a blood supply, but in the adult only 10-25% of the periphery of the meniscus is vascular. The anterior and posterior horns are covered by vascular synovium and have a good blood supply (Arnoczky and Warren, 1983). The peripheral vessels are within the deeper cartilage substance, the surface receiving its main nutrition via diffusion from the synovial fluid. A few myelinated and non-myelinated nerve fibres are found in the outer third of the menisci, but no nerve endings.

Because the menisci are held more firmly centrally, they are able to alter their shape and move forwards and backwards over the tibial plateau. The lateral meniscus has a greater amount of movement, and is often 'pulled away from trouble' leaving the medial meniscus to be more commonly injured in association with the MCL and ACL to which it has attachments.

In flexion, the lateral meniscus is carried backwards, onto the steep posterior slope of the lateral tibial plateau, and with extension, it moves forwards again. In flexion/extension the medial meniscus is held firm until the last 20° of extension when the knee begins to rotate (screw home mechanism p. 150). As this happens, the medial meniscus is carried backwards. In extension, the menisci are squeezed and elongated in an anteroposterior direction, and in flexion, they become wider.

The menisci enlarge the tibio-femoral contact area, thus spreading the pressure taken by the sub-chondral bone (Fig. 11.9a). It has been estimated that the menisci disperse between 30% and 55% of the load across the knee (Kelley, 1990). When only a portion of the meniscus is removed,

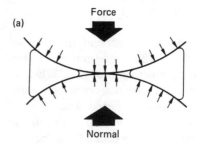

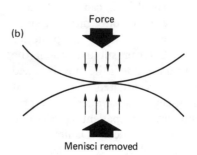

**Figure 11.9** The effect of cartilage removal (menisectomy) on the knee. (a) Forces on the normal knee. (b) Menisci removed. The bones take more jarring strain.

the joint surface contact forces may increase by 350% (Seedhom and Hargreaves, 1979). The menisci contribute substantially to knee stability. In the ACL deficient knee, the anterior drawer test may be positive in only 35% of knees with an intact medial meniscus, but in 83% when the meniscus is removed (Levy, Torzilli and Warren, 1982). The menisci limit sagittal gliding of the femur over the tibial plateau, a movement greatly increased in patients who have undergone menisectomy. In addition, they allow a dual movement to occur, normally only possible in joints which are far more lax. The menisci also aid joint lubrication by spreading the synovial fluid over the surface of the articular cartilage.

## Injury

It has been estimated that meniscal injury occurs with a frequency of 61 per 100 000 individuals. The condition is three times more prevalent in males than females, with the medial meniscus being injured four times as often as the lateral (Kelley, 1990).

The history of injury is usually one which combines twisting on a semiflexed knee with the foot fixed on the ground. The onset is sudden, and pain is felt deep within the knee, the patient often saying they 'felt something go'. Effusion may be extensive after injury, and haemarthrosis may result if the injury occurs in combination with ACL or MCL damage. Tears may occur to the periphery or body of the meniscus, running horizontally or vertically. A longitudinal tear (Bucket handle) of the medial meniscus may allow its lateral portion to slip over the dome of the medial femoral condyle causing blocked extension (true locking).

On examination, effusion is apparent and tenderness is often found over the joint line, most usually medially. A capsular pattern may be noticeable (Table 2.2), and terminal extension is often blocked with a springy end feel if muscle spasm is not present. Various tests are used to assess the problem, of which the two most common are McMurray's and Apley's.

McMurray's test requires full flexion of the knee and so is not suitable for the acute joint. The medial joint line is palpated and, from the fully flexed position, the knee is externally rotated and extended, as a slight varus strain is applied. If positive, a painful click is felt over the medial meniscus. The lateral meniscus is similarly tested by extending the knee with internal rotation and a valgus strain. In each case only the posterior portion of the meniscus is tested, and so a negative McMurray's sign does not preclude meniscal damage, but when positive the test is clinically revealing.

Apley's grinding test involves placing the patient in a prone lying position, flexing the knee to 90° rotating the tibia and compressing it against the femur in an attempt to elicit a popping or snapping sensation. It is important not to force the movements too far, as this may further tear the already damaged meniscus (Garrick and Webb, 1990). The intention with this test is to help differentiate between meniscal and MCL damage at the joint line. Symptoms will be present as the knee is compressed when the meniscus is damaged, but not if the MCL alone is injured, because this

structure will be relaxed by the compression force (Apley and Solomon, 1989). Conversely, a distraction force stretches the ligament but disengages the meniscus, thus giving pain when MCL damage has occurred in isolation (Fig. 11.10).

The results of meniscal tests combined with the clinical history will indicate if damage is likely, in

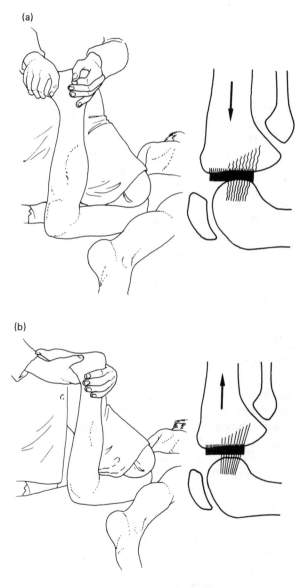

(a)

(b)

**Figure 11.10** Apley grinding test. (a) Compression stresses the menisci, but relaxes the collateral ligaments. (b) Traction disengages the menisci and places stress on the collateral ligaments.

which case arthroscopy is called for to confirm the findings.

## Management

If a meniscal tear is present, the choice is either non-operative management or surgical intervention involving removal or repair of the injured meniscus.

### Non-operative management

Henning (1988) argued that meniscal tears of less than 10 mm in length, and partial thickness injuries involving 50% or less of the vertical height of the meniscus could be treated non-operatively, provided that the ACL was undamaged. Weiss et al. (1989) reported that stable vertical longitudinal tears in the vascular outer area of the meniscus had a good potential for healing, whereas stable radial tears did not. They performed a repeat arthroscopy on 32 patients (on average 26 months after the first procedure), and found that 17 longitudinal tears had healed completely. Five radial tears showed no evidence of healing and one had extended. No degenerative changes were found in the adjacent articular cartilage of the stable lesions.

### Meniscal repair

The peripheral part of the meniscus has a blood supply sufficient to support healing. Initial healing in this region is by fibrosis with vessels from the capillary plexus and synovial fringe penetrating the area. Fibrous healing may be complete within 10 weeks, and the scar tissue can be remodelled into normal fibrocartilage within several months (Hammesfahr, 1989). The mid-portion of the meniscus is avascular and has traditionally been thought not to heal. However, Arnoczky and Warren (1983) demonstrated healing in canine tissue by cutting an access channel from the peripheral region to the midpoint of the meniscus. The peripheral vessels proliferated through the channel into the lesion, giving fibrovascular scarring throughout both areas.

The peripheral tear may be sutured, and healing improved by abrading the parameniscal synovium.

Henning (1988) argued that healing may be further enhanced by injecting an exogenous blood clot into the injury site. Results are good when repair is limited to the vascular area of the meniscus and to vertical tears (Ryu and Dunbar, 1988). Weight bearing or full range motion will deform the menisci and so pull on the scar site. For this reason rehabilitation of the repaired meniscus is much less intense than that of a patient who has undergone menisectomy.

DeHaven et al. (1989) reported follow-up results on 80 repaired menisci on average 4.6 years after surgery. Of these, 11% had torn again (only three at the repair zone), and these authors recommended meniscal repair in view of the degenerative changes following menisectomy.

### Menisectomy

The preceding descriptions of non-operative management and meniscal repair make it apparent that menisectomy is not the first choice in many cases of meniscal tearing. Degenerative changes which have been described after total menisectomy include joint narrowing, ridging and flattening (Fairbank, 1948). However, where the meniscus is grossly damaged, and the knee is unstable, a partial or total menisectomy may be required. The minimum amount of tissue should be removed to reduce the biomechanical impairment to the joint.

The traditional method for menisectomy (O'Donoghue, 1976) is with the patient supine, and the knee flexed to 90° over the table end. For a medial menisectomy a straight incision is often used, starting proximal to the lower pole of the patella and medial to the patellar tendon, and stretching parallel to the tendon. The retinaculum is split and the joint washed out (lavaged) with warm saline to remove any blood. The whole cartilage may be visible if the knee can be sprung open medially, but usually only palpation with forceps is possible. The bony attachment of the meniscus is dissected and the meniscus itself removed.

Arthroscopic removal of all or part of the meniscus is commonplace nowadays. An anterolateral or anteromedial approach may be taken, depending on which compartment of the knee the lesion is in. The knee is held in 10° flexion and the joint is gapped by applying a valgus or varus stress. The joint is distended with fluid, to allow easier inspection of the tissue surfaces. An initial incision is made into the anterior part of the meniscus, and the incision is then extended into the middle and posterior segments. The posterior horn is released, followed by the anterior horn and the meniscus is removed. In cases where only part of the meniscus is removed, the edge of the remaining tissue is trimmed.

Arthroscopy, although commonplace, is not without risk of complication. The committee on complications of arthroscopy of North America (1985) found a 0.8% complication rate in over 100 000 procedures, while Sherman et al. (1986) reported a complication rate of 8.2%. Neurological injury, poor wound healing, instrument breakage, intra-articular infection, knee ligament injury, and pulmonary embolism resulting in death have all occurred. The patient's age and the length of time that a tourniquet is used have been found to be the most significant factors in predicting problems (Sherman et al., 1986).

The use of arthroscopy with local anaesthesia is steadily increasing (Ngo et al., 1985; Besser and Stahl, 1986; Buckley, Hood and MacRae, 1989), and obviously removes the risk inherent in any procedure involving a general anaesthetic. The skin puncture sites are injected with lignocaine or similar, and the joint is distended with saline and anaesthetic solution. Arthroscopic surgery of this type allows the patient to be discharged significantly earlier than when general anaesthesia is used.

## Jumper's knee

Jumper's knee is an anterior knee pain affecting the teno-osseous junctions of the quadriceps tendon where it is attached to the superior pole of the patella, and the patellar tendon where it is attached to the inferior pole of the patella and tibial tuberosity. It is therefore an insertional tendonopathy resulting in derangement of the bone–tendon unit (Colosimo and Bassett, 1990).

The injury is often described as patellar or quadriceps tendinitis, although these conditions represent an inflammation of the tendon itself, rather than isolated damage to the teno-osseous junction. In a strict sense the conditions should be considered separately, but they are generally accepted as a single entity. However, it should be remembered that tendinitis does not necessarily mean that the teno-osseous junction is affected, but when the tendon insertion itself is damaged, the tendon will almost always be inflamed.

Jumper's knee occurs more frequently in athletes who regularly impose rapid eccentric loading (traction) on the extensor mechanism of the knee, especially on hard surfaces.

The condition affects the inferior pole of the patella in 80% of cases and is most common at this site in athletes over 40 years of age. The insertion of the quadriceps is more commonly affected in the over 40s, and the tibial tuberosity is the most common sight for jumper's knee in children (David, 1989).

Repetitive stress on the teno-osseous junction causes microtearing over time, and an insidious onset of pain. The condition progresses in a series of stages. Initially, pain is experienced only after intense activity, as a well-localized dull ache without a history of trauma. With time, pain occurs at the onset of activity, and disappears when the athlete is warmed up, only to reappear when the sport has finished. Eventually, pain is constant with consequent impairment of performance, and as a final, but rare, scenario the tendon may rupture completely.

On examination, quadriceps wasting is apparent in long-standing cases, and pain occurs to resisted extension with slight soreness to full passive flexion. Some swelling may be noticed around the patellar tendon in acute cases, with fluctuance present if the condition is severe. A non-capsular pattern is found.

Palpation is performed with the knee in full extension to relax the patellar tendon. Palpation to the lower pole of the patella is best performed by pressing with the flat of the hand onto the upper surface of the patella to tilt it. This brings the lower pole into prominence and enables the practitioner to reach the part of the teno-osseous junction which lies on the under-surface of the angular lower pole.

Radiographic changes are usually apparent if symptoms have been present for more than 6 months (Colosimo and Bassett, 1990). An elongation of the involved pole of the patella may be seen with calcification of the affected tendon matrix. Bone scan has indicated increased blood pooling and concentration of radioactive tracer in the inflamed area (Kahn and Wilson, 1987).

Both intrinsic and extrinsic factors have been implicated as possible causes. Intrinsic factors include biomechanical alterations in the extensor mechanism, such as hypermobility, altered Q angle and genu valgum or genu recurvatum. Changes in the HQ ratio and hamstring flexibility may also have a part to play and should be examined. Extrinsic factors include frequency and intensity of training, training surface and footwear. Feretti (1986) showed a correlation between jumper's knee and both hardness of playing surface and training frequency. Thirty seven percent of players (matched for sport, playing position and training type) using cement surfaces in his study suffered from the condition, compared with only 5% of those using softer surfaces. In addition, the percentage of players affected by the condition escalated as the number of training sessions per week increased.

As with any overuse syndrome, part of the management of the condition involves avoidance or modification of training. Athletes should be encouraged to warm up adequately, and practise flexibility exercises to both the quadriceps and hamstrings. Strength must be developed symmetrically, and footwear should incorporate shock-absorbing materials.

In the early stages of the condition these modifications combined with ice application when pain is acute are usually sufficient. Later, transverse frictional massage is the treatment of choice. Frictions to the teno-osseous junctions attaching to the patella are only effective if the patella is tilted and pressure from the therapist's finger is directed at a 45° angle to the long axis of the femur rather than straight down.

In chronic conditions, where scar tissue has formed at the teno-osseous junctions, limitation in flexion may be apparent. Flexibility exercises will increase the range of movement, but more by stretching the quadriceps than the scar tissue. Where this is the case, soft tissue manipulation may be required in an attempt to rupture the adherent scarring. If this procedure fails to produce a complete result surgery may be required. Various procedures have been described, some of which attempt to alter underlying malalignment and others to excise abnormal tissue.

## Sinding–Larsen–Johansson disease

In this condition the secondary ossification centre on the lower border of the patella is affected in adolescents. The epiphysis is tractioned, leading to inflammation and eventual fragmentation. Avascular necrosis is not usually present, but a temporary osteoporosis has been described (Traverso, Baldari and Catalani, 1990) during the adolescent growth spurt. This may weaken the inferior pole of the patella making avulsion more likely.

Sinding–Larsen–Johansson disease can easily be confused with chondromalacia on first inspection as it causes pain in the lower pole of the patella, especially when kneeling. However, on closer examination the differences are soon apparent, and X-ray confirms the bony change. The condition may exist with Osgood–Schlatter's syndrome (Traverso, Baldari and Catalani, 1990), and the conservative management of the two syndromes is largely the same, involving the use of pain relieving/anti-inflammatory modalities, and training modification. Surgical removal of the lower pole of the patella has been recommended in persistent cases (Williams and Sperryn, 1976).

## Osgood–Schlatter's syndrome

This condition affects adolescents, especially males. Most often the patient is an active sportsperson who has recently undergone the adolescent growth spurt. With Osgood–Schlatter's syndrome traction is applied to the tibial tubercle, eventually causing the apophysis of the tubercle to separate from the proximal end of the tibia. Initially, fragmentation appears, but with time the fragments coalesce and further ossification leads to an increase in bone. This gives the characteristic prominent tibial 'bump' often noticeable when the knee silhouette is compared with that of the unaffected side.

The infrapatellar tendon shows increased vascularization and, particularly where radiographic changes are not apparent, soft tissue swelling and infrapatellar fat pad involvement is noted. Pain is highly localized to the tibial tubercle and exacerbated by activities such as running, jumping and descending stairs. The condition may coalesce with patellar malalignment faults, such as patella infera and patella alta. Patellar tendon avulsion can occur following this condition, and Levi and Coleman (1976) reported 26% of those seen with this type of fracture to have had a previous history of Osgood–Schlatter's disease.

Initial management is by limiting activity. Pain relief and reduction of inflammation may be obtained using electrotherapy modalities alone or iontophoresis with an anti-inflammatory medication and local anaesthetic (Antich and Brewster, 1985). Injection of the tibial tubercle with hydrocortisone has been described (Grass, 1978). The use of an infra-patellar strap to reduce the pull of the quadriceps onto the tibial tubercle has been used with some success (Levine and Kashyap, 1981).

Assessment of the lower limb musculature often reveals hypertrophy and inflexibility of the quadriceps. When passive knee flexion is tested, intense pain precludes the use of quadriceps stretching. However, when pain has subsided, flexibility of this muscle group must be regained. If prolonged rest has given rise to muscle atrophy, strengthening exercises are indicated. Ice packs may be used to limit pain or inflammation following activity.

## Synovial plica

The synovial plica is a remnant of the septum which separates the knee into three chambers until the fourth intrauterine month. The plica, placed supra-medially, may be present in some 20–60% of knees (Amatuzzi, Fazzi and Varella, 1990), but does not necessarily cause symptoms. In a series of 3250 knee disorders, Koshino and Okamoto (1985)

found only 32 patients to have the complaint (1%). The structure separates the knee joint into two reservoirs, one above the patella and the other constituting the joint cavity proper. The normal plica is a thin, pink, flexible structure, but when inflamed it becomes thick, fibrosed and swollen, losing its elasticity and interfering with patellofemoral tracking.

These tissue changes are often initiated by trauma that results in synovitis, and is more common in athletes. Pain is usually intermittent and increases with activity. Discomfort is experienced when descending stairs and may mimic anterior knee pain. However, pain of plical origin normally subsides immediately when the knee is extended. In addition, the 'morning sign' may be present. This is a popping sensation which occurs as the knee is extended, particularly on rising, but disappears throughout the day. The popping may be accompanied by giving way, and is caused by the thickened plica passing over the medial femoral condyle. As the day progresses, joint effusion pushes the plica away from the condyle. This sign may be reproduced with some patients by extending the knee from 90° flexion while internally rotating the tibia and pushing the patella medially. The pop is usually experienced at between 45° and 60° flexion.

Conservative treatment has been found to be effective in 60% of cases (Amatuzzi, Fazzi and Varella, 1990) and aims to reduce the compression over the anterior compartment of the knee, by using stretching exercises. The length of the hamstrings, quadriceps and gastocnemius muscles should be assessed, and these muscles stretched if noticeable shortening is found. Where conservative treatment fails, and symptoms limit sport or daily living, surgery may be warranted. Koshino and Okamoto (1985) reported pain and symptom relief in 90% of knees treated surgically by plical resection, but did not quote figures for long-term follow up.

## Tendinitis

Tendinitis around the knee occurs most commonly within the patellar tendon (jumper's knee, see above) the semi-membranosus, and the popliteus.

Semi-membranosus tendinitis gives a persistent ache over the posteromedial aspect of the knee. It occurs as the semi-membranosus tendon slides over the medial corner of the medial femoral condyle, and is distinct from semi-membranosus bursitis which affects the area of the medial tibial condyle. Pain may occur within the tendon substance itself, or over the teno-osseous junction, when an insertional tendinitis is present. Increased tracer uptake has been noted on bone scan with this latter condition (Ray, Clancy and Lemon, 1988).

Popliteus tendinitis is related to increased pronation of the STJ and excessive internal rotation of the tibia (Brody, 1980). The increased internal rotation causes traction on the popliteus attachment to the lateral femoral condyle. The popliteus acts with the PCL to prevent forward displacement of the femur on the flexed tibia, and so will be overworked with downhill running (Baylis and Rzonca, 1988). On examination, tenderness is revealed over the popliteus, just anterior to the fibular collateral ligament. The patient is examined in a supine position, with the injured knee in the 'figure of four' position, that is affected hip flexed, abducted and externally rotated, knee bent to 90° and foot placed on the knee of the contralateral leg. The condition is differentiated from ITB friction syndrome by testing resisted tibial internal rotation with the knee flexed, and palpating the popliteus as internal rotation is resisted in extension (Allen and Ray, 1989).

Treatment for tendinitis involves rest, anti-inflammatory modalities, and training modification. The flexibility of the knee musculature and the biomechanics of the lower limb should be assessed and corrected as necessary.

## Bursitis

The knee joint has on average 14 bursae (see Table 11.2) in areas where friction is likely to occur, between muscle, tendon, bone and skin. Any of these can become inflamed and give pain when compressed through muscle contraction or direct palpation. Those most commonly injured in sport include the pre-patellar, pes anserine, and semi-membranosus.

The pre-patellar bursa is usually injured by falling onto the anterior aspect of the knee, or by prolonged kneeling (housemaid's knee). Haemorrhage into the bursa can cause an inflammatory reaction and increased fluid volume. Enlargement is noticeable and the margins of the mass are well defined, differentiating the condition from general knee effusion or subcutaneous haematoma. Knee flexion may be limited, the bursa being compressed as the skin covering the patella tightens.

Septic bursitis may result from secondary infection if the skin over the bursa is broken by laceration or puncture wound. If the condition becomes chronic, the bursa may collapse and the folded walls of the thickened bursa sac appear as small hardened masses on the anterior aspect of the knee. In these cases, erythema and exquisite tenderness is usually present.

Minor cases normally respond to rest and ice, but more marked swelling requires aspiration. Aspiration is carried out under sterile conditions, and a compression bandage applied.

Semi-membranosus bursitis gives rise to pain and swelling over the lower posteromedial aspect of the knee. Pain may be made worse by hamstring or gastrocnemius contraction against resistance, and in activities involving intense action of these muscles, such as sprinting and bounding.

Pes anserine bursitis gives pain and swelling over the metaphyseal area of the tibia, sometimes referred to the medial joint line (Baylis and Rzonca, 1988). The bursa may be injured by direct trauma (hitting the knee on a hurdle) or by overuse of the pes anserine tendons.

With both of the latter causes of bursitis, rest and anti-inflammatory modalities are required. Biomechanical assessment of the lower limb and analysis of the athlete's training regime are called for where there is no history of injury.

One condition often referred to as 'bursitis' is a Baker's cyst. This is actually a posterior herniation of the synovial membrane into the bursa lying between semi-membranosus and the medial head of gastrocnemius. The mass bulges into the popliteal space, and occurs particularly in rheumatoid arthritis. The posterior knee ligaments weaken and fail to support the joint capsule, allowing the herniation to occur. The cyst can be palpated over

**Table 11.2    Bursae around the knee**

| Bursa | Lying between |
|---|---|
| Subcutaneous pre-patellar | Lower patella/skin |
| Deep infrapatellar | Upper tibia/patellar ligament |
| Subcutaneous infrapatellar | Lower tibial tuberosity/skin |
| Suprapatellar | Lower femur/deep surface of quadriceps (communicates with joint) |
| No specific name | Lateral head of gastrocnemius/capsule |
|  | Lateral collateral ligament/tendon of biceps femoris |
|  | Lateral collateral ligament/popliteus |
|  | Popliteus tendon/lateral condyle of femur |
|  | Medial head gastrocnemius/capsule |
|  | Medial head of gastrocnemius/semi-membranosus |
| Pes anserine | Superficial to medial collateral ligament/sartorius, gracilus, semi-tendinosus |
| No specific name | Deep medial collateral ligament/femur, medial meniscus |
| Semi-membranosus | Semi-membranosus/medial tibial condyle, gastrocnemius |
| No specific name | Semi-membranosus/semi-tendinosus |

the medial side of the popliteal space beneath the medial head of gastrocnemius.

When painless, the condition may be managed conservatively, but if the enlargement compromises venous return or causes severe pain, aspiration is called for.

## Fat pads

Fat pads consist of fat cells (adipose tissue) packed closely together and separated from other tissues by fibrous septa. They have an abundant blood supply, and are well innervated. Most significant to the knee is the infrapatellar fat pad, lying beneath the patellar tendon, and in front of the femoral condyles. The fat pad is intracapsular but extrasynovial, and a piece of synovial membrane (ligamentum mucosum) passes from the pad to the intracondylar notch of the femur. When the knee is fully flexed, the infrapatellar fat pad fills the anterior aspect of the intercondylar notch. As the knee extends, the fat pad covers the trochlear surface of the femur within the patellar groove (Hertling and Kessler, 1990).

The usual pathology of the infrapatellar fat pad is an enlargement causing increased pressure with resultant pain. Direct trauma can cause haemorrhage and local oedema, and swelling may also occur as a result of pre-menstrual water retention. Space occupying lesions, such as osteochondrotic fragments, may also cause enlargement, and Smillie (1974) described a case where a displaced bucket handle tear of the medial meniscus was forced into the infrapatellar fat pad of the knee.

Enlargement and entrapment of the patellar fat pad has been described by Finsterbush, Frankl and Mann (1989). The entrapped pad was shown to be in various stages of tissue degeneration, including fat necrosis and replacement of the fatty tissue with fibrinoid material. Complete fibrosis was later seen. Silver and Campbell (1985) described persistent inflammation of the knee fat pads as a cause of delayed recovery in dancers with knee injuries. Surgical removal of the pad resulted in restoration of full range motion at the knee. Tsirbas, Paterson and Keene (1990) described excision of the fat pad tip to relieve patello-femoral pain. Patients presented with a history of pain inferomedial, and sometimes inferolateral, to the patella. On examination, impingement pain occurred deep to the inferior pole of the patella at 20° flexion with resisted quadriceps contraction.

## Knee rehabilitation

Exercise begins in a non-weight-bearing starting position and progresses to partial and full weight-bearing movements. Straight leg raising progresses to limited range movements with short lever arms. The quadriceps, hamstrings, hip abductors, hip adductors and knee rotators are all worked. Free exercise progresses to resisted exercise using rubber bands, sand bags and weights.

The progression to partial and then full weight-bearing from non-weight-bearing changes the movement from an open to a closed kinetic chain action. Rotation and shearing stresses are imposed upon the knee, and these forces increase as the speed and range of motion increases, and also as combined movements are used. Sagittal plane movements (flexion/extension) are progressively combined with horizontal plane (rotation/translation) and frontal plane (abduction/adduction) actions. Examples of progressions for free exercises performed in full weight-bearing are listed below.

Walk on the spot
Walk forwards/backwards
Side step
Circle walk
Single leg dips, gradually increasing range of motion

Lunge onto affected leg, gradually increasing range of motion
Single leg squat, gradually increasing range of motion
Dip and cross legs forwards and backwards

Jogging on the spot
Jogging forwards/backwards
Side step
Circle run
Figure of eight run
Carioca
Running on camber
Running up/down slope

Double leg standing on balance board
Single leg standing on balance board
Bench stepping
Bench rib walking
Step down from bench
Step over bench
Side step over bench

Lunge from floor to balance board
Walk over series of balance boards (in parallel bars)
Squat while standing on balance board

Bench support alternate leg thrust
Bench support jump over (both legs)
Bench support jump over (single leg)

Jumping forwards/backwards
Side jumps
Ski-training machine
Jump and twist
Increase depth of above
Hopping as above
Hop and hold position for 2 seconds
Plyometric progressions

The exercise progressions dictate the level of training that the athlete should be allowed to use in his or her own sport. For example, no athlete should be allowed to run on turf until he or she is able to hop and twist without pain, as this movement may occur in an uncontrolled training situation. The final decision of competitive fitness will depend on the athlete's performance with advanced stage rehabilitation exercises, and the assessment of skills by his or her coach (see p. 69).

## References

Allen, M.E. and Ray, G. (1989) Popliteus tendinitis, a new perspective. *Sports Training and Medical Rehabilitation*, **1**, 219–226

Amatuzzi, M.M., Fazzi, A. and Varella, M.H. (1990) Pathologic synovial plica of the knee. *American Journal of Sports Medicine*, **18**, (5) 466–469

Antich, T.J. and Brewster, C.E. (1985) Osgood–Schlatter disease: Review of literature and physical therapy management. *Journal of Orthopaedic and Sports Physical Therapy*, **7**, (1) 5–10

Apley, A.G. and Solomon, L. (1989) *Concise System of Orthopaedics and Fractures*, Butterworth–Heinemann, Oxford

Arno, S. (1990) The A angle: a quantitative measurement of patella alignment and realignment. *Journal of Orthopaedic and Sports Physical Therapy*, **12**, (6) 237–242

Arnoczky, S. and Warren, R. (1983) Microstructure of the human meniscus. *American Journal of Sports Medicine*, **11**, (3) 131–140

Baylis, W.J. and Rzonca, E.C. (1988) Common sports

injuries to the knee. *Clinics in Podiatric Medicine and Surgery*, 5, 3

Beckman, M., Craig, R. and Lehman, R.C. (1989) Rehabilitation of patellofemoral dysfunction in the athlete. *Clinics in Sports Medicine*, 8, (4) 841–860

Besser, M.I.B. and Stahl, S. (1986) Arthroscopic surgery performed under local anaesthesia as an outpatient procedure. *Archives of Orthopaedic Trauma and Surgery*, 105, 296–297

Brody, D.M. (1980) Running injuries. *Clinical Symposia*, 32,(4) Ciba Pharmaceutical Company

Buckley, J.R., Hood, G.M. and Macrae, W. (1989) Arthroscopy under local anaesthesia. *Journal of Bone and Joint Surgery*, 71B, 126–127

Colosimo, A.J. and Bassett, F.H. (1990) Jumpers knee – diagnosis and treatment. *Orthopaedic Review*, 19, (2), 139–149

Committee on complications of arthroscopy association of North America (1985) Complications of arthroscopy and arthroscopic surgery: results of a national survey. *Arthroscopy*, 1, 214–220

Cox, A.J. (1990) Biomechanics of the patello-femoral joint. *Clinical Biomechanics*, 5, 123–130

Daniel, D.M., Stone, M.L., Barnett, P. and Sachs, R. (1988) Use of the quadriceps active test to diagnose posterior cruciate ligament disruption and measure posterior laxity of the knee. *Journal of Bone and Joint Surgery*, 70A, 386–391

David, J.M. (1989) Jumper's knee. *Journal of Orthopaedic and Sports Physical Therapy*, 11, (4) 137–141

de Andrade, J.R., Grant, C. and Dixon, A. (1965) Joint distention and reflex muscle inhibition in the knee. *Journal of Bone and Joint Surgery*, 47, (A) 313–322

DeHaven, K.E., Black, K.P. and Griffiths, H.J. (1989) Open meniscus repair: technique and two to nine year results. *American Journal of Sports Medicine*, 17, 788–795

DiVeta, J. A. and Vogelbach, W. D. (1992) The clinical efficacy of the A-angle in measuring patellar alignment. *Journal of Orthopaedic and Sports Physical Therapy*, 16, (3) 136–139

Donaldson, W.F., Warren, R.F. and Wickiewicz, T. (1985) A comparison of acute anterior cruciate ligament examinations. *American Journal of Sports Medicine*, 13, 5–10

Evans, P. (1986) *The Knee Joint: a Clinical Guide*, Churchill Livingstone, London

Exler, Y. (1991) Patella fracture: review of the literature and five case presentations. *Journal of Orthopaedic and Sports Physical Therapy*, 13,(4) 177–183

Fairbank, T.J. (1948) Knee joint changes after meniscectomy. *Journal of Bone and Joint Surgery*, 30B, (4) 664–670

Ferretti, A. (1986) Epidemiology of jumper's knee. *Sports Medicine*, 3, 289–295

Finsterbush, A. Frankl, U. and Mann, G. (1989) Fat pad adhesion to partially torn anterior cruciate ligament: a

cause of knee locking. *American Journal of Sports Medicine*, 17, (1)

Fowler, P.J. and Messieh, S.S. (1987) Isolated posterior cruciate ligament injuries in athletes. *American Journal of Sports Medicine*, 15, 553–557

Fulkerson, J.P. (1982) Awareness of the retinaculum in evaluating patello-femoral pain. *American Journal of Sports Medicine*, 10, 147–149

Garrick, J.G. and Webb, D.R (1990) *Sports Injuries: Diagnosis and Management*, W.B. Saunders, London

Gose, J.C. and Schweizer, P.(1989) Iliotibial band tightness. *Journal of Orthopaedic and Sports Physical Therapy*, 10, (10) 399–407

Grass, A.L. (1978) Treatment of Osgood–Schlatter injury. *Journal of the American Medical Association*, 240, 212–213

Gruber, M.A. (1979) The conservative treatment of chondromalacia patellae. *Orthopedic Clinics of North America*, 10, (1) 105–115

Hammesfahr, R. (1989) Surgery of the knee. In *Orthopaedic Physical Therapy*, (ed. R. Donatelli and M.J. Wooden), Churchill Livingstone, London

Henning, C.E. (1988) Semilunar cartilage of the knee: function and pathology. *Exercise and Sports Science Review*, 16, 205–213

Hertling, D. and Kessler, R.M. (1990) *Management of Common Musculoskeletal Disorders*, J.B. Lippincott, Philadelphia

Insall, J. (1979) Chondromalacia patellae: patellar malalignment syndrome. *Orthopedic Clinics of North America*, 10, 117–127

Jensen, K. (1990) Manual laxity tests for anterior cruciate ligament injuries. *Journal of Orthopaedic and Sports Physical Therapy*, 11, (10) 474–481

Jerosch, J.G., Castro, W.H.M. and Jantea, C. (1989) Stress fracture of the patella. *American Journal of Sports Medicine*, 17, 4

Kahn, D. and Wilson, M. (1987) Bone scintigraphic findings in patellar tendinitis. *Journal of Nuclear Medicine*, 28, 1768–1770

Keene, J.S. (1990) Ligament and muscle tendon unit injuries. In *Orthopaedic and Sports Physical Therapy*, 2nd edn, (ed. J.A. Gould), Mosby, St Louis, pp. 137–165

Kelley, M.J. (1990) Meniscal trauma (of the knee) and surgical intervention. *Journal of Sports Medicine and Physical Fitness*, 30, (3) 297–306

Key, J., Johnson, D., Jarvis, G. and Ponsonby, D. (1989) Knee and thigh injuries. In *Sports Medicine of the Lower Extremity*, (ed. S.I. Subotnick), Churchill Livingstone, London

Koshino, T. and Okamoto, R. (1985) Resection of painful shelf (Plica synovialis mediopatellaris) under arthroscopy. *Arthroscopy*, 1, 136–141

Levi, J.H. and Coleman, C.R. (1976) Fractures of the tibial tubercle. *American Journal of Sports Medicine*, 4, 253–263

Levine, J. and Kashyap, S. (1981) A new conservative treatment of Osgood-Schlatter's disease. *Clinical Orthopaedics and Related Research*, **158**, 126–128

Levy, I.M., Torzilli, P.A. and Warren, R.F. (1982) The effect of medial meniscectomy on anterior-posterior motion of the knee. *Journal of Bone and Joint Surgery*, **64**, 883–888

McConnell, J. (1986) The management of chondromalacia patella: a long term solution. *Australian Journal of Physiotherapy*, **31**, 214–223

Ngo, I.U., Hamilton, W.G., Wichern, W.A. and Andree, R.A. (1985) Local anesthesia with sedation for arthroscopic surgery of the knee: a report of 100 consecutive cases. *Arthroscopy*, **1**, 237–241

Noyes, F.R., Mooar, L.A., Moorman, C.T. and McGinnis, G.H. (1989) Partial tears of the anterior cruciate ligament: progression to complete ligament deficiency. *Journal of Bone and Joint Surgery*, **71B**, 825–833

Noyes, F.R., Mangine, R.E. and Barber, S. (1987) Early motion after open and arthroscopic anterior cruciate ligament reconstruction. *American Journal of Sports Medicine*, **15**, 149–160

Noyes, F.R., Butler, D.L. and Grood, E.S. (1984) Biomechanical analysis of human ligament grafts used in knee ligament repairs and reconstructions. *Journal of Bone and Joint Surgery*, **66A**, 344–352

O'Donoghue, D.H. (1976) *Treatment of injuries to athletes*, W.B. Saunders, Philadelphia

Palastanga, N., Field, D. and Soames, R. (1989) *Anatomy and Human Movement*, Heinemann Medical, Oxford

Palmitier, R.A., An. K., Scott, S.G. and Chao, E.Y.S. (1991) Kinetic chain exercise in knee rehabilitation. *Sports Medicine*, **11**, (6) 402–413

Parolie, J.M. and Bergfeld, J.A. (1986) Long term results of nonoperative treatment of isolated posterior cruciate ligament injuries in the athlete. *American Journal of Sports Medicine*, **14**, 53–38

Ray, J.M., Clancy, W.G. and Lemon, R.A. (1988) Semimembranosus tendinitis: an overlooked cause of medial knee pain. *American Journal of Sports Medicine*, **16**, (4), 347–351

Ryu, R.K.N. and Dunbar, W.H. (1988) Arthroscopic meniscal repair with two-year follow-up: a clinical review. *Arthroscopy*, **4**, 168–173

Sachs, R.A., Daniel, D.M., Stone, M.L. and Garfein, R.F. (1989) Patellofemoral problems after anterior cruciate ligament reconstruction. *American Journal of Sports Medicine*, **17**, 760–765

Sandberg, R., Nilsson, B. and Westlin, N. (1987) Hinged cast after knee ligament surgery. *American Journal of Sports Medicine*, **15**, 270–274

Saunders, H.D. (1989) *Assessing Flexibility and Strength in Industrial Workers*, Educational Opportunities, Bloomington

Seedhom, B.B. and Hargreaves, D.J. (1979) Transmission of the load in the knee joint with special reference to the role of the menisci. Part II: Experimental results, discussion and conclusions. *Engineering Medicine*, **8**, 220–228

Sherman, O.H., Fox, J.M., Snyder, S.J., Pizzo, W.D., Friedman, M.J., Ferkel, R.D. and Lawley, M.J. (1986) Arthroscopy- 'No problem surgery'. An analysis of complications in two thousand six hundred and forty cases. *Journal of Bone and Joint Surgery*, **68A**, 256–265

Shino, K., Kimura, T., Hirose, H., Inoue, M. and Ono, K. (1986) Reconstruction of the anterior cruciate ligament by allogenic tendon graft: an operation for chronic ligamentous insufficiency. *Journal of Bone and Joint Surgery*, **68B**, 739–746

Silver, D.M., Campbell, P. (1985) Arthroscopic assessment and treatment of dancers knee injuries. *Physician and Sportsmedicine*, **13**, (11) 74–82

Smillie, I.S. (1974) *Diseases of the Knee Joint*, Churchill Livingstone, London

Speakman, H.G.B. and Weisberg, J. (1977) The vastus medialis controversy. *Physiotherapy*, **63**, (8) 249–254

Stokes, M. and Young, A. (1984) The contribution of reflex inhibition to arthrogenous muscle weakness. *Clinical Science*, **67**, 7–14

Tiberio, D. (1987) The effect of excessive subtalar joint pronation on patellofemoral mechanics: a theoretical model. *Journal of Orthopaedic and Sports Physical Therapy*, **9**, (4) 160–165

Torg, J.S. (1989) In *Year Book of Sports Medicine*, (ed. R.J. Shephard, J.L. Anderson, E.R. Eichner et al.) Yearbook Medical Publishers, Chicago, pp. 186

Traverso, A., Baldari, A. and Catalani, F. (1990) The coexistence of Osgood–Schlatter's disease with Sinding–Larsen–Johansson's disease. *Journal of Sports Medicine and Physical Fitness*, **30**,(3) 331–333

Tsirbas, A., Paterson, R.S. and Keene, G.C.R. (1991) Fat pad impingement; a missed cause of patellofemoral pain? *Australian Journal of Science and Medicine in Sport*, **23**, (1) 24–26

Warwick, R. and Williams, P.L. (1973) *Gray's Anatomy*, 35th edn. Longman, Harlow

Weiss, C.B., Lundberg, M., Hamberg, P., DeHaven, K.E., and Gillquist, J. (1989) Non-operative treatment of meniscal tears. *Journal of Bone and Joint Surgery*, **71A**, 811–822

Williams, J.G.P. and Sperryn, P.N. (1976) *Sports Medicine*, Edward Arnold, London

Wilson, W.J., Lewis, F. and Scranton, P.E. (1990) Combined reconstruction of the anterior cruciate ligament in competitive athletes. *Journal of Bone and Joint Surgery*, **72A**, (5) 742–748

# 12 Shin pain

The term 'shin splints' is often used as a blanket description of any persistent pain occurring between the knee and the ankle in an athlete. More accurate descriptions are provided by the various 'compartment syndromes' which identify the anatomical structures affected. The anterior compartment contains the tibialis anterior, extensor hallucis longus and extensor digitorum longus. The lateral compartment contains the peronei. The superficial posterior compartment contains the gastrocnemius and soleus and the deep posterior compartment contains the tibialis posterior, flexor digitorum longus and flexor hallucis longus (Fig. 12.1).

## Anterior compartment syndrome

Anterior compartment syndrome involves pain in the anterior lower leg, which is increased in resisted dorsiflexion. There is usually a history of a sudden increase in training intensity, frequently involving jumping or running on a hard surface. The anterior compartment muscles swell, and in some cases hypertrophy occurs. The fascia covering the muscles may be too tight and inflexible to accommodate the increase in size. As a consequence, when the muscles relax, their intramuscular pressure remains high and fresh blood is unable to perfuse the tissues freely. This decrease in blood

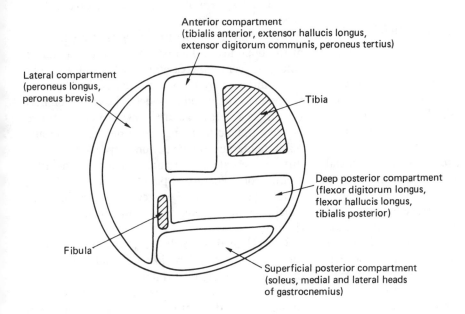

Anterior compartment
(tibialis anterior, extensor hallucis longus,
extensor digitorum communis, peroneus tertius)

Lateral compartment
(peroneus longus,
peroneus brevis)

Tibia

Deep posterior compartment
(flexor digitorum longus,
flexor hallucis longus,
tibialis posterior)

Fibula

Superficial posterior compartment
(soleus, medial and lateral heads
of gastrocnemius)

**Figure 12.1**   Compartments of the lower leg.

flow leads to ischaemia with associated pain and impairment of muscle function.

Usually, when a muscle contracts, its blood flow is temporarily stopped. Arterial inflow occurs once more between the muscle contractions as the intramuscular pressure falls. Normal resting pressure within the tibialis anterior in the supine subject is about 5–10 mm Hg, increasing to as much as 150–250 mm Hg with muscle contraction. Muscle relaxation pressure, that which occurs between repeated contractions, is between 15–25 mm Hg in the normal subject, but in athletes with anterior compartment syndrome pressures may rise to 30–35 mm Hg and take up to 15 minutes to return to normal values (Styf, 1989).

The exact cause of the condition is not known. Hypertrophy may be one factor, as the condition occurs frequently when training intensity is increased. However, bodybuilders rarely suffer from the condition, so the rate, rather than the amount, of muscle hypertrophy may be important. Microtrauma and excessive stress to the blood capillaries and lymphatics may give rise to inflammation and, in some cases, myositis in the area (Styf, 1989).

## Lateral compartment and superficial peroneal nerve

This is an unusual cause of shin pain and occurs when the peronei muscles are affected, usually by hyperpronation (Brody, 1980). The condition may have existed for some time, but is brought to the fore when running begins. Again, there is ischaemia and pain, but in addition the superficial peroneal nerve may be compressed as it emerges from the lateral compartment.

The nerve lies deep to the peroneus longus and then passes forwards and downwards between the peronei and the extensor digitorum longus. It pierces the fascia in the distal third of the leg, where it divides into medial and lateral branches to enter the foot. Entrapment may occur if muscle herniation or fascial defect exist. In addition, ankle sprain, fasciotomy, and an anomalous course of the nerve have been suggested as contributory factors (Styf, 1989). Clinically, the patient presents with

loss of sensation over the dorsum of the foot, especially the second to fourth toes. Certain resting positions may compress the nerve and bring on the symptoms. To test the nerve, it is compressed over the anterior intermuscular septum 8–15 cm proximal to the lateral malleolus while the patient actively dorsiflexes and everts the foot. Tinel's sign, involving local percussion over the compression site, may be positive.

## Posterior compartment

The superficial compartment contains the soleus and gastrocnemius. These muscles are usually affected by trauma, rather than ischaemia, and are dealt with separately below.

The deep posterior compartment contains the tibialis posterior, flexor digitorum longus and flexor hallucis longus, and is the most common site for shin pain. Pain in this region is usually experienced over the distal third of the tibia and represents 'medial tibial stress syndrome' (Mubarak et al., 1982). The exact site of pain will vary depending on the specific structures affected. Detmer (1986) described a system of classification involving three types of chronic condition.

Type I involves microfractures or stress fracture of the bone itself. The patient is usually a runner who has recently increased his or her mileage. The stress imposed by the sport exceeds the ability of the bone to adapt and remodel. The condition may present as a stress fracture showing a concentrated positive uptake in a single area on bone scan and point tenderness to palpation (type IA), or as a diffuse area along the medial edge of the tibia giving more generalized pain (type IB). In chronic conditions which have existed for some time, the tibial edge may be uneven due to new bone formation.

Type II medial tibial stress syndrome involves the junction of the periosteum and fascia, and occurs particularly in sprinters, and those involved in jumping activities. Pain is maximal just posterior to the bone, and has often persisted for a number of years. Initially, pain occurs only with activity, but as the condition progresses discomfort is felt with walking and even at rest. In this condition compartment pressures may not be elevated, and the periosteum is unchanged. One explanation is that the periosteum is traumatically avulsed from the bone by the action of the soleus through its attachment to the fascia. During the chronic stage of this condition, adipose tissue has been found, during surgery, between the periosteum and underlying bone (Detmer, 1986). In the early stages of the condition the periosteum may heal back with rest, but when the condition becomes chronic, it is unable to heal, and continues to cause pain when stressed by activity.

The type III condition involves ischaemia of the distal deep posterior compartment, and presents as a dull aching over the posterior soft tissues brought on by exercise. Intramuscular pressures are elevated, as in anterior compartment syndrome (see above), and remain elevated after exercise.

## Management

Initial management of shin pain involves a reduction of the stresses which caused the condition. This involves accurately identifying the structures affected and taking a thorough history of causal factors, particularly stresses imposed during training. Biomechanical assessment of the lower limb is mandatory and prescription of orthotics should be made where necessary. Initially, rest and anti-inflammatory modalities are used to allow the acute inflammation to settle, but external compression and elevation of the limb may exacerbate the problem (Di Manna and Buck, 1990). If training stresses can be modified and the condition has been identified early enough this may be all that is required.

In chronic conditions in which conservative management has failed, decompression by fasciotomy may be called for. Here, the fascia of the affected compartment is surgically split along its length. The procedure is often performed on an out-patient basis, with two incisions being made, at the junction of the proximal and middle third of the leg and the middle and distal third. Athletes mobilize early and are often able to resume running after 3 weeks.

If fasciotomy is not successful, it may be the case that the epimysium over the tibialis posterior has been missed at surgery. Hannaford (1988) argued that the tibialis posterior should be classified as a condition independent from that affecting the other deep posterior muscles.

## Osteogenic causes of shin pain

The tibia and fibula are common sites for stress fractures, especially in runners. Posteromedial pain can occur in the tibia as a result of stress fracture (Devas, 1958). Pain may be mild at first, but increases in intensity as training is continued, until eventually the athlete is forced to rest. Pain typically occurs at the end of a run. As time goes on symptoms occur with daily activities, and eventually even during rest. Pain initially occurs without radiographic changes, although a bone scan may be revealing. However, the bone scan itself may be positive in the absence of symptoms (Groshar et al., 1985) so a number of factors must be considered before an accurate diagnosis can be made.

Accuracy in palpation when assessing bone pain is perhaps the most useful measure. The tenderness of a stress fracture is usually well localized, whereas that of compartment syndrome is more diffuse. The usual history is of a recent change in activity. It is obviously important to determine the mechanism of injury if a recurrence is to be prevented. The athlete will commonly limp, and swelling may be evident in the later stages of the condition if the bony surface is superficial.

Rest is the most important component of treatment of this condition. This should be total, because even allowing an athlete to train the upper body will often result in him or her 'just trying the leg out' in the gymnasium. Training should not resume until the athlete has been totally pain-free for 10 days. It should be emphasized to the athlete that this means that at the end of each day they should go to bed having felt no pain over the injured area in that entire day. When activity is resumed, the athlete should be closely monitored, and activities stopped if any pain occurs.

The return to sport should be progressive and varied. Different speed, running surfaces and activities should all be used to spread the emphasis of training. Alternative training should be used, to reduce the weight bearing on the limb. Swimming and cycling may be utilized to restore cardiopulmonary fitness for example.

Following lower limb fracture, a bony link may form between the tibia and fibula (tibiofibular synostosis). Pain typically occurs after an injury, and increases during vigorous activity, mimicking stress fracture. The synostosis is revealed by X-ray and removed surgically (Flandry and Sanders, 1987).

## Tennis leg

Of the sural muscles, it is the gastrocnemius which is usually injured. The soleus is infrequently affected being a single-joint muscle, but is more usually the victim of temporary ischaemia, giving rise to superficial posterior compartment syndrome.

Tennis leg is a strain of the gastrocnemius, normally involving the medial head at its musculotendinous junction with the Achilles tendon. The history of injury is usually a sudden propulsive action, such as a lunge or jump as the athlete pushes off from the mark. Women are more commonly affected, and the athlete is usually over 30 years of age (Garrick and Webb, 1990). The condition is often described as a rupture of the plantaris, more by tradition than anything else, because this muscle is rarely the cause of symptoms.

The athlete often feels something 'go' in the back of the leg as though he or she were hit from behind. Pain and spasm occur rapidly, preventing the athlete from putting his or her heel to the ground. Later, swelling and bruising develop distal to the injury site, peaking at 48 hours after injury. There is local tenderness over the medial head of gastrocnemius, at the junction between the middle and proximal third of the calf. Pain to passive stretch is worse with the knee straight than with it flexed.

Initial treatment is to immobilize the calf to prevent further tissue damage. Some authorities recommend a plantarflexed position with a 2–4 cm

heel lift (Cyriax, 1982), while others claim that a 90° neutral ankle position gives a better result by preventing contraction and tightening the fascia to limit the spread of bruising (Garrick and Webb, 1990). Pain and the amount of tissue damage is usually the deciding factor. Partial ruptures are best immobilized non-weight-bearing in plantarflexion to approximate the tissue, whereas less serious injuries can be prevented from shortening by adopting a neutral resting position.

Compression from an elastic bandage limits the formation of swelling, and strength and flexibility is maintained by starting rehabilitation early. Massage involving calf kneading and transverse frictions ensures adequate broadening of the muscle fibres. Stretching to the gastrocnemius begins in the long sitting position. A towel or band is placed over the foot and the athlete gently pulls the foot into dorsiflexion. Stretching with the toes on a block in a partial, and later full weight-bearing position is the exercise progression. Strength is regained by utilizing a comparable long sitting position but substituting an elastic band for the strap. The foot is pressed into plantarflexion against the resistance of the band. Heel raises are performed in a standing position, initially from the floor and later with the heel on a 2–3 cm block.

Gait re-education is used to encourage equal stride length and the adoption of a normal heel–toe rhythm avoiding external rotation of the leg. When the calf is pain free, strength activities give way to power movements. Gentle jogging, jumping and skipping are used and progressed to toe springing (knees braced) and leg drives from a mark.

## Achilles tendon

The Achilles tendon is some 15 cm long and about 2 cm thick. It originates from the musculotendinous junction of the calf muscles, the soleus inserts lower down on the deep surface of the tendon. The Achilles tendon gradually becomes more rounded as it travels distally, and flares out to insert into the posterior aspect of the calcaneum. The tendon is separated from the calcaneum by the retrocalcaneal bursa and from the skin by the subcutaneous calcaneal bursa.

The whole tendon rotates through 90° as it descends, so that the medial fibres become posterior by the time the tendon attaches to the calcaneum. This rotation is thought to account in part for the elastic properties of the tendon, giving it an elastic recoil when stretched. In the running action, as the lower limb moves from heel strike to midstance, the Achilles tendon is stretched, storing elastic energy. At toe off, the tendon recoils, releasing its stored energy and reducing the work required from the calf muscles to propel the body forwards.

The Achilles tendon is surrounded by a soft membranous paratenon which is continuous proximally with the muscle fascia and distally with the calcaneal periosteum. The blood supply to the tendon is from either end and from the paratenon itself, but a relatively avascular zone exists between 2 and 6 cm proximal to the tendon insertion. Under normal circumstances, blood vessels do not travel from the paratenon to the tendon substance, and removal of the paratenon does not seem to compromise the blood supply (Williams, 1986). Tendon tissue in general has a low metabolic rate, and this, coupled with the poor blood supply to the tendon, means that the structure has a slow rate of healing.

Injuries to the Achilles tendon fall broadly into one of two categories. First, those which affect the tendon substance (partial or complete rupture), and, secondly, injury to the surface of the tendon and its covering (tendinitis or peritendinitis).

### Tendinitis

Tendinitis presents as a swelling of the Achilles tendon of gradual onset. The main change is a disruption of the ground substance, causing the tendon fibres to separate, which in turn leads to degeneration.

In peritendinitis the paratenon is inflamed and thickened, and there is local oedema and crepitus. Kager's triangle (the space between the inner surface of the Achilles tendon, the deep flexors and the calcaneus) is obliterated. Hard, scarred bands appear within the paratenon and adhesions develop between the Achilles tendon and surrounding tissue. Kvist et al. (1988) showed that the fatty tissue surrounding the tendon was still thickened and swollen, after nearly two years in subjects with paratenonitis (peritendinitis). Connective tissue had increased, and local blood vessels had degenerated or been obliterated, suggesting the presence of immature scar tissue.

Initial management of tendinitis or peritendinitis is aimed at reducing local oedema. Rest and ice are used in conjunction with electrotherapy modalities aimed at reducing pain and resolving inflammation. Transverse friction massage has been used extensively (Cyriax and Cyriax, 1983), for both the teno-osseous junction and the tendon itself. The teno-osseous junction may be frictioned with the patient prone and the foot plantarflexed. The therapist uses the side of his or her flexed forefingers to impart the friction, pulling the hands distally against the curved insertion of the Achilles tendon into the calcaneum. The musculotendinous junction is frictioned with the foot dorsiflexed and the tendon gripped from above between the finger and thumb. The movement is perpendicular to the tendon fibres. The tendon sheath may be treated by placing the length of the finger alongside the tendon and pressing inwards. The forearm is pronated/supinated to impart the friction.

A heel raise is used to reduce the stretch on the tendon, and the calf may be strapped in plantarflexion. If pain is intense the patient should initially be non-weight-bearing.

### Tendon substance

Focal degeneration may occur in the Achilles tendon in athletes in their early 30s. The onset is usually gradual, giving highly localized pain. Microscopically there is proliferation of capillary cells and lacunae along the tendon fibres leading to a loss of the normal wavy alignment of collagen.

Tendon rupture generally occurs later in an athlete's life, being more common from the late 30s to mid-40s. With partial rupture, a few fibres or nearly all of the tendon may be affected. The characteristic history is one of sudden onset. There is swelling, pain on resisted movement, and the patient is unable to support his or her weight through the toes of the affected foot.

In complete rupture there is usually a single incident in which the patient feels a sudden sharp 'give' in the tendon as though he or she had been struck from behind. Immediately afterwards there may be little pain but gross weakness. The patient is again unable to take his or her weight through the toes. Active plantarflexion is minimal, being accomplished by the peronei and posterior tibial muscles only. With the patient in a prone position, Simmond's test may be performed. The calf is squeezed, and the foot fails to plantarflex. Closer examination reveals a depression (the Toygar angle) which is visible in the normal smooth contour of the Achilles tendon. If the athlete is not examined until a number of days after injury, this hollow will have been bridged by haematoma and scar tissue, giving a raised fibrous area unless the tendon ends have retracted. Without surgery, the tendon will heal, but very slowly. Granulation tissue forms poorly, partly due to repeated use, and partly as a result of the anticoagulant effect of synovial fluid contained by the unruptured paratenon (Williams, 1986).

Lesions of the tendon may be differentiated from those of the paratenon by using the 'painful arc' sign (Williams, 1986). The point of maximum tenderness is palpated as the foot is dorsiflexed and plantarflexed. When only the tendon is affected, the painful area will move up and down as the tendon moves. However, when the paratenon is affected, as the tendon slides within its sheath, the area of maximum pain remains fixed (Fig. 12.2).

When examining the patient it must be remembered that the Achilles tendon is normally painful to palpation, so the intensity of discomfort must always be compared with that of the contra-lateral limb.

Surgical management of Achilles tendon injuries carries a high rate of complication. Williams (1986) described complications in 64 out of 461 surgical procedures (13.9%). These included mainly wound dehiscence (bursting), scar hypertrophy, and wound infection. Surgery may be necessary if conservative management has failed and symptoms have persisted for more than 3 months.

Achilles tendon repair is the subject of considerable debate. Many authors claim that conservative treatment does not allow direct realignment of the torn tendon fibres and so the repair is less secure. In addition, they claim that re-rupture of surgically treated injuries is less likely (Turbo and Spinella, 1987). Others argue that the risk of surgical complications is too great, and that the sophistication of rehabilitation is as important to the eventual outcome of the condition as whether the surgical or non-surgical route was chosen (Garrick and Webb, 1990). A number of repair methods have been described, including direct suture, reinforcement with plantaris or peroneus brevis tendon, and reconstruction using carbon fibre or polypropylene mesh.

Whatever the surgical method used, following immobilization the main problem is initially lack of flexibility, to the Achilles tendon, ankle, and subtalar joint in particular. Intense rehabilitation of the foot, ankle and leg is needed to regain full function.

## Rehabilitation following surgery

To begin with stretching procedures are begun non-weight-bearing. It is usually sufficient to hook a towel over the forefoot and gently pull it into dorsiflexion. Partial weight-bearing activities in a sitting position are used to begin the closed kinetic chain exercises, with the athlete gently pressing into dorsiflexion using varying foot angles. The same starting positions are chosen for early static and later dynamic strength training using straps and elastic bands. Isokinetics is used for the calf specifically and the lower limb in general.

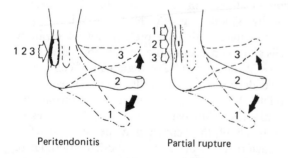

Peritendonitis          Partial rupture

**Figure 12.2** The 'painful arc' in diagnosis of Achilles tendon pain. If the lesion is in the tendon, the point of maximum tenderness moves with excursion into dorsi- or plantar-flexion. In peritendinitis it remains fixed. From Williams (1986), with permission.

Walking re-education using parallel bars or sticks introduces functional movements and introduces skill work. When full weight-bearing activities are begun the flexibility and strength work is progressed and augmented with skill training involving balance and co-ordination exercises (see ankle rehabilitation p. 206) and further walking re-education.

Both static and dynamic flexibility training is used from the earliest stages, and eccentric actions are begun as soon as possible (often in the swimming pool to limit weight-bearing) to mimic the true function of the Achilles tendon. When function has improved sufficiently, walking pace is increased and speed walking introduced, followed by on-the-spot and, later, small-step jogging. Straight running, zig-zags, and circle running are all used. Thick-heeled training shoes are used, and gradually the heel is lowered. Toe walking progresses to jogging on the toes, springing, and finally hopping, skipping and jumping.

General fitness is maintained throughout the programme by cardiopulmonary activities in the swimming pool (assuming good healing of the scar) and, later, static cycle riding, until the intensity of rehabilitation itself is sufficient to challenge aerobic fitness. Pain is the rate limiting factor for both exercise intensity and progression.

Assuming that the surgery has been totally successful, the final stages of training must include the use of plyometric exercise to develop elastic strength. Poor results can be expected if the rehabilitation programme is stopped at the stage of heavy isotonic exercise and not progressed in terms of speed.

## Aetiology

A number of factors may combine to cause Achilles tendon pain, including training alterations, footwear and flexibility. Alterations in training type or intensity, such as a sudden increase in the distance run over a holiday period, or more intensive training in the lead-up to a competition, can both produce problems.

Footwear is an important factor. Inadequate shock-absorbing properties stress the Achilles tendon during eccentric loading, a situation which is aggravated if an athlete has a rigid cavus foot. Good shock-absorption of the shoe heel is important for athletes who exercise on a hard surface. In addition to reducing the impact at heel strike, the height of the heel will also reduce the stretch on the Achilles tendon. A rigid sole lengthens the ankle to forefoot lever arm, affecting the Achilles tendon mechanics, but may be necessary to protect the first toe (see p. 212). If the heel counter of a sports shoe is hard, it can abrade the Achilles tendon as the foot plantarflexes at toe off. A negative heel counter, or a soft tab, is to be encouraged.

Lack of flexibility in the calf and Achilles tendon may contribute greatly to injury. When flexibility is limited, the tendon loses some of its elastic recoil, making it more susceptible to damage due to rapid eccentric loading of the calf in mid-stance. Flexibility exercises should be used for prevention and management of the sub-acute injury. Stretching may be performed with the forefoot on an angled block. The heel is kept on the ground and the hip is pressed forward, bringing the knee over the forefoot and increasing dorsiflexion. The exercise is first performed with the knee locked to stretch the gastrocnemius, and then with the knee flexed to 20° to stress the Achilles tendon and soleus. A static stretch is used and held for 20–30 seconds. The range of motion is generally greater when the tendon is warm, after a hot shower or bath for example.

Malalignment of the lower limb is probably a contributory factor to Achilles tendon pain, although as these faults have generally been present for some time before the Achilles tendon condition started they are unlikely to be the sole cause. Increased pronation of the foot stresses the medial aspect of the Achilles tendon. A 30° increase in rearfoot position has been shown to lengthen these fibres by 10% (Nichols, 1989). In addition, excessive tibial rotation caused by hyperpronation will twist the Achilles tendon fibres together 'wringing them out'. This will close any blood vessels between the tendon fibres, temporarily reducing an already poor blood supply. In an interesting survey of 109 runners with Achilles tendon problems, Clement, Taunton and Smart (1984) found 75% showed training errors, 56% demonstrated hyperpronation, 39% suffered inflexibility of the calf, and 10% wore improper footwear.

The effect of corticosteroids on ligament failure has been discussed on p. 42. Inhibition of collagen synthesis, reduction in the speed of tendon repair, lower elastic limit, and fatty degeneration have all been described (Nichols, 1989). Various studies have shown an increased likelihood of Achilles tendon rupture after injection (Chechick et al., 1982; Kleinman and Gross, 1983; Urban, 1989). Cyriax (1982) argued that Achilles tendon rupture only occurred when an incorrect injection technique was used, the corticosteroid being introduced into the tendon substance rather than along its surface. However, Williams (1986) claimed that both techniques had been shown to precipitate rupture, and further argued that the benefits of such injections were relatively short-lived. In addition, he contested that in acute peritendinitis, similar results could be obtained using a local anaesthetic and hyaluronidase.

## Retrocalcaneal pain

### Sever's disease

Calcaneal apophysitis (Sever's disease) may occur in adolescents during the rapid growth spurt, sometimes in association with Achilles tendon pain itself. Sever's disease is more common in boys than girls, and occurs at the time of fusion of the apophysis to the calcaneum, between the ages of 11 and 15 years. The condition is inappropriately named, as rather than a disease entity it is a traction injury.

On examination, there is tenderness to medial and lateral heel compression, but no noticeable skin changes. Radiographically, sclerosis and irregularity of the calcaneal apophysis is seen as a result of avascular necrosis (Caspi, Ezra and Horoszowski, 1989). Associated Achilles tendon tightness has been described, with the affected side showing 4–5° less passive dorsiflexion than the unaffected side (Mitcheli and Ireland, 1987).

Initially, total rest is called for to allow the condition to settle. Later, any sporting activity which exacerbates the pain is avoided, and shock-absorbing heel pads are used in all shoes. Achilles tendon stretching is taught to restore dorsiflexion range.

### Haglund's syndrome

Haglund's syndrome is present when an exostosis is found over the posterior lateral aspect of the calcaneum. Radiographically, a spur of bone is seen coming from the calcaneal insertion of the Achilles tendon, showing as a prominence of the posterior superior calcaneal angle (Wooten and Chandler, 1990). Assessment of radiographs may be made by comparing 'parallel pitch lines' (Pavlov et al., 1982). The first line joins the anterior and posterior calcaneal tubercles. A second line is drawn parallel to the first, but this time starting from the posterior lip of the talar articulation (Fig. 12.3). If the posterior superior calcaneal angle stands prominent to this second line, the diagnosis is positive.

In addition to the bony changes, a painful soft tissue swelling (pump bump) is noted at the insertion of the Achilles tendon. This swelling can vary in size and shape depending on the stage of the condition. Haglund's syndrome commonly exists in association with retrocalcaneal bursitis, the inflamed bursa becoming visible on X-ray when low penetrating radiation is used (Rossi et al., 1987).

Contributory factors to the formation of Haglund's syndrome include a hard edge to the posterior aspect of the shoe (heel tab) and a rearfoot varus. As the foot is plantarflexed, the hard heel tab will abrade the posterior aspect of the calcaneum. If a rearfoot varus exists, compensatory pronation will cause the heel to twist in the shoe and soft tissue pressure occurs over the posterior calcaneum. Although soft tissue changes could be expected from abrasion of this type, bony changes are less likely. The bony change itself could be the result of a secondary ossification centre in the calcaneus (Horn and Subotnick, 1989).

Management of retrocalcaneal pain is by pain relief until the condition settles. A horseshoe pad made from non-compressible rubber is placed over the painful calcaneal area, and held in place by an ankle sock. A heel raise may be used to reduce stress through the tendon on to the calcaneus, and

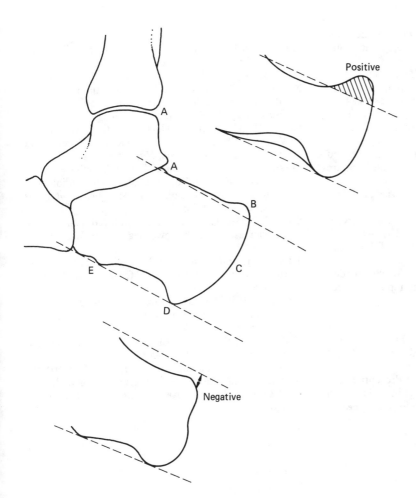

**Figure 12.3** Parallel pitch lines to determine the position of the posterior superior calcaneal angle. A, posterior lip of talar articulation; B, posterior superior calcaneal angle; C, posterior calcaneal tuberosity; D, medial calcaneal tuberosity; E, anterior calcaneal tuberosity. After Rossi et al. (1987).

gentle tendon stretching is taught. Electrotherapy modalities are used to alleviate pain and reduce inflammation.

## References

Brody, D.M. (1980) Running injuries. *Clinical Symposia*, **32**, (4) Ciba Pharmaceutical Company, New Jersey

Caspi, I., Ezra, E. and Horoszowski, H. (1989) Partial apophysectomy in Sever's disease. *Journal of Orthopaedic and Sports Physical Therapy*, **10**, (9) 390–373

Chechick, A., Amit, Y., Israli, A. and Horoszowki, H. (1982) Recurrent rupture of the achilles tendon in-duced by corticosteroid injection. *British Journal of Sports Medicine*, **16**, 89–90

Clement, D.B., Taunton, J.E. and Smart, G.W. (1984) Achilles tendinitis and peritendinitis: aetiology and treatment. *American Journal of Sports Medicine*, **12**, 179–184

Cyriax, J.H. and Cyriax, P.J. (1983) *Illustrated Manual of Orthopaedic Medicine*, Butterworth, London

Cyriax, J. (1982) *Textbook of Orthopaedic Medicine* Vol. one, 8th edn, Baillière Tindall, London

Detmer, D.E. (1986) Chronic shin splints: classification and management of medial tibial stress syndrome. *Sports Medicine*, **3**, 436–446

Devas, M.B. (1958) Stress fractures of the tibia or 'shin soreness'. *Journal of Bone and Joint Surgery*, **40**, 227–239

Di Manna, D.L. and Buck, P.G. (1990) Chronic compartment syndrome in athletes: Recognition and treatment. *Athletic Training*, **25**, 1

Flandry, F. and Sanders, R.A. (1987) Tibiofibular synostosis: An unusual cause of shin splint-like pain. *American Journal of Sports Medicine*, **15**, 280–284

Garrick, J.G. and Webb, D.R (1990) *Sports Injuries: Diagnosis and Management*, W.B. Saunders, Philadelphia

Groshar, D., Lam, M., Even-Sapir, E., Israel, O. and Front, D. (1985) Stress fractures and bone pain: are they closely associated? *Injury*, **16**, 526–528

Hannaford, P.G.H. (1988) Shin splints re-visited. *Excel*, **4**, (4) 16–19

Horn, L.M. and Subotnick, S.I (1989) Surgical intervention. In *Sports Medicine of the Lower Extremity*, (ed. S.I. Subotnick), Churchill Livingstone, Edinburgh, pp. 461–566

Kleinman, M. and Gross, A.E. (1983) Achilles tendon rupture following steroid injection: report of three cases. *Journal of Bone and Joint Surgery*, **65A**, 1345–1346

Kvist, M.H., Lehto, M.U.K., Jozsa, L., Jarvinen, M. and Kvist, H.T. (1988) Chronic achilles paratenonitis. *American Journal of Sports Medicine*, **16**, (6) 616–622

Micheli, L.J. and Ireland, M.L. (1987) Prevention and management of calcaneal apophysitis in children: an overuse syndrome. *Journal of Paediatric Orthopaedics*, 7, 34–38

Mubarak, S.J., Gould, R.N., Lee, Y.F. and Schmidt, D.A. (1982). The medial tibial stress syndrome. *American Journal of Sports Medicine*, **10**, 201–205

Nichols, A.W. (1989) Achilles tendinitis in running athletes. *Journal of the American Board of Family Practice*, **2**, (3) 196–203.

Pavlov, H., Henegan, M., Hersch, A., Goldman, A. and Vigorita, V. (1982). The Haglund syndrome: initial and differential diagnosis. *Radiology*, **144**, 83–8.

Rossi, F., La Cava, F., Amato, F. and Pincelli, G. (1987) The Haglund syndrome: clinical and radiological features and sports medicine aspects. *Journal of Sports Medicine*, **27**, 258–265

Styf, J. (1989) Chronic exercise-induced pain in the anterior aspect of the lower leg. *Sports Medicine*, **7**, 331–339

Turco, V.J. and Spinella, A.J. (1987) Achilles tendon ruptures: Peroneus brevis transfer. *Foot and Ankle*, **7**, 253–259

Urban, K (1989) Partial rupture of the achilles tendon in athletes. *Acta Chirurgiae Orthopaedicae et Traumatologiae Cechoslovaca*, **56**, (1) 30–38

Williams, J.G.P. (1986) Achilles tendon lesions in sport. *Sports Medicine*, **3**, 114–135

Wooten, B. and Chandler, J. (1990) Use of an orthotic device in the treatment of posterior heel pain. *Journal of Orthopaedic and Sports Physical Therapy*, **11**, (9) 410–413

# 13 The ankle joint

The joint mechanics of the ankle and foot have been described on pp. 150–152. The ankle joint is the articulation between the trochlear surface of the talus and the distal ends of the tibia and fibula. The synovial membrane of the joint is loose and travels superiorly between the tibia and fibula as far as the interosseous ligament.

## Collateral ligaments

The joint is strengthened by a variety of ligaments, the collateral ligaments being the most important from the point of view of injury. Both medial and lateral collateral ligaments travel from the malleoli, and have bands attaching to the calcaneus and talus.

The medial (deltoid) ligament (Fig. 13.1) is triangular in shape. Its deep portion may be divided into anterior and posterior tibiotalar bands. The more superficial part is split into tibionavicular and tibiocalcaneal portions, which attach in turn to the spring ligament. The lateral ligament (Fig. 13.2) is composed of three separate components, and is somewhat weaker than its medial counterpart. The anterior talofibular (ATF) ligament is a flat band that travels from the anterior tip of the lateral malleolus to the neck of the talus, and

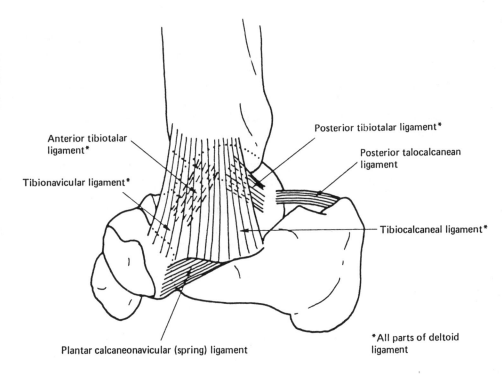

Anterior tibiotalar ligament*

Tibionavicular ligament*

Posterior tibiotalar ligament*

Posterior talocalcanean ligament

Tibiocalcaneal ligament*

Plantar calcaneonavicular (spring) ligament

*All parts of deltoid ligament

**Figure 13.1** The deltoid ligament of the ankle.

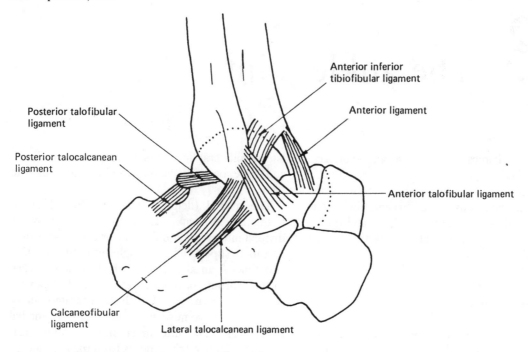

Posterior talofibular ligament

Posterior talocalcanean ligament

Anterior inferior tibiofibular ligament

Anterior ligament

Anterior talofibular ligament

Calcaneofibular ligament

Lateral talocalcanean ligament

**Figure 13.2**   The lateral ligaments of the ankle. From Palastanga, Field and Soames (1989), with permission.

may be considered the primary stabilizer of the ankle joint (Palastanga, Field and Soames, 1989). The posterior talofibular (PTF) ligament travels almost horizontally from the fossa on the bottom of the lateral malleolus to the posterior surface of the talus. Lying between the ATF and PTF ligaments is the calcaneofibular ligament, arising from the front of the lateral malleolus to pass down and back to attach on to the lateral surface of the calcaneum. The role of the collateral ligaments in maintaining talocural stability is summarized in Table 13.1.

## Injury

The most common injury to the ankle is damage to the ATF ligament with or without involvement of the peroneus brevis. The sub-tabloid and mid-tarsal joints may be involved, but these will be dealt with separately for clarity. The typical history of ankle injury is one of inversion, sometimes coupled with plantarflexion. The athlete 'goes over' on the ankle, usually on an uneven surface. One of three

grades of ligament injury may occur (see pp. 40–42). There is usually an egg-shaped swelling in front of, and around, the lateral malleolus. The lateral malleolus should be palpated gently to assess whether bone pain is present; if it is, an X-ray may be required. If palpation reveals tenderness below, rather than over, the lateral malleolus and the athlete is able to bear weight, there is a high probability of soft tissue injury alone (Vargish and Clarke, 1983). Any fracture that is missed by this type of close palpation is likely to be an avulsion or non-displaced hairline type that will respond favourably to management as a sprain (Garrick and Webb, 1990).

Stress tests to the ankle are useful to assess the degree of instability in the sub-acute phase, and to give a differential diagnosis. Acute injuries may be exacerbated by full range motion with overpressure. The capsule of the ankle joint itself is assessed by passive dorsiflexion and plantarflexion only, the capsular pattern presenting as a greater limitation of plantarflexion. However, as the ankle ligaments span the sub-taloid and mid-tarsal joints, inversion/

**Table 13.1  Role of the collateral ligaments in ankle stability**

| Movement | Controlled by |
| --- | --- |
| Abduction of talus | Tibiocalcaneal and tibionavicular bands |
| Adduction of talus | Calcaneofibular ligament |
| Plantarflexion | ATF ligament and anterior tibiotalar band |
| Dorsiflexion | Posterior tibiotalar band and PTF ligament |
| External rotation of talus | Anterior tibiotalar and tibionavicular bands |
| Internal rotation of talus | As above with ATF ligament |

From Palastanga et al. (1989).

eversion and adduction/abduction are also included in ankle joint examination.

The ATF ligament is placed on maximum stretch by passive inversion, plantarflexion, and adduction. The heel is held with the cupped hand and the sub-taloid joint inverted. The opposite hand grasps the forefoot from above and swings it into plantarflexion and adduction. In addition, anterior glide of the talus on the tibia should be assessed with the foot in a neutral position. The heel is again held in the cupped hand, but this time the palm of the opposite hand is over the anterior aspect of the lower tibia. The calcaneus and talus are pulled forward as the tibia is pushed back. Movements are compared with that of the uninjured side for range and quality.

The calcaneocuboid ligament is stressed by combined supination/adduction and the calcaneofibular ligament by inversion in a neutral position. The medial collateral ligament is stressed by combined plantarflexion/eversion/abduction (anterior fibres) or eversion alone (middle fibres). Resisted eversion will not be painful unless the peronei are affected (see below).

## Management

Immediate management consists of the RICE protocol, with electrotherapy modalities as appropriate. Intermittent pneumatic compression (IPC) used in conjunction with cooling is effective. In the sub-acute phase, massage, especially finger kneading around the malleolus is of value in preventing the development of pitting oedema. Transverse frictions may be used to encourage the development of a mobile scar, and as a prelude to manipulation for scar tissue rupture in a chronic injury. Grade two and three injuries present with marked swelling and are protected non-weight-bearing (severe injury) or preferably partial weight-bearing with a compression bandage. Where minimal swelling indicates a grade one injury, an eversion strapping may be applied to protect the ligament from inversion stresses and to shorten it. A felt wedge is placed beneath the heel to evert the sub-taloid joint, and a U-shaped pad is placed over the sub-malleolar depressions to prevent pockets of oedema forming and to apply even compression when the ankle is strapped. Adhesive strapping is applied after skin preparation or underwrap, initially to lock the sub-taloid joint and then to passively evert the foot. The athlete can then walk partial weight-bearing in a well-supporting shoe.

Early mobility is essential to increase ligament strength and restore function. Non-weight-bearing ankle exercise is instigated within the pain-free range, and fitness is maintained by general exercise. Strapping is replaced by a tubular elastic bandage as pain subsides.

# Rehabilitation of the injured ankle

As with any joint, rehabilitation of the ankle aims to restore mobility, strength and function. With the ankle, however, the restoration of normal proprioception is of particular concern.

Resisted exercise using rubber powerbands is used for inversion, eversion, dorsiflexion and plantarflexion, together with combinations of these movements. Maximum repetitions are used to restore muscle endurance, while strength is developed using maximal resistance. Eversion movements are performed with the band placed over both forefeet. For other movements, one end of the band is placed around a table leg, and the other over the foot. Various thicknesses of band are used as the exercises progress.

Static stretching exercises include calf and Achilles tendon stretching (see above), and inversion/eversion movements applied manually by the athlete. The starting position for these latter movements is sitting with the injured leg crossed over the contralateral limb. The exercise mimics the stability test for the ligaments outlined above.

Partial, and then full, weight-bearing exercises are used to develop strength in a closed kinetic chain position and to restore proprioception. In single leg standing (with wall-bar support) trunk movements are performed to throw stress onto the ankle, in addition exercises such as heel raising, toe lifts, and inversion/eversion are performed. A balance beam (flamingo balance) is used, and again trunk and hip movements of the contralateral limb throw stress onto the injured ankle. The foot may be placed along the beam, or with the beam travelling transversely and only the toes supported. Intense muscle activity is seen around the ankle as the athlete attempts to maintain his or her balance. By varying the athlete's footwear, and performing the exercises in bare feet the stresses imposed are altered.

A balance board with a single transverse rib is used for sagittal movements, and a longitudinal rib for frontal plane actions. A board with a domed central raise (wobble board or ankle disk) is used to combine movements for circumduction. In addition to trunk movements, actions such as throwing and catching while standing on the balance board are helpful as these take the athlete's attention away from the ankle, and so are a progression in terms of skill. When balance board exercises are performed blindfolded, and therefore visual input is eliminated, improved proprioception has been shown in the ankle (De Carlo and Talbot, 1986).

Running, hopping and jumping activities are all used, on varying surfaces including sand, grass, and a mini-trampoline. Running in a circle, figure-of-eight and on hills/cambers all change the stress on the ankle, and hopping and jumping develop power rather than strength.

The importance of proprioceptive training in preventing the development of chronic instability ('giving way' in normal usage) is of great importance. Freeman, Dean and Hanham (1965) compared ligament injuries to the foot and ankle treated by immobilization, 'conventional' physiotherapy, and by proprioceptive training, which consisted of balance board exercises. After treatment, 7% of the proprioceptive group showed instability, compared with 46% of those treated by other means. Balance ability was measured using a modified Rhomberg test, which assesses the ability to maintain single leg standing with the eyes closed. Lentell, Katzman and Walters (1990) assessed the strength of the ankle musculature in 33 subjects with instability and found that there was no significant difference between the injured and uninjured sides. However, when balance ability was measured the majority of subjects exhibited a deficit between the two extremities. Konradsen and Ravn (1990) measured the time taken for peroneal contraction to occur in response to a sudden inversion stress in chronically unstable ankles. Their results showed the peroneal reaction time to be prolonged in unstable ankles, indicating a proprioceptive deficit.

As the ankle ligaments and capsule are torn, articular nerve fibres are also likely to be damaged, leading to a partial de-afferentiation of the joint. This, in turn, will decrease the athlete's motor control and inhibit reflex stabilization of the foot and ankle. Proprioceptive training should therefore be incorporated into a general rehabilitation training. Where chronic instability is seen, the modified Rhomberg test should be used to assess the degree of proprioceptive deficit.

## Ankle taping

Reduction of excessive inversion-eversion stress in the previously injured athlete, or as a preventive measure is widely used, more so in the USA than in Europe. Taping has traditionally been used, but semi-rigid orthoses are becoming increasingly popular. These allow dorsiflexion-plantarflexion but limit inversion-eversion and so should have a less detrimental effect on overall lower limb mechanics.

Orthoses have been shown to be as effective as taping at reducing inversion-eversion movement, but have the advantage that this support is more effectively maintained throughout training. Greene and Hillman (1990) compared several ankle orthotics with taping and found that after 20 minutes of exercise the taping revealed maximal losses of restriction, while the orthoses demonstrated no mechanical failure. Rovere et al. (1988) showed ankle stabilizers to be more effective than taping at reducing ankle injuries.

In addition to support characteristics, the effect on lower limb mechanics is important. Taping has been shown to throw stress onto the forefoot as the foot compensates for the reduction of dorsiflexion in mid-stance in walking subjects (Carmines, Nunley and McElhaney, 1988). Where an ankle orthosis allows normal dorsiflexion, the forefoot is likely to receive less compensatory stress.

The combination of forefoot stress and loss of restriction capabilities may make the use of ankle orthoses preferable to taping in certain circumstances. The contribution of taping to proprioception, providing an increased skin stimulation to movement may also be of importance. Restoration of full ankle function with a combination of strength and balance activities must always be the main consideration, with ankle supports used as an interim measure wherever possible.

## Impingement syndromes

Repeated forced dorsiflexion, such as occurs with dismounts in gymnastics, may cause anterior impingement of the talus on the tibia. Pain occurs over the front of the ankle, and is exacerbated by dorsiflexion with overpressure. Radiographs may reveal talar osteophytes, but these do not usually contribute to the impingement. Forced plantarflexion, for example repeated karate kicks or football, may cause posterior impingement giving pain over the back of the ankle without tenderness to the Achilles tendon.

Both conditions show slight swelling, and represent a repeated impaction of the joint surfaces, leading to compression of the cartilage and subchondral bone. These structures do not show great sensitivity, and will not be the primary source of pain. Instead, pain must come either from the periosteum, joint capsule, or more likely from chemical irritation and mechanical stress caused by the inflammatory response itself. Impingement syndromes respond to rest, anti-inflammatory modalities and training modification.

If the impingement force persists, an exostosis may form, on the back or front of the lower tibia depending on the type of stress involved. The exostosis may be up to 1 cm long in some cases (O'Donoghue, 1976), and should this break off it will float in the joint as a loose body. In cases where the exostosis causes symptoms, it should be surgically removed.

Rapid, forceful dorsiflexion, such as may occur in a fall on to the feet, can force the talus up with enough force to stress the distal tibiofibular ligament. The joint is tender to palpation within the sulcus between the tibia and fibula, and pain is elicited to passive dorsiflexion but not to inversion or eversion. Treatment involves strapping the foot to limit dorsiflexion, and using a heel raise.

On the posterior aspect of the talus the flexor hallucis longus travels in a small groove. If the bone lateral to this point is extended it is called Stieda's process. When this piece occurs as a separate bone (ossicle) attached to the talus by fibrous tissue, it is known as the os trigonum. Between 8 and 13% of the population have one of these bony configurations (Brodsky and Khalil, 1987) (Fig. 13.3). Repeated plantarflexion may compress the os trigonum and give impingement pain, requiring surgical removal of the ossicle.

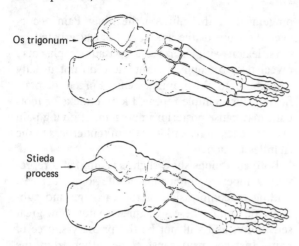

Os trigonum →

Stieda process →

**Figure 13.3** Lateral view of the ankle, showing the os trigonum and Stieda's process. From Brodsky and Khalil (1987), with permission.

## The peronei

One complication of ankle sprain is a strain or avulsion of the peroneus brevis where it attaches to the base of the fifth metatarsal. There may be local bruising, and pain is reproduced by resisted eversion. Point tenderness proximal to the base of the fifth metatarsal indicates the tendon, while bone pain may indicate avulsion. Radiographs are required to differentiate avulsion from a fracture to the fifth metatarsal itself (Jones' fracture). Treatment is similar to that of an ankle injury, with frictions performed to the tendon while the foot is inverted, and exercises to restore strength and flexibility of the peroneus brevis.

Peroneal tendon dislocation may occur if the tip of the lateral malleolus is fractured with forced dorsiflexion (skiing) or a direct blow (soccer). Local pain is present and the tendons dislocate as the foot is dorsiflexed and reduce as it is plantarflexed. As they do so, more movement is evident than on the uninjured ankle and a 'snapping' sensation is felt as the tendons move over the bone. If function is impaired, surgical repair may be required.

## Sub-taloid joint

The sub-taloid joint (STJ) has a thin capsule strengthened by the medial, posterior and lateral talocalcanean ligaments. The joint cavity is isolated from that of the ankle and mid-tarsal joints, and its stability is largely maintained by the interosseous talocalcanean ligament running from the sinus tarsi to the talus.

Subtaloid mobility is often reduced following ankle sprain or fracture of the calcaneus from a fall onto the heel. Movement may also be reduced by impaction when jumping on a hard surface in adequate footwear. The lack of mobility sometimes goes unnoticed, unless the patient is assessed by a physiotherapist.

Some distraction may be given to the STJ in supine with one hand cupping the calcaneum laterally and applying a caudal force while the other hand stabilizes the dorsomedial aspect of the mid-foot. In the prone position, with the patients foot slightly plantarflexed, and the toes over the couch end, a distraction force may be implanted by pushing caudally with the heel of the hand onto the posterior aspect of the calcaneum near the achilles insertion. Pronation and supination of the STJ may be mobilized by cupping the heel in both hands and performing an inversion/eversion action, while pulling the calcaneum caudally and anteriorly to dorsiflex the foot. Following injury, rearfoot position should be assessed as posting may be required.

## Mid-tarsal joint

The mid-tarsal joint is composed of the calcaneocuboid joint (lateral), and the talocalcaneonavicular joint (medial). The calcaneocuboid joint forms part of the lateral longitudinal arch of the foot and so takes the whole bodyweight. The joint is strengthened by the dorsal and plantar calcaneocuboid ligaments, and the part of the bifurcate ligament attaching to the cuboid. More superficially, support is provided by the long plantar ligament stretching over the length of the lateral aspect of the foot. The talocalcaneonavicular joint is strengthened by the spring (calcaneonavicular) ligament, the dorsal talonavicular ligament and the portion of

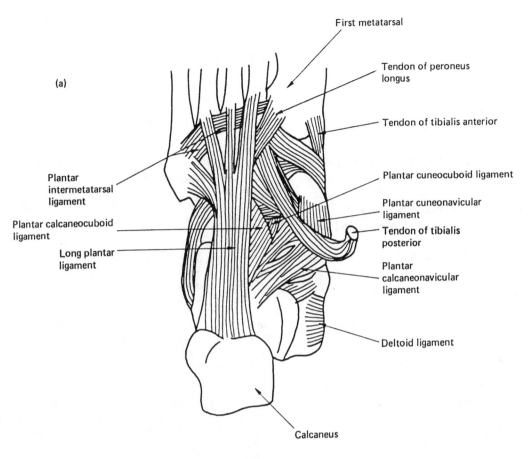

(a)

First metatarsal

Tendon of peroneus longus

Tendon of tibialis anterior

Plantar intermetatarsal ligament

Plantar cuneocuboid ligament

Plantar cuneonavicular ligament

Plantar calcaneocuboid ligament

Tendon of tibialis posterior

Long plantar ligament

Plantar calcaneonavicular ligament

Deltoid ligament

Calcaneus

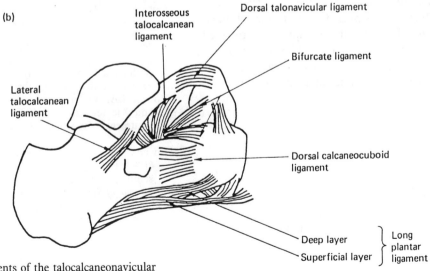

(b)

Interosseous talocalcanean ligament

Dorsal talonavicular ligament

Bifurcate ligament

Lateral talocalcanean ligament

Dorsal calcaneocuboid ligament

Deep layer

Superficial layer

Long plantar ligament

**Figure 13.4**   Ligaments of the talocalcaneonavicular joint. (a) From below. (b) Lateral view. From Palastanga, Field and Soames (1989), with permission.

the bifurcate ligament attaching to the navicular.

The calcaneocuboid joint may be injured at the same time as the ATF ligament by an inversion and plantarflexion stress. On examination, pain is reproduced by fixing the rearfoot in dorsiflexion and eversion, and inverting and adducting the forefoot. Often the condition goes unnoticed at the time of injury as the AFT sprain is the dominant pain. In time, chronic pain results and the dorsal calcaneocuboid ligament may be tender to palpation. The ligament is most easily found by identifying the tubercle on the base of the fifth metatarsal, and coming one finger breadth posteriorly and superiorly. Transverse frictions may be given to the ligament by adducting the foot and aiming the friction sweep vertically. Mobilization of the calcaneocuboid joint may be achieved in supine by gripping the lateral aspect of the foot, with one hand stabilising the calcaneus and the other the cuboid. The hands work against each other to impart a superior-inferior gliding motion.

The talocalcaneonavicular joint may be injured by excessive foot pronation or, more rarely, at the same time as medial ligament injury to the ankle. In chronic foot sprain, caused by hyperpronation, the spring ligament lengthens and becomes tender, as does the plantarfascia when the medial longitudinal arch flattens. Treatment is by correction of hyperpronation and strengthening to the plantar musculature. The talocalcaneonavicular joint may be moblized in a similar fashion to the calcaneocuboid joint. This time the therapist grips the medial aspect of the athlete's foot, stabilising the navicular and talus. Again the hands work against each other to create a superior-inferior gliding motion.

# References

Bowers, K.D. and Martin, R.B. (1976) Turf toe: a shoe-surface related football injury. *Medicine and Science in Sports and Exercise*, **8**, 81–83

Brodsky, A.E. and Khalil, M.A. (1987) Talar compression syndrome. *Foot and Ankle*, **7**, 338–344

Carmines, D.V., Nunley, J.A. and McElhaney, J.H. (1988) Effects of ankle taping on the motion and loading pattern of the foot for walking subjects. *Journal of Orthopaedic Research*, **6**, 223–229

Clanton, T.O., Butler, J.E. and Eggert, A. (1986) Injuries to the metatarsophalangeal joints in athletes. *Foot and Ankle*, **7**, 162–176

De Carlo, M.S. and Talbot, R. W. (1986) Evaluation of ankle joint proprioception following injection of the anterior talofibular ligament. *Journal of Orthopaedic and Sports Physical Therapy*, **8**, (2) 70–76

Freeman, M.A.R., Dean, M.R.E. and Hanham, I.W.F. (1965) The etiology and prevention of functional instability of the foot. *Journal of Bone and Joint Surgery*, **47B**, (4) 678–685

Garrick, J.G. and Webb, D.R. (1990) *Sports Injuries: Diagnosis and Management*, W.B. Saunders, London

George, F.J. (1989). In *Year Book of Sports Medicine*, (ed. R.J. Shephard), pp. 75, Year Book Medical Publishers, Chicago

Greene, T.A. and Hillman, S.K. (1990) Comparison of support provided by a semirigid orthosis and adhesive ankle taping before, during, and after exercise. *American Journal of Sports Medicine*, **18**, (5) 498–506

Konradsen, L. and Ravn, J.B. (1990) Ankle instability caused by prolonged peroneal reaction time. *Acta Orthopaedica Scandinavica*, **61**, (5) 388–390

Lentell, G.L., Katzman, L.L. and Walters, M.R. (1990) The relationship between muscle function and ankle stability. *Journal of Orthopaedic and Sports Physical Therapy*, **11**, (12) 605–611

O'Donoghue, D.H. (1976) *Treatment of Injuries to Athletes*, W.B. Saunders, Philadelphia

Palastanga, N., Field, D. and Soames, R. (1989) *Anatomy and Human Movement*, Butterworth–Heinemann, Oxford

Rodeo, S.A., O'Brian, S.J. and Warren, R.F. Turf toe: an analysis of metatarsophalangeal joint sprains in professional football players. *American Journal of Sports Medicine*, to be published.

Rodeo, S.A., O'Brian, S.J., Warren, R.F., Barnes, R. and Wickiewicz, T.L. (1989) Turf toe: diagnosis and treatment. *Physician and Sportsmedicine*, **17**, (4) 132–147

Rovere, G.D., Clarke, T.J., Yates, C.S. and Burley, K. (1988) Retrospective comparison of taping and ankle stabilizers in preventing ankle injuries. *American Journal of Sports Medicine*, **16**, 228–233

Vargish, T. and Clarke, W.R. (1983) The ankle injury—indications for the selective use of X-rays. *Injury*, **14**, 507–512

# 14 The foot

The foot is the athlete's main contact area with the ground, which in part accounts for the very high number of conditions affecting this area in sport. An athlete's foot may have to withstand forces two or three times greater than bodyweight, and this may be repeated more than 5000 times every hour when running. Most sports involve some sort of running or jumping, and so the foot is continually called upon to provide both stability and shock attenuation.

## The first metatarsophalangeal joint

The first metatarsal bone joins proximally to the first cuneiform to form the first ray complex. Distally, the bone forms the first metatarsophalangeal (MP) joint with the proximal phalanx of the hallux. The first MP joint is reinforced over its plantar aspect by an area of fibrocartilage known as the volar plate (plantar accessory ligament). This is formed from the deep transverse metatarsal ligament, and the tendons of flexor hallucis brevis, adductor hallucis, and abductor hallucis. It has within it two sesamoid bones which serve as weight-bearing points for the metatarsal head.

Movement of the joint is carried out by flexor hallucis longus and brevis, extensor hallucis longus and the medial tendon of extensor digitorum brevis, and abductor and adductor hallucis. This fairly complex structure is often taken for granted but does give rise to a number of important conditions.

### Turf toe

Turf toe is a sprain involving the plantar aspect of the capsule of the first MP joint. It is most often seen in athletes who play regularly on synthetic surfaces, and results from forced hyperextension (dorsiflexion) of the first MP joint. The condition is quite common in some sports; studies of American football players have shown that 45% of athletes had suffered from turf toe at some stage (Rodeo, O'Brian and Warren, 1989).

Forced hyperextension of the first MP joint causes capsular tearing, and sometimes disruption of the components of the medial sesamoid. Examination reveals a hyperaemic swollen joint with tenderness over the plantar surface of the metatarsal head. Local bruising may develop within 24 hours. Differential diagnosis must be made from sesamoid stress fracture (insidious onset) and metatarsal or phalangeal fractures (site of pain and radiograph).

Treatment aims to reduce pain and inflammation and to support the joint by taping. The first MP joint is held in neutral position and strips of 2.5 cm inelastic tape are applied in a figure-of-eight fashion crossing over the joint. The strips begin on the plantar aspect of the foot, go over the top and around the toe to finish on the dorsum of the foot. An oval piece of felt or foam with a hole in the middle is placed beneath the toe, the hole corresponding to the metatarsal head.

A number of factors may predispose the athlete to turf toe. The condition is more common with artificial playing surfaces than with grass (Bowers and Martin, 1976). Artificial turf is less shock-absorbing, and so transmits more force directly to the first MP joint. Sports shoes also have an important part to play. Lighter shoes tend to be used with artificial playing surfaces. These shoes are more flexible around the distal forefoot, and allow the MP joints to hyperextend. In addition, shoes which are fitted by length alone, rather than width, may cause problems for athletes with wider feet, who must buy shoes which are too long to accommodate their foot width. Such shoes increase the leverage forces acting on the toe joints and allow the feet to slide forwards in the shoes, increasing the speed of movement at the joints.

Preventive measures include wearing shoes with more rigid soles, to avoid hyperextension of the injured joint. In addition, semi-rigid (spring steel or heat-sensitive plastic) insoles may be used. Some authors recommend the use of rigid insoles as a preventive measure when playing on all-weather surfaces for all athletes with less than 60° dorsiflexion at the first MP joint (Clanton, Butler and Eggert, 1986). An increased range of ankle dorsiflexion has been suggested as a risk factor which may predispose an athlete to turf toe (Rodeo, O'Brian and Warren, 1989). However, in walking subjects, when the ankle is strapped to reduce dorsiflexion, the heel actually lifts up earlier in the gait cycle, causing the range of motion at the metatarsal heads to increase (Carmines, Nunley and McElhaney, 1988). This increased range may once again predispose the athlete to turf toe (George 1989), so the amount of dorsiflexion itself may not be that important. If injury has recently changed the range, the athlete may not have had time to adapt fully to the altered movement pattern, and the altered foot/ankle mechanics in total may be the problem.

As with many soft tissue injuries, if incorrectly managed the condition may predispose the athlete to arthritic changes in later life. In the case of turf toe, this may occur as calcification of the soft tissues around the injury site, presenting as hallux valgus or hallux rigidus.

### Hallux valgus

Hallux valgus usually occurs when the first MP joint is hypermobile, and the first ray is shorter than the second (Morton foot structure). When this is the case, the second metatarsal head takes more pressure than in a non-Morton foot (Rodgers and Cavanagh, 1989) (Fig. 14.1). In addition, hallux valgus is more common in athletes who hyperpronate. As the first MP joint dorsiflexes during the propulsive phase of running, the instability allows the hallux to deviate from its normal plane. Adduction and axial rotation occur, and the long flexors, which normally stabilize the joint, now

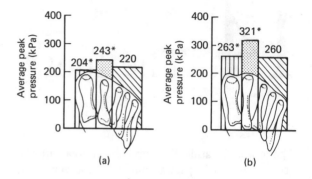

**Figure 14.1** Pressure distribution in (a) Morton and (b) non-Morton feet. From Rodgers and Cavanagh (1989), with permission.

themselves become deforming influences. As the first metatarsal head adducts, the sesamoids sublux and eventually erode the plantar aspect of the first metatarsal head—this is one source of pain. Compensatory stress is placed on the joints proximal and distal to the first MP joint and further pain arises through synovial inflammation and capsular distraction. Eventually, secondary osteoarthritis occurs in the first MP joint and sesamoids. Bunion formation to the side of the first metatarsal head is common.

Management of this condition is initially to stabilize the first MP joint by correcting faulty foot mechanics (especially hyperpronation) and advising on correct athletic footwear. If conservative management fails, surgery may be required. If the deformity is purely soft tissue in nature, the bunion may be removed, and the dynamic structures around the first toe realigned. If bony deformity is present, osteotomy or arthroplasty may be necessary.

### Hallux limitus/rigidus

A reduction in movement of the first MP joint, hallus limitus, may progress to complete immobility or hallux rigidus. The condition is more common when the first metatarsal is longer than the second. Pain is generally worse during sporting activities, and occurs especially when pushing off. On examination the joint end feel is usually firm, and limitation of movement is noted to dorsiflexion. To differentiate between a tight flexor hallucis longus and joint structures, the foot is assessed both with the foot dorsiflexed and everted (tendon on stretch) and then plantarflexed and inverted (tendon relaxed). Limitation of motion through muscle tightness responds well to stretching procedures, while joint limitation which is soft tissue in nature is treated by joint mobilization. Distal distraction, and gliding mobilizations with the metatarsal head stabilized are particularly useful (Cibulka, 1990). Where bony deformity is present, surgery is indicated.

A number of surgical procedures are available for hallux conditions, and the interested reader is referred to Horn and Subotnick (1989) for an excellent review.

## Plantar fasciitis

Inflammation of the plantar fascia is common in sports which involve repeated jumping, and with hill running. The fascia consists of a dense fibrous band running forwards from the calcaneal tuberosity to the metatarsal heads. Overuse may cause microtears and inflammation of the fascial insertion, and nodules from the fascial granuloma can occasionally be felt (Tanner and Harvey, 1988).

Normally, during mid-stance, the foot is flattened, stretching the plantar fascia and enabling it to store elastic energy to be released at toe off. However, a variety of malalignment faults may increase stress on the fascia. Excessive pronation will lower the arch and overstretch the fascia, and a reduction in mobility of the first metatarsal may also contribute to the condition (Creighton and Olson, 1987). In addition, weak peronei, often the result of incomplete rehabilitation following ankle sprains, will reduce the support on the arch, thus stressing the plantar fascia. Congenital problems, such as pes cavus, will also leave an athlete more susceptible to plantar fasciitis.

As the foot is plantarflexed with the toes on the ground, the fascia is stretched over the metatarsal heads, raising the longitudinal arch and making the foot more rigid (Fig. 14.2). Plantar fasciitis is therefore exacerbated if the Achilles tendon is tight, or if high-heeled shoes are worn. Pain is often

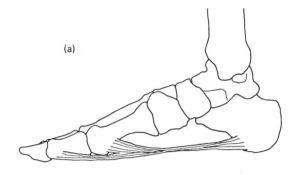

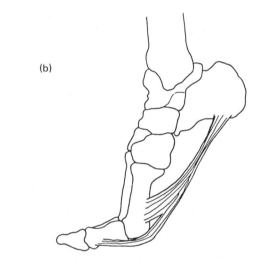

**Figure 14.2** Plantarfascia stretch. (a) Foot flat, normal tension in fascia. (b) Raising on to the toes tightens the plantar fascia and raises the longitudinal arch. From Hertling and Kessler (1990), with permission.

worse when taking the first few steps in the morning until the Achilles tendon is stretched.

Sports shoes play an important part in the course of this condition. Inadequate rearfoot control may fail to eliminate hyperpronation, and a poorly fitting heel counter will allow the calcaneal fat pad to spread at heel strike, transmitting extra impact force to the calcaneus and plantar fascia. On a hard surface, the shock absorbing qualities of the shoe are important, and a patient's footwear should always be examined.

Pain usually occurs over the calcaneal attachment of the fascia or its medial edge. Pain may be localized to the heel as though the athlete is 'stepping on a stone', or may present as a burning pain over the arch. The problem must be differentiated from rheumatoid conditions, which often give bilateral pain, and from Sever's disease, which gives pain to the insertion of the Achilles tendon.

Taping the foot may often give surprisingly rapid relief. The foot is locked in the neutral position (p. 158) and an anchor strap is placed just behind the metatarsal heads. Strips of inelastic adhesive strapping are then fastened from the fifth metatarsal, across the plantar aspect of the foot to the medial side of the calcaneus. From here they travel around the back of the heel and across the foot once more to the first metatarsal, so forming an incomplete figure-of-eight. Additional strips may be placed transversely across the foot from the metatarsal heads to the calcaneal tubercle. As well as supporting both the longitudinal and transverse arches of the foot, this strapping will also help to hold the STJ in a more neutral position and reduce hyperpronation. In addition, the head of the first metatarsal is stabilized.

More permanent management may require rearfoot posting to control excessive pronation. In addition, strengthening the intrinsic foot musculature is important. Although the plantar fascia is inert, stress on the structure may be increased when the intrinsic foot musculature is weak. Foot strengthening, including actively increasing the arch height, may have a re-education effect on plantar proprioception. The action is to try to 'shorten' the foot and raise the medial longitudinal and transverse arches.

## Morton's neuroma

Morton's neuroma affects the plantar interdigital nerve between the third and fourth metatarsal heads. Symptoms may occur spontaneously and are often described as feeling like 'electric shocks' along the sensory nerve distribution. The condition is more common in runners (particularly when sprinting and running uphill) and dancers, and is often aggravated by wearing narrow, high-heeled shoes. The sustained dorsiflexed position of these activities stretches the digital nerve, causing inflammation. Once swollen, the nerve is open to entrapment between the metatarsal heads, and eventually the nerve is scarred and permanently enlarged to form a neuroma.

Pain may be reproduced by direct pressure over the neuroma while compressing the forefoot medially and laterally. If the condition is caught in its oedematous stage, alteration of footwear, ice application and ultrasound are effective. Injection with corticosteroid and local anaesthetic is also used. Once the neuroma has formed, surgical excision under local anaesthesia is usually required. There may be a permanent loss of sensation over the plantar aspect of the foot supplied by the digital nerve, but in some cases regeneration occurs between 8 and 12 months after surgery.

## Metatarsalgia

The term 'metatarsalgia' is often used to describe any pain in the forefoot. Such pain may occur in a variety of conditions, including those affecting the hallux, a digital neuroma, or even stress fractures. However, in this description, the term refers to 'functional metatarsalgia', where altered foot function causes abnormal mechanical stress in the forefoot, which is symptomatic.

The transverse arch of the foot (Fig. 14.3) is supported at the level of the cuneiforms by the peroneus longus, which pulls the medial and lateral edges of the foot together. More distally, the arch is formed by the metatarsal heads, the highest point, or 'keystone' being the second metatarsal. In midstance, the arch flattens and the five metatarsal heads come to lie in the same transverse plane to take the bodyweight. The first metatarsal takes weight through its sesamoid bones, and it and the fifth metatarsal are more mobile than the other three. Stability is provided to the metatarsal heads both passively by the transverse metatarsal ligament, and actively by adductor hallucis, and to a lesser extent, the intrinsics. Normally, these structures keep the metatarsals together. However, in cases of hypermobility, such as excessive pronation or hallux valgus, the metatarsal heads may splay apart, effectively increasing the width of the fore-

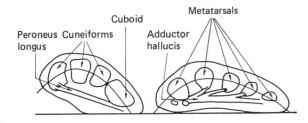

**Figure 14.3** The transverse arch of the foot at different levels. From Palastanga, Field and Soames (1989), with permission.

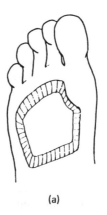 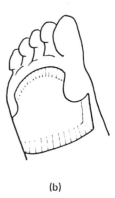

(a)                                  (b)

**Figure 14.4** Plantar metatarsal padding. (a) Basic PMP. (b) Double-winged PMP for first and fifth metatarsal heads.

foot, and allowing the central metatarsal heads to take too much weight.

Hypermobility may cause abnormal shearing forces, especially in an ill-fitting shoe, leading to plantar keratosis. As the metatarsal heads splay, the transverse ligament and intrinsic muscles are subjected to tensile stress, causing pain. Rigidity of the foot may also cause problems. If any of the metatarsals are fixed, or if the toes are 'clawed', plantar compression will occur, again giving keratoma (Neale and Adams, 1989).

Clearly, successful management of the condition relies to a large extent on the identification of any underlying biomechanical abnormality in the foot. Short-term relief may be obtained by using anti-inflammatory modalities, and padding and strapping to relieve the stress on the forefoot tissues. An adhesive plantar metatarsal pad (PMP), made from orthopaedic felt, is contoured to cover the heads and upper shafts of the three central metatarsals, lifting them above ground level on weight bearing (Fig. 14.4). The pad is cut around the head of the first metatarsal to avoid excessive pressure at this point. To prevent metatarsal splaying, inelastic strapping is placed around the forefoot, encircling the metatarsals just beneath the first and fifth metatarsal heads. If the metatarsals are immobile, a metatarsal bar may be built into the shoe. This has the effect of transferring the bodyweight to the metatarsal shafts and away from the painful metatarsal head.

Coupled with strapping and padding, strengthening of the intrinsic muscles is essential. Simple exercises, such as 'shortening' the foot in bare feet, are effective at building isometric strength and endurance of the intrinsic muscles.

Eccentric strength is similarly developed by initially tensing the intrinsic muscles of the foot and increasing the arch with the leg non-weight-bearing. The bodyweight is then taken onto the foot and the arch is gradually allowed to flatten under control.

## Skin and nail lesions

### Subungual haematoma

In this condition, a haematoma forms directly below the nail plate as a result of direct trauma. Pressure builds up in the space between the nail and nailbed, causing acute pain and throbbing. In some cases the pressure may be great enough to loosen the nail from its bed. Subungual haematoma is often referred to as 'black toe' or 'runners toe'. Ill-fitting shoes are a common cause, if the toe box is too small the nail may rub, especially when running downhill.

When the problem is acute, the haematoma is often decompressed by the athlete penetrating the nail with a red-hot needle or paperclip to release the blood (Subotnick, 1989). A less hazardous approach is for the therapist to use a sterile needle. The best treatment for chronic haemorrhage is to remove the cause, and buy shoes which allow enough room for the toes to spread on weight-bearing and expand with warmth. When standing, a sports shoe should allow one thumb's breadth between the end of the shoe and the athlete's longest toe.

## Onychocryptosis

Onychocryptosis, or ingrown toe-nail, is particularly common in the hallux of athletes, especially males. It may occur secondarily to ill-fitting sports shoes, or to incorrect toe-nail cutting. Shoes are often too narrow, leading to lateral pressure on the hallux, and athletes often cut the toe-nails too short, causing the underlying soft tissues to protrude. Cutting across the corners of the nail is another common fault in footcare, allowing the nail to embed itself into the nail grooves. Frequently, excessive sweating (hyperhidrosis) causes skin softening, a condition exacerbated by prolonged hot bathing.

A splinter of nail grows into the subcutaneous tissue and, with time, acute inflammation occurs, possibly with infection (paronychia). The skin becomes red, tight and shiny, and the toe swells. There is throbbing pain and acute tenderness to palpation. Normal healing will not take place as long as the nail splinter remains, and so hypergranulation occurs. The combination of granulation tissue and the swollen nail-fold overlaps the nail plate itself.

When the condition occurs without infection, the nail splinter may be removed with a nail knife, avoiding further damage to the sulcus. The edge of the nail is smoothed and the area treated with hydrogen peroxide. The nail edge is then packed with sterile gauze, allowing some to rest under the nail plate itself. The area is protected with a sterile dressing, and regularly inspected.

When the condition is accompanied by infection, a local anaesthetic is injected at the base of the toe away from the infected area. The foot may be soaked in hot magnesium sulphate solution to ease removal of the nail splinter. Hypergranulation tissue is excised. If this procedure is ineffective,

nail surgery involving partial or complete nail avulsion is required (Neale and Adams, 1989).

Prevention of the problem relies on the use of correctly fitting sports shoes, and on cutting the nails to the shape of the end of the toe, while avoiding splintering the nail sides. It is good practice to address basic footcare at the beginning of the season, especially with athletes new to the squad.

## Blisters

Blisters occur as a result of compression or shearing on the skin. A narrow toe box may cause blisters over the medial aspect of the fifth toe, and between the first and second toes in the case of hallux valgus. Blisters over the plantar aspect of the foot are common when sports shoes are loose. Shoes should be fitted correctly and friction reduced wherever possible. Petroleum jelly used between the toes is helpful, and proper foot hygiene, which may include powder or astringents to dry the foot, should be observed.

Acute blisters may be drained through a puncture hole. A sterile needle is used and enters the blister at the side, the needle being held parallel to the skin. This will leave a skin flap intact for protection. The underlying cause of the blister should be addressed.

## Athlete's foot

Tinea pedis or 'athlete's foot' is the most common fungal infection of the feet, and is particularly rampant in communal washing areas in sport, and where standards of hygiene are poor. Sports shoes create moisture and warmth between the toes, conditions in which the complaint thrives. Three types of tinea pedis are generally seen. First, the lateral toe spaces become macerated, due to three organisms, *Trichophyton rubrum*, *Trichophyton interdigitale* and *Epidermophyton floccosum*. Secondly, the condition may spread to the soles of the feet, where vesiculation occurs as a result of *T. interdigitale* and *E. floccosum*, and finally a diffuse 'moccasin type' scaling appears, usually due to *T. rubrum*. The condition may also spread to the nails and hands in some cases.

Treatment initially aims to remove the scaling tissue by the application of ointments, such as phenyl mercuric acetate. When the scaling has cleared, antifungal dusting powders, such as tolnaftate, are used. Sprays containing clotrimazole and dusting powders are used by the athlete, and socks and footwear should be changed daily and preferably disinfected. While the infection remains, athletes should not go barefoot in public areas (changing rooms and swimming baths), and should not share towels, socks or footwear.

## Hyperkeratosis

Keratinization is a normal physiological process which turns the stratum corneum of the skin into a hard protective cover. The process becomes overactive if the skin is continually subjected to mechanical stress, for example on the hands of heavy manual workers, or the feet of athletes. Hyperaemia occurs, stimulating a proliferation of epidermal cells, and at the same time the rate of desquamation reduces. This type of keratoma or callus on the foot has a protective function, and providing it is asymptomatic it should be left in place. However, when the bulk of such tissues becomes excessive and causes pain or deformity, treatment is required.

The size and shape of the hyperkeratosis is largely dictated by the stress imposed on the skin. A callus is a diffuse area of thickened skin resulting from stress over a fairly wide area, while a corn is a smaller concentrated area which has formed into a nucleus. Corns typically seen in sports medicine are either soft or hard, although vascular and neurovascular types do exist. Soft corns are common in the cleft between the fourth and fifth toes, and appear macerated due to sweat retention. The corn nucleus is generally ring-shaped and the centre of the lesion is very thin. Hard corns occur on the plantar aspect of the foot beneath the metatarsal heads, or on the dorsum of the interphalangeal joints. They develop because of concentrated pressure due to bodyweight and ground reaction forces. The corn nucleus is often associated with surrounding callus due to shearing stress.

The corn or callus may be removed with a scalpel by a therapist and the corn nucleus eradicated. Antiseptic agents, such as cetrimide and chlorhexidine, are then applied. Loss of moisture from the skin is prevented by applying a fleecy web dressing. Moist skin is treated with an astringent, such as salicylic acid in spirit, and excessively dry skin managed with an emollient, such as lanolin or soft white paraffin. It is important to remove the underlying cause of the keratoma so that it does not simply return. Examination of foot biomechanics and sports footwear is therefore essential.

## Verruca

Verruca pedis is a lesion caused by one of the human papilloma viruses (HPV), of which about 15 have been identified. A benign epithelial tumour, which is self-limiting, is produced in the plantar skin. The wart is covered by hyperkeratotic tissue, and contains brown or black specks caused by intravascular thromboses within its dilated capillaries. Where the wart is over a weight-bearing site, it is forced into the dermis leaving just the hyperkeratotic area on the surface. For this reason athletes often assume that a verruca is simply a corn or callus. However, close inspection will usually reveal the papillary appearance of the verruca. A number of other factors differentiate the two. A wart has a far more rapid onset than an area of callus, and may occur in an area of skin not associated with mechanical stress. In addition, bleeding can occur if the verruca is cut because of capillary dilation, whereas a callus is avascular.

The virus normally enters the body through broken skin in the foot, especially if the foot has been wet and the skin macerated. Unfortunately, the virus spreads quickly through a population before the plantar wart becomes obvious. The aim of treatment is to destroy all the cells within the lesion by chemical cautery or cryosurgery. Various preparations are used. The skin surrounding the area is protected, and a liquid or paste of salicylic acid (or mono-chloroacetic acid) is applied. An aseptic necrosis is produced, and destroyed tissue is removed one week later.

Cryosurgery aims to freeze the verruca with carbon dioxide snow, nitrous oxide, or liquid nitrogen applied through a probe. Tissue necrosis with blister formation occurs when the skin is cooled to $-20°C$ and bluish colouration results. The rapid cooling causes ice crystals to form in the body cells and interstitial fluids, which in turn ruptures the cells. Liquid nitrogen is perhaps the most common of the cryosurgery techniques, applied by dipping a cotton-tipped stick into the liquid. This is applied to the verruca for about 30–60 seconds. The lesion is protected by a cavity pad if it is over a weight-bearing area.

If the verruca is not painful, treatment may not be required as the lesion will regress naturally in some months (Neale and Adams, 1989). However, cross-infection must still be guarded against by the use of plastic waterproof socks in public areas.

## The sports shoe

The design of sports shoes has received a great deal of attention over the last two decades. This interest has to a large extent been market-led due to the massive increase in the number of people jogging. Manufacturers vie with each other to produce a shoe feature which can act as a unique selling point to give them an increased market share.

There is little doubt that shoe design has improved, and that athletes have benefited from this. However, many developments are simply variations on the same theme and give little substantial improvement in overall shoe design. In addition, the mounting cost of sports shoes makes it imperative that athletes receive the right advice concerning the shoe which will best suit their foot and be appropriate to their sport.

As most sports involve running, more emphasis will be given to the features of running shoes, as many of these features are carried over into other sports footwear.

### Forces acting on the foot

During the stance phase of running, the foot must accommodate to three phases, heel strike, mid-

stance and toe off, during which the biomechanics of the foot changes considerably. At heel strike the single force of the foot moving downwards and forwards may be resolved into two components. The first is an impact stress acting vertically, and the second a horizontal shearing force, creating friction. Not all athletes strike the ground with the heel when running. For some 80% the initial contact point is at the heel (Frederick, Clarke and Hamill, 1984). The ground reaction force curve in this case shows an initial (passive) peak at heel strike of about half bodyweight, occurring 20-30 ms after heel-strike. A secondary (active) peak occurs approximately 100 ms after heel contact as the centre of pressure moves over the ball of the foot prior to toe off (Fig. 14.5).

Other runners show a centre of pressure over the mid foot or rear foot (Fig. 14.6). The magnitude of the force acting on the foot can be as much as three times bodyweight.

The rear foot runner strikes the ground with his or her knee locked, and consequently will require more shock attenuation from the sports shoe. The mid foot or fore foot striker has his or her knee slightly flexed, and so part of the contact shock is absorbed by the elasticity of the knee structures. In some cases, the heel does not touch the ground at all, leaving the stance phase under the control of the posterior leg muscles. In this type of runner, the shock-absorbing function of a heel wedge will be under-utilized.

During mid-stance there can be 5° of abduction of the foot, causing friction between the shoe and running surface. This creates a torsion force, which tends to rotate the upper part of the shoe in relation to the sole (Cavanagh, 1989).

### Components of a running shoe

The outer sole (Fig. 14.7) of a shoe is generally a carbon rubber material with treads or studs cut into it. The outer sole must provide a combination of four features: grip (traction), durability, flexibility and light weight. Studs provide better cross-country grip, while bars are more durable on hard surfaces and so are better suited to road shoes. However, the thicker studs or cleats of a cross-

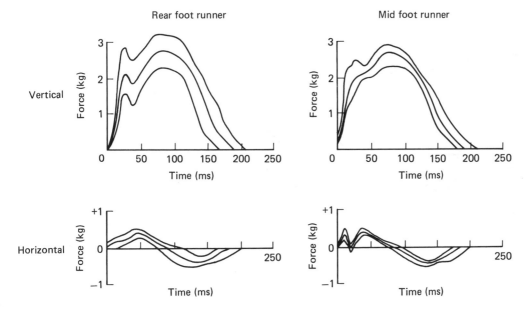

**Figure 14.5**   Ground reaction forces in rear foot and mid foot runners. From Segresser and Pforminger (1989), with permission.

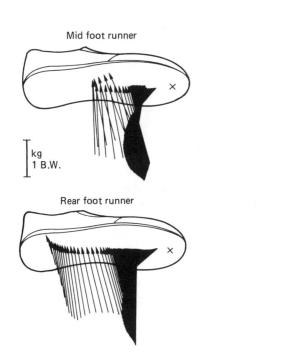

**Figure 14.6**   Force vector curves for rear foot and mid foot runners. From Segresser and Pforminger (1989), with permission.

country or fell running shoe will also add weight, so faster road racing shoes tend to have thin, smoother soles.

Beneath the sole is the midsole, extending the full length of the shoe, and the wedge which begins behind the metatarsal heads and extends back to the heel. These take the place of the wooden 'shank' of the traditional street shoe. Both the midsole and wedge are designed for cushioning, giving good elastic recoil, but they must also maintain good foot control. There are usually two or three layers of different foam materials, such as ethyl vinyl acetate (EVA), or more expensive polyurethane. Thicker materials tend to give better cushioning, but they will also raise the foot off the ground, creating greater leverage forces if the foot contacts the ground at the side of the sole.

On top of the midsole is the insole board, again running the whole length of the shoe. This semi-rigid board prevents the foot from twisting and so provides stability. The edge of the shoe upper is usually fastened below the insole board, and the board itself may be chemically treated to resist

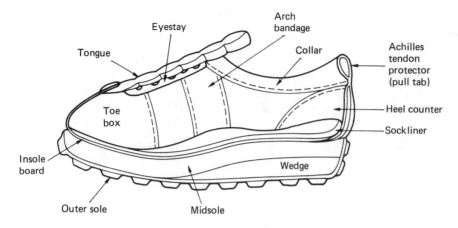

**Figure 14.7**   Parts of the sports shoe.

deterioration from moisture or micro-organism growth.

The heel counter provides rear foot stability, helping to prevent over-pronation and is usually a hard thermoplastic, which will keep its rigidity. Poorer quality shoes may have cardboard heel counters which will feel stiff when the shoe is new, but quickly soften and allow excessive rearfoot motion. Often the heel counter itself will have an additional support.

The shoe upper is contoured to the foot, and made from three sections. The 'vamp' covers the fore foot, and the mid foot and hind foot are covered by the medial and lateral quarters, respectively. The nylon upper provides lightness and breathability, and is supported by the eyestay and arch bandage. The eyestay will normally have eyelets for lacing, and the arch bandage is positioned at the highest point of the longitudinal arch of the foot.

The foot rests within the shoe, directly on top of the sock liner. This should be removable for washing and can also have further padding, such as gel or air sacs, incorporated into it. The liner is designed primarily to reduce friction and absorb sweat, and may be removed when an orthotic device is placed into the shoe.

The ankle collar should be heavily padded and soft, and the heel tab (pull tab) should be notched to prevent friction on the Achilles tendon during toe off. Some older designs of sports shoes still have so called 'Achilles tendon protectors'. Unfortunately the effect of these is usually to injure rather than protect. As the foot is plantarflexed, the Achilles tendon tab will press onto the Achilles tendon cuasing friction, one cause of Haglund's syndrome (see p. 200). Shoes of this type may be modified by cutting a slot down each side of the tab or simply cutting the tab off, providing neither of these solutions interferes with the overall shoe structure.

Many shoes have variable lacing systems to accommodate different foot widths and ensure that the shoe fits the foot snugly. With reference to shoe width, it is important to encourage athletes to stand and walk around/jog in sports shoes before they buy them. Obviously the foot spreads with weight-bearing, so if the shoe is tried on when sitting it will not give an accurate impression of fit.

### Shoe function

Cushioning effects of shoes have been shown to reduce initial impact at heel strike by as much as 50% (Light, McLellan and Klenerman, 1980; Subotnick, 1989). The aim is to reduce or 'attenuate' the peak forces to levels which are well tolerated by the human body, and which do not result either in trauma or overuse injury. At the same time, the forces produced at toe off have to be conserved to maintain running efficiency.

Heel materials which are too soft will compress or 'bottom out', while those which are too hard reduce cushioning. In addition, the construction of the shoe will also affect shock absorption. A stiff insole board for example, cemented to a soft mid-sole will give the shoe a functional hardness usually found only with much firmer midsole materials (Frederick, 1989).

The overhand or 'flare' of the sole of a running shoe creates leverage force which exaggerates pronation and foot slap (Fig. 14.8). When running bare foot, the sub-talar joint axis lies over the ground contact point as does the ankle joint axis (Fig. 14.8a). Whilst wearing a typical running shoe, the leverage force created by the heel flare places the ground contact point further away from the sub-talar joint axis, thus increasing the leverage effect by a factor of three (Fig. 14.8b). In the sagittal plane, the heel flare moves the ground contact point back, further from the ankle joint, thus increasing the leverage effect. To compensate, the anterior tibial muscles have to work harder. By altering the heel to a more rounded design, and using a shoe with a dual density midsole, over-pronation can be limited.

The sole of a sports shoe should bend at a point just proximal to the metatarsal heads, to an angle of about 30°. Bending a stiffer sole may increase energy expenditure, and could therefore lead to local muscle fatigue. A lighter shoe is more energy conserving. Frederick (1985) showed that carrying 100 g excess weight on the foot increased energy expenditure by 1%; enough, he claimed, to add 1 or 2 minutes on to the time of a competitive marathon runner. Similarly, softer soled shoes are more energy conserving. The same author showed

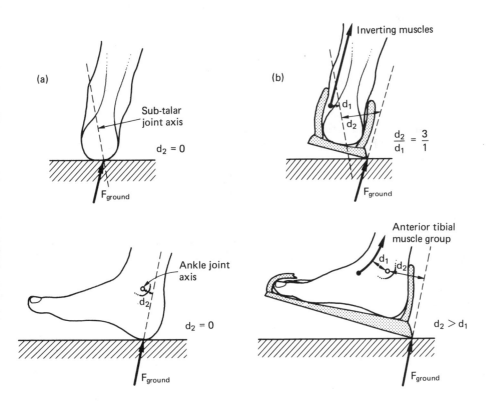

**Figure 14.8** Effect of leverage in running shoes. (a) Running barefoot, the sub-talar joint axis lies over the ground contact point, as does the ankle joint. (b) The 'overhang' of the shoes moves the ground contact point further from the sub-taloid and ankle joints, increasing the leverage effect. Muscle action is required to compensate. From Subotnick (1989), with permission.

a 2.8% reduction in energy expenditure for subjects wearing soft-soled shoes while running a marathon.

The ideal combination of features in a running shoe is unfortunately not possible to obtain. There is always a compromise because many of the attributes are contradictory. Cushioning conflicts with qualities of stability and flexibility. Decreasing the hardness of the sole can increase pronation, so to get adequate cushioning, a thicker more shock-absorbing sole is chosen rather than a softer one.

By combining data from various sources, Frederick (1989) analysed the relationship between heel height, maximum pronation, and hardness of a sole to find an 'ideal' combination. He concluded that optimum cushioning and rear-foot control are obtained in a shoe with a heel height of 25–35 mm with cushioning values of 40–55 shore A. Hardness is quantified by measuring the resistance of a material to the penetration of a defined object. The shore A scale runs from 0 (softest) to 100 (hardest).

This combination would, however, give a reduction in sole flexibility, as highly flexible soles are usually soft and thin. Figure 14.9 demonstrates the stresses produced when a sole is bent. The top of the sole is compressed, and the bottom tensioned. To make the sole more flexible, while still maintaining its cushioning effect, a bar of softer material is placed in the top layer of the sole just behind the

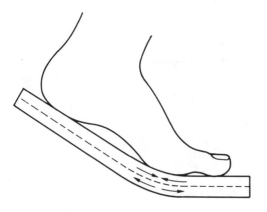

**Figure 14.9** Stresses produced when the sole is flexed. The bottom layers are in tension, while the top layers are compressed. From Segresser and Pforminger (1989), with permission.

metatarsal heads. In addition, grooves are cut in the bottom of the sole at the point of bending.

### Is a running shoe necessary?

Robbins and Hanna (1987) argue that habitually unshod humans are not susceptible to chronic overloading of the foot. Locomotion in barefoot adapted subjects (those who regularly run unshod) differs considerably from that of normally shod subjects. When walking, unshod subjects attempt to grip the ground with their toes, and when running the medial longitudinal arch flattens completely during mid-stance. Foot flattening when running unshod is probably a result of eccentric muscle action and elastic deformation of the intrinsic foot musculature and plantar fascia. Robbins and Gouw (1990) claimed that this response is behaviourly induced in the barefoot adapted runner. They argued that the subject was attempting to minimize discomfort by transferring forefoot load from the MP joints to the distal digits. This process, they claimed, results in hypertrophy of the intrinsic musculature, and relaxes the plantar fascia (Fig. 14.10).

Robbins and Gouw (1990) argued that this shock moderating behaviour of the foot is related to plantar sensibility. The subject attempts to minimize discomfort by increasing the activity of the intrinsic muscles. However, a running shoe with a thick soft sole, will mask sensation to the plantar surface of the foot, and so the subject will not use his or her intrinsic muscles to their full extent.

The above authors therefore recommend that runners run barefoot, after a progressive period of adaptation. If a runner is not able to do this each day, or if safety factors prevent it, Robbins and Gouw advised a less yielding shoe which provides adequate sensory feedback.

Although many practitioners will find Robbins and Gouw's conclusions unsatisfactory, their work does raise a number of interesting points. It illustrates the importance of the inherent shock absorbing mechanisms of the foot, rather than seeing the foot simply as a 'passive falling object'. Furthermore, the often forgotten significance of sensory feedback from the plantar surface of the foot is stressed.

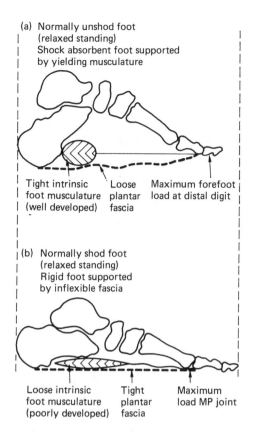

(a) Normally unshod foot
(relaxed standing)
Shock absorbent foot supported
by yielding musculature

Tight intrinsic | Loose | Maximum forefoot
foot musculature | plantar | load at distal digit
(well developed) | fascia |

(b) Normally shod foot
(relaxed standing)
Rigid foot supported
by inflexible fascia

Loose intrinsic | Tight | Maximum
foot musculature | plantar | load MP joint
(poorly developed) | fascia |

**Figure 14.10** Function of intrinsic musculature in (a) unshod and (b) shod foot. From Robbins and Gouw (1990), with permission.

## The court shoe

In running, foot movements occur cyclically, but in court games such as tennis, squash and badminton, the movements are more varied both in direction, and speed. The casual tennis player makes contact mostly with the heel, and less with the ball of the foot. However, when a player is under pressure the situation is reversed. Now, contact is more frequently made with the ball of the foot than the heel, and contact with the medial and lateral edges of the foot is increased (Nigg, Luthi and Bahlsen, 1989).

Movement most commonly occurs in the forward direction, but when under pressure the tennis player moves laterally more frequently. This movement is often combined with contact on the forefoot.

A court shoe must allow all of these movements. The same heel-toe mechanism found in a running shoe is required, but in addition, force attenuation from forefoot contact is needed. The frictional characteristics of the shoe to surface are important. Both translational and rotational movements are needed, translation less so in surfaces which permit some degree of sliding, such as indoor courts or sand/granules.

Because the demands placed on the foot when playing court games are so different to those encountered in road running, athletes must be discouraged from wearing the same shoes for both sports unless they use specifically designed 'cross training' footwear. During lateral movements in particular, the leverage involved with the higher (flared) heel of the running shoe makes injury much more likely. Similarly, tennis shoes do not give adequate rearfoot control or shock attenuation for running.

## The soccer boot

In football, the ball may reach velocities of 140 km/h (Masson and Hess, 1989). This speed, combined with the weight of the ball, especially when wet, leads to deformation of both the boot and foot with kicking. Forces generated may lead to microtrauma to the foot and ankle. Soccer footwear must therefore be as light as possible to minimize any excessive forces created by kicking. At the same time, the shoe must provide both support and protection for the foot.

Combinations of rotation and flexion with the foot fixed to the ground are particularly taxing on the knee structures. Most boots unfortunately compound this problem by the use of cleats or studs, which although improving grip on a wet surface, will also increase rotation forces by reducing 'give'. Indoor surfaces in some cases offer greater grip with similar problems, and shoes need a sole with a greater number of smaller studs to compensate for this.

Shoes must allow the increased range of movement required in soccer, and be flexible enough to accommodate fore foot rocking. Any studs must be placed so as to avoid pressure irritation to the plantar aspect of the foot. Studs on the heel are placed towards the outside of the shoe to avoid rocking or buckling on weight-bearing.

## The sports surface

Ground reaction forces may be resolved into both horizontal and vertical components. The vertical component occurs because of gravity, and the horizontal component is a result of friction. The hardness (ability to withstand distortion) of the ground surface or the sports shoe greatly influences the vertical component of the reaction force on landing (impact force). The playing surface will distort in one of two ways, known as point elasticity and area elasticity (Fig. 14.11). Point elasticity refers to a surface's ability to compress under weight, while area elasticity is a measure of its ability to flex as a whole.

Frictional characteristics occur as a result of the interaction between the shoe and the playing surface. The friction that occurs will be influenced by moisture and floor treatments, and surfaces with different frictional properties will impose different loads on the body. As a consequence, performance characteristics such as energy expenditure and muscle work will change with different sports surfaces, and so will the type and frequency of injury. High amounts of friction may produce excessive forces on the knees and ankles (Ekstrand and Nigg, 1989) while too little friction can cause slipping which could result in trauma. Both trans-

lational (straight line) and rotational (twisting) friction is important. Translational friction is needed for athletes to stop and start, but as it increases so does the possibility for abrasion injuries. Higher levels of rotational friction may increase the likelihood of injury when a player is tackled with his or her weight-bearing leg fixed to the ground. Clearly, there are optimal levels for both types of friction, and simply increasing the amount of friction by changing the shoe or sports surface to give the player 'more grip' is not satisfactory. Frictional characteristics may also be important for the development of arthritis in later life. In one study (quoted in Nigg and Segesser, 1988) from a group of individuals suffering hip arthritis, a greater number were found to be athletes, and 70% of these had participated on surfaces where the foot was 'locked' to the surface.

While the number of non-severe injuries, such as abrasions, seen on artificial surfaces is increased, the frequency of severe injuries remains about the same. Importantly, the number of abrasions suffered on an artificial surface can be reduced by accustomizing players to the new surface (Nigg and Segesser, 1988; Ekstrand and Nigg, 1989). In addition, because artificial surfaces have different frictional characteristics from grass surfaces, the footwear worn by athletes must also be different. Torg and Quedenfeld (1971) showed that both frequency and severity of injury were greater when athletes used conventional shoes with seven cleats (19 mm) than when they used shoes with 14 smaller (9.5 mm) cleats on an artificial playing surface.

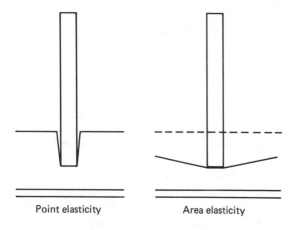

Point elasticity          Area elasticity

**Figure 14.11** Distortion of a playing surface.

### Surface construction

Sports were traditionally performed on grass playing-fields outside, and wooden floors indoors. Later, sprung wooden flooring became the norm for indoor surfaces, while cinder became increasingly popular outdoors. The 1960s saw the development of synthetic resins which could be produced and applied on site at ambient temperatures, to create a playing surface. These new artificial playing surfaces had the advantage of much lower operating and maintenance costs. The maintenance costs of an artificial playing surface for soccer for example is 15% of the cost for a traditional grass surface (Ekstrand and Nigg, 1989).

Outdoor surfaces are most commonly of single layer or sandwich construction, with a variety of porous and non-porous materials being used. Indoor surfaces include spring boards mounted crosswise over wooden slats (area elastic), and elastic base layers with a PVC covering (point elastic).

# References

Bowers, K.D. and Martin, R.B. (1976) Turf toe: a shoe-surface related football injury. *Medicine and Science in Sports and Exercise*, **8**, 81–83

Carmines, D.V., Nunley, J.A. and McElhaney, J.H. (1988) Effects of ankle taping on the motion and loading pattern of the foot for walking subjects. *Journal of Orthopaedic Research*, **6**, 223–229

Cavanagh, P.R. (1989) The biomechanics of running and running shoe problems. In *The Shoe in Sport*, (ed. B. Segesser and W. Pforringer), Year Book Medical Publishers, Wolfe, London

Cibulka, M.T. (1990) Management of a patient with forefoot pain: A case report. *Physical Therapy*, **70**, (1) 55–58

Clanton, T,O., Butler, J.E. and Eggert, A. (1986) Injuries to the metatarsophalangeal joints in athletes. *Foot and Ankle*, **7**, 162–176

Creighton, D.S. and Orson, V.L (1987) Evaluation of range of motion of the first metatarsophalangeal joint in runners with plantar fasciitis. *Journal of Orthopaedic and Sports Physical Therapy*, **8**, 357–361

Ekstrand, J. and Nigg, B.M. (1989) Surface-related injuries in soccer. *Sports Medicine*, **8**, (1) 56–62

Frederick, E.C., Clarke, T.E. and Hamill, C.L. (1984) The effect of running shoe design on shock attenuation. In *Sports Shoes and Playing Surfaces*, (ed. E.C. Frederick), Human Kinetics Publishers, Champaign, Illinois, pp. 190–198

Frederick, E.C. (1989) The running shoe: dilemmas and dichotomies in design. In *The Shoe in Sport*, (ed. B. Segesser and W. Pforringer), Year Book Medical Publishers, Wolfe, London

Frederick, E.C. (1985) The energy cost of load carriage on the feet during running. In *Biomechanics IX*, (ed. D.A. Winter et al.), Human Kinetics Publishers, Champaign, Illinois

George, F.J. (1989) In *Year Book of Sports Medicine*, (ed. R.J. Shephard), Year Book Medical Publishers, Chicago, p. 75

Horn, L.M. and Subotnick, S.I. (1989) Surgical intervention. In *Sports Medicine of the Lower Extremity* (ed. S.I. Subotnick), Churchill Livingstone, Edinburgh

Light L.H., McLellan G.E. and Klenerman, K. (1980). Skeletal transients on heel strike in normal walking with different footwear. *Journal of Biomechanics*, **13**, 477

Masson, M. and Hess, H. (1989) Typical soccer injuries —their effects on the design of the athletic shoe. In *The Shoe in Sport*, (ed. B. Segesser and W. Pforringer), Year Book Medical Publishers, Wolfe, London

Neale, D. and Adams, I.M. (1989) *Common Foot Disorders*, Churchill Livingstone, London

Nigg, B.M., Luthi, S.M. and Bahlsen, H.A. (1989) The tennis shoe — biomechanical design criteria. In *The Shoe in Sport*, (ed. B. Segesser and W. Pforringer), Year Book Medical Publishers, Wolfe, London

Nigg, B.M. and Segesser, B. (1988) The influence of playing surfaces on the load on the locomotor system and on football and tennis injuries. *Sports Medicine*, **5**, 375–385

Palastanga, N., Field, D. and Soames, R. (1989) *Anatomy and Human Movement*, Heinemann Medical, Oxford

Robbins, S.E. and Gouw, G.J (1990) Athletic footwear and chronic overloading. *Sports Medicine*, **9**, (2) 76–85

Robbins, S.E. and Hanna, A.M. (1987) Running related injury prevention through barefoot adaptations. *Medicine and Science in Sports and Exercise*, **19**, 148–156

Rodeo, S.A., O'Brian, S.J., Warren, R.F., Barnes, R. and Wickiewicz, T.L. (1989). Turf toe: diagnosis and treatment. *Physician and Sportsmedicine*, **17**, (4) 132–147

Rodgers, M.M. and Cavanagh, P.R. (1989) Pressure distribution in Morton's foot structure. *Medicine and Science in Sports and Exercise*, **21**, 23–28

Rovere, G.D., Clarke, T.J., Yates, C.S. and Burley, K. (1988) Retrospective comparison of taping and ankle stabilizers in preventing ankle injuries. *American Journal of Sports Medicine*, **16**, 228–233

Segesser, B. and Pforringer, W. (1989) *The Shoe in Sport*, Year Book Medical Publishers, Wolfe, London

Subotnick, S.I (1989) *Sports Medicine of the Lower Extremity*, Churchill Livingstone, London

Tanner, S.M. and Harvey, J.S. (1988) How we manage plantar fasciitis. *Physician and Sportsmedicine*, **16**, (8) 39–47

Torg, J.S. and Quedenfeld, T. (1971) Effect of shoe type and cleat length on incidence and severity of knee injuries among high school football players. *Research Quarterly*, **42**, 203–211

# 15 The lumbar spine

Spinal problems are amongst the most common conditions encountered by the physiotherapist or physical medicine practitioner. More working days are lost because of back pain than any other single condition, and sport does not escape this epidemic. Although an in-depth study of back pain is outside the scope of this book, it is necessary to look at a number of features of spinal injury which are important in the context of sport.

## The spinal disc

There are 24 intervertebral discs lying between successive vertebrae, making the spine an alternatively rigid then elastic column. The amount of flexibility present in a particular spinal segment will be determined by the size and shape of the disc, and the resistance to motion of the soft tissue support to the spinal joints. The discs increase in size as they descend the column, the lumbar discs having an average thickness of 10 mm, twice that of the cervical discs. The disc shapes are accommodated to the curvature of the spine, and the shapes of the vertebrae. The greater anterior widths of the discs in the cervical and lumbar regions reflect the curvature of these areas. Each disc is made up of three closely related components, the annulus fibrosus, nucleus pulposus and cartilage end plates.

The annulus fibrosus is composed of layers of fibrous tissue arranged in concentric bands (Fig. 15.1). Each band has fibres arranged in parallel, and the various bands are angled at 45° to each other. The bands are more closely packed anteriorly and posteriorly than they are laterally, and those innermost are the thinnest. Each disc has about 20 bands in all, and fibre orientation, although partially determined at birth, is influenced by torsional stresses in the adult (Palastanga, Field

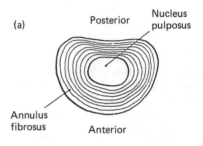

(a)

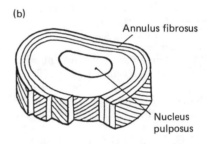

(b)

**Figure 15.1** (a) Concentric bands of annular fibres. (b) Horizontal section through a disc. From Oliver and Middleditch (1991), with permission.

and Soames, 1989). The posterolateral regions have a more irregular make-up, and this may be one reason why they become weaker with age, predisposing them to injury.

The annular fibres pass over the edge of the cartilage end plate of the disc, and are anchored to the bony rim of the vertebra and to its periosteum and body. The attaching fibres are actually interwoven with the fibres of the bony trabeculae of the vertebral body. The outer layer of fibres blends with the posterior longitudinal ligament, but the anterior longitudinal ligament has no such attachment (Vernon-Roberts, 1987).

The hyaline cartilage end plate rests on the surface of the vertebra. This is approximately 1 mm thick at its outer edge and becomes thinner towards its centre. The central portion of the end plate acts as a semipermeable membrane to facilitate fluid exchange between the vertebral body and disc. In addition, it protects the body from excessive pressure. In early life the end plate is penetrated by canals from the vertebral body, but these disappear after the age of 20–30 years. After this period the end plate starts to ossify and become more brittle, the central portion thinning and in some cases being completely destroyed.

The nucleus pulposus is a soft hydrophilic (water attracting) substance taking up about 25% of the total disc area. It is continuous with the annulus, but the nuclear fibres are far less dense. The spaces between the collagen fibres are filled with proteoglycan, giving the nucleus its water-retaining capacity, and making it a mechanically plastic material. The area between the nucleus and annulus is metabolically very active and sensitive to physical force and chemical and hormonal influence (Palastanga, Field and Soames, 1989). The proteoglycan content of the nucleus decreases with age, but the collagen volume remains unchanged. As a consequence, the water content of the nucleus reduces. In early life the water content may be as high as 80–90%, but this decreases to about 70% by middle age.

The lumbar discs are the largest avascular structures in the body. The nucleus itself is dependent upon fluid exchange by passive diffusion from the margins of the vertebral body and across the cartilage end plate. Diffusion takes place particularly across the centre of the cartilage end plate, which is more permeable than the periphery. There is intense anaerobic activity within the nucleus (Holm et al., 1981), which could lead to lactate build up and a low oxygen tension, placing the nuclear cells at risk. Inadequate ATP supplies could lead to cell death.

## Discal biomechanics

In sport, the most important area to consider when discussing the mechanics of the disc is the lumbar spine. The major function of the disc is to allow the spine to twist and bend. The nucleus attracts water by osmosis, creating a high internal fluid pressure able to withstand compressive loads, similar in effect to the air in a car tyre. As the nucleus is compressed, it would tend to bulge, a force contained by the annulus. Compression of the spine is also taken up by the cancellous bone of the vertebrae themselves. As the bone is compressed, blood flows from it, decreases the cancellous bone volume, and dissipates energy without bone damage (contrast bone fracture). The blood returns slowly as the force is reduced, leading to a time-dependent reaction to compression.

Torsional stress is accommodated by the annular fibres. As the disc is twisted, only the fibres facing in one direction are stretched and they are therefore able to resist the stretching force. When the twisting force is reversed, the opposite annular fibres are placed under stretch, so that at any one time only half of the annular fibres are available to resist the torsion. In addition, with torsion the fibres of the outer lamellae are stretched more than those of the inner lamellae, whereas with compression it is the inner fibres that deform to a greater extent (Hukins, 1987).

Discal pressure varies tremendously with alterations in posture. For a 70 kg subject, the pressure in the L3 disc has been found to be about 500 N (Nachemson, 1987). Taking this value as 100%, and comparing different postures to it, lying supine reduces discal pressure to 25%, but sitting increases it to 140%, and bending forwards from this position increases the pressure still further to 275%. Lifting again increases intradiscal pressure, with values of 220% for a forward stooping position. Incorrect lifting techniques which involve bending the spine and keeping the legs straight greatly increase the stress on the intervertebral discs. Pressure variation in different postures are shown in Fig. 15.2

Performing a squat exercise is potentially a dangerous movement for the lumbar spine in sport. Athletes may lift more than twice their own bodyweight in this exercise, causing compression loads of 6–10 times bodyweight on the L3–L4 segment (Cappozzo et al., 1985). During any lift from ground level one of the main back support mechanisms is the thoraco-lumbar fascia (TLF), working in conjunction with the ligamentous and muscular

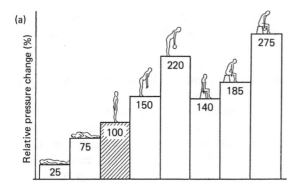

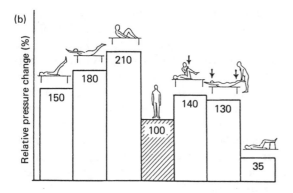

**Figure 15.2** Relative pressure changes in the third lumbar disc. (a) In various positions. (b) In various muscle strengthening exercises. From Nachemson (1976), with permission.

systems. Intra-abdominal pressure (IAP) increases the tension of the TLF, resisting the flexion moment created by the weight of the object and trunk combined (Sullivan, 1989).

To reduce the likelihood of lumbar injury in a squat exercise, two mechanisms exist. First, limiting the forward angulation of the trunk to reduce lumbar compression loading (Cappozzo et al., 1985) and lumbar shear (Russell and Phillips, 1989). Secondly, increasing the IAP by using a weight lifting belt with maximal lifts (Harman et al., 1989). However, athletes must be cautious when using a tight weight-lifting belt, as heart rate and systolic pressure have been shown to increase during this activity (Hunter et al., 1989).

Compression of the lumbar spine with a pressure which exceeds the osmotic pressure within the nucleus will cause water to be exuded through the disc wall, resulting in a loss of disc height. Leatt,

Reilly and Troup (1986) showed an average height loss of 5.4 mm over roughly 25 minutes of weight training. In addition, a 6 km run showed a mean height loss of 3.25 mm. Tyrrell, Reilly and Troup (1985) showed static loading with a bar-bell to increase loss of disc height in a linear fashion to 11.2 mm for a 40 kg weight held for 20 minutes. Reversal of discal shrinkage, by the adoption of the Fowler position or the use of gravity inversion, may be used to unload the spine (Leatt et al., 1986).

In addition to spinal loading, circadian rhythms play an important part in disc height reduction. Peak height reduction occurs within 2–3 hours of rising, with values of 19.3 mm being quoted by Reilly, Tyrrell and Troup (1984), indicating that the spine may be more vulnerable to injury from loading in the evening when it has already lost appreciable disc height.

Lumbar compression and shear forces have also been shown to vary considerably during the performance of different abdominal muscle strengthening exercises. Reductions of 18% for compressive forces and 97% in shear forces were shown by Johnson and Reid (1991) during the performance of a sit-up exercise with the knees and hips flexed to 90° (bench curl-up or abdominal crunch) using an assessment by computer simulation. Greatest tension is developed in the iliopsoas during supine lying when the muscle is in its resting position. As the muscle is shortened by adopting a bench curl-up position, tension in the iliopsoas will reduce. With 45° hip flexion tension development is 70–80% of its maximum, while with the hips and knees flexed to 90° this figure reduces to 40–50% (Johnson and Reid, 1991).

## Discal injury

During flexion, extension and lateral flexion, one side of the disc is compressed and the other stretched. In flexion, the axis of motion passes through the nucleus, but with extension the axis moves forwards (Klein and Hukins, 1983). This fact, coupled with the increased range of motion during flexion, makes it the more dangerous movement. Combinations of torsion and flexion place the disc at particular risk from plastic deformation, which stretches the annular fibres irreversibly, and may cause fibre damage.

A single movement of flexion will stretch and thin the posterior annulus (Oliver and Middleditch, 1991), but it is repeated flexion, especially under load, which is likely to give the most serious pathological consequences. Discal injury occurs most frequently through repeated flexion movements, and when a flexion/rotation strain is placed on the spine during lifting.

When hyperflexion takes place, the supraspinous and interspinous ligaments will overstretch, reducing the support to the lumbar spine. Circumferential tearing will occur to the disc annulus, posterolaterally, usually at the junction between the disc lamina and end plate (Oliver and Middleditch, 1991). The outer annular fibres are innervated, a possible cause of the 'dull ache' in the lumbar spine which often precedes disc prolapse. Rotational strain will increase the likelihood of these injuries. Although rotation is limited in the lumbar spine, it is increased significantly as a result of facet joint degeneration, and during flexion as the facets are separated.

Posterolateral radial fissuring occurs later, and connects the disc nucleus to the circumferential tear, allowing the passage of nuclear material towards the outer edge of the disc. This type of injury has been produced experimentally during discal compression in a combined flexed and laterally flexed posture (Adams and Hutton, 1982). An annular protrusion can occur, when the pressure of the displaced nuclear material causes the annulus to

bulge. Eventually, nuclear material is extruded (herniated) through the ruptured annular wall (Fig. 15.3).

The discal injury may occur gradually as a result of repeated bending, giving symptoms of gradually worsening pain. Pain occurs initially in the lower back, and with time the symptoms are peripheralized into the buttock and lower limbs. Sudden pain may occur from a seemingly trivial injury which acts as the 'last straw' to cause the disc herniation. Loads of sufficient intensity may give rise to an abrupt massive disc herniation. The stress is usually one of weight combined with leverage during a lifting action. Hyperflexion of the spine occurs, due in part to overstretching of the posterior lumbar ligaments.

Radiographic investigations of discal movement have been made by inserting metal pins into the lumbar nucleus pulposus and asymmetrically loading the disc (reported in McKenzie, 1990). These have shown that the disc migrates towards the area of least load. When the asymmetrical load was removed, the nucleus remained displaced, but its relocation was accelerated by compression in the opposite direction or by traction.

## Spinal ligaments

Six spinal ligaments are involved in the biomechanics of the lumbar spine; the anterior and posterior longitudinal ligaments, the intertransverse ligament, the ligamentum flavum, the interspinous and supraspinous ligaments, and the capsular ligaments of the facet joint. A general reduction in energy absorption of all the ligaments has been found with age (Tkaczuk, 1968). The stiffest is the posterior longitudinal ligament and the most flexible the supraspinous (Panjabi, Hult and White, 1984). Interestingly, the ligamentum flavum in the lumbar spine is pre-tensioned (resting tension) when the spine is in its neutral position, a situation which compresses the disc. This ligament has the highest percentage of elastic fibres of any tissue in the body (Nachemson and Evans, 1968), and contains nearly twice as much elastin as collagen. The anterior longitudinal ligament and joint capsules have been found to be the strongest, while the

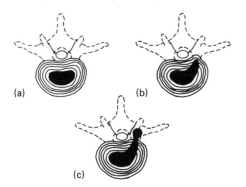

**Figure 15.3** Stages of disc herniation. (a) Normal disc. (b) Nuclear bulge with annulus intact. (c) Ruptured annulus, nuclear protrusion onto nerve root.

interspinous and posterior longitudinal ligaments are the weakest (Panjabi, Hult and White, 1987).

The ligaments act rather like rubber bands, resisting tensile forces but buckling under compressive loads (Fig. 15.4). They must allow adequate motion and fixed postures between vertebrae, enabling a minimum amount of muscle energy to be used. In addition, they protect the spine by restricting motion and in particular protect the spinal cord in traumatic situations, when high loads are applied at rapid speeds. In this situation, the ligaments absorb large amounts of energy.

The longitudinal ligaments are viscoelastic materials, which are stiffer when loaded rapidly, and they exhibit hysteresis as they do not store the energy used to stretch them. When loaded repeatedly, they become stiffer, and the hysteresis is less marked, making the longitudinal ligaments more prone to fatigue failure (Hukins, 1987). The supraspinous and interspinous ligaments are further from the flexion axis, and therefore need to stretch more than the posterior longitudinal ligament when they resist flexion.

## Posture and the spine

A posture is simply a body position. Static posture is a position at rest, while dynamic postures are the various stances which occur with movement. A good posture is one which involves the minimum amount of muscle work, and places little strain on the body tissues. A particular posture is maintained by both inert and contractile structures. The inert structures, such as the bones, fascia and joint structures, support the body, while the muscles, being contractile, move the body from one posture to another. Posture may be discussed in terms of the relationship of the various body segments to the line of gravity. To maintain equilibrium, the line of gravity must either fall directly through the axis of rotation of a joint, or a counter force (inert or contractile) must exist to balance the effect of gravity.

In a balanced standing posture, the line of gravity passes through the bodies of the lumbar and cervical vertebrae, requiring only minimal muscle work from the erector spine as the body sways. Body sway is counteracted by eccentric muscle

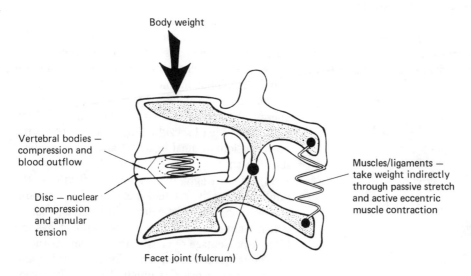

Body weight

Vertebral bodies — compression and blood outflow

Disc — nuclear compression and annular tension

Facet joint (fulcrum)

Muscles/ligaments — take weight indirectly through passive stretch and active eccentric muscle contraction

**Figure 15.4** The spinal segment as a leverage system. From Kapandji (1974), with permission.

action. When the body and line of gravity move forwards, the spinal extensors are stretched and they contract to resist the forward motion and so pull the body back. Backwards sway is similarly resisted by the trunk and hip flexors, while lateral movement is balanced by contralateral muscle action. Persistently poor posture may cause adaptive shortening, leading to dysfunction, and muscle weakness through overstretch or loss of elasticity (Kisner and Colby, 1990).

## Common postural faults

### Lumbar region

The pelvis may be thought for simplicity to balance on the hip joints like a see-saw. Pelvic tilt is controlled by the muscular action of the abdominal muscles, hip flexor, hip extensor, and spinal extensor muscles. Alteration of strength or resting length of these muscles will also change the angle of pelvic tilt and, in turn, the lumbar curvature. Increased lordosis will result from a forward tilt of the pelvis occurring due to weak abdominal muscles, while a reduction in lordosis is a result of reduced pelvic tilt. The lordotic posture is one in which the lumbosacral angle is increased and the pelvis tilts forwards. The condition may exist in parallel with increased thoracic kyphosis and a forward-held head.

The anterior longitudinal ligament will be lengthened, the posterior lumbar disc space narrowed, and the facet joint approximated with accompanying dural compression and synovial irritation. Hip flexors are tight, as are the lumbar extensors, while the abdominals are weak and stretched. Such postures are common following pregnancy, during obesity and following abdominal surgery.

A slouched or swayback posture is one in which the whole pelvis is shifted anteriorly and the hips are forced into extension. To compensate, the thorax is flexed, increasing the lordosis and kyphosis, although the pelvic tilt remains unchanged. The iliofemoral ligaments are stretched, as are the anterior longitudinal ligament of the lower spine and the posterior longitudinal ligament of the upper lumbar and thoracic spines. If the posture is asymmetrical, and weight is taken onto only one leg, the ITB band is also tightened on the straight leg side.

The discs and facets react as they do with the lordotic posture, and the upper abdominal muscles may be tightened while the lower abdominal muscles are stretched or weak. This is a temporary posture, normally caused by fatigue, or in some cases by muscle weakness.

The flat-back posture is characterized by a reduction in lumbosacral angle and posterior tilting of the pelvis. The lordosis is lost and an extension dysfunction is present. The trunk flexors are tight, and the spinal extensors are stretched and weakened. The nucleus of the disc will move backwards. This is the classic posture of the sedentary office worker, in whom prolonged sitting is the norm. In addition, repeated flexion of the spine or disc derangement may also be the cause.

Frontal plane deviations causing secondary scoliosis may occur following discal lesions, or through unilateral sports involving the upper limb. Overstretch of muscle occurs at the side of the convexity and tightness on the side of concavity. Alterations in leg length or pelvic torsions are also a causal factor.

### Thoracic region

The most common postural faults here are a rounded back (increased kyphosis) and a flattened back. Increased kyphosis linked with protracted scapulae is common in relaxed postures, and with an overemphasis on shoulder protraction exercises (bench press) and flexion exercises in exercise classes. The anterior muscles of the thorax are tight, especially the intercostal and pectorals while the scapular retractors and thoracic extensors are weak.

An exaggeration of the normal upright posture, such as occurs in the military stance, may lead to a flat upper back. The thoracic curve is reduced, and the scapulae depressed. Fatigue comes from excess muscle work, and approximation of the clavicle and ribs may give rise to thoracic outlet syndrome in extreme cases. The thoracic extensors and scapular rotators are tight and shoulder movement may be limited.

## Cervical region

The most common fault in the cervical region is that of head protraction, occurring as an occupational condition or with prolonged leaning forwards (for example, in spectators). There is increased flexion in the lower cervical and upper thoracic regions, with increased extension at the occiput and upper cervical spine. Stress may occur in the anterior longitudinal ligament of the upper cervical and posterior longitudinal ligaments of the lower cervical spines. Facet irritation or subluxation may occur with narrowing of the intervertebral foramen of the upper cervical spine. This, in turn, may impinge on the vertebral arteries and/or nerve roots, causing pain, dizziness, headache and nausea. The anterior cervical muscles are tight, and the upper trapezius may be shortened if the scapulae are elevated. Frontal plane asymmetry may occur with tightness to the upper trapezius or sternomastoid, giving torticollis.

Again, exaggeration of the upright posture may occur, reducing the cervical curve and increasing flexion in the upper cervical spine. Stress occurs to the overstretched ligamentum nuchae and neck musculature.

### Postural assessment and correction

Static posture may be assessed by comparing body alignment with a plumb-line reference in the frontal and sagittal planes. Spine, shoulder and pelvic positions are assessed, and marked according to the score chart shown in Fig. 15.5. Forward flexion of the trunk, viewed from behind (Adam's position) is also added to obtain a tangential view of the scapulae and rib cage and check for a rib hump consequent to scoliosis. Dynamic posture in different sporting positions is assessed using video-playback. Important dynamic postures include, for example, lifting positions in weight training, lower limb kinematics in runners, and upper limb mechanics in throwing athletes.

Correction is by identifying and strengthening weak muscle and stretching adaptively shortened tissues. Mechanical therapy is useful for dysfunction of the spinal curves, and shoulder stretching procedures for the pectorals and upper trapezius are particularly worthwhile. Re-alignment of the body segments in static postures is then progressed to simple and then more complex dynamic postures.

## Low back pain

The exact structure which is affected in low back pain is open to discussion, with whole careers in some cases being built on the belief that one tissue is, or is not, the most likely source of pain. To a large extent, the precise anatomical location becomes irrelevant as long as the patient is made better. The situation is made considerably easier if, instead of focusing attention on the injured structure, we attend to the loss of function and our need to restore this.

To this end, the approach taken by McKenzie (1981) is extremely useful. Back pain may be classified as mechanical or chemical (non-mechanical) in origin. Mechanical pain is produced by deformation of structures containing nociceptive nerve endings, and there is a clear correlation between certain body positions and the patient's symptoms.

Conversely, non-mechanical pain is of a constant nature. This may be exacerbated by movement or position, but importantly, no position will be found which completely relieves the symptoms. This category encompasses both inflammatory and infective processes. Inflammation will occur following trauma, and the accumulation of chemical irritant substances will affect the nociceptive fibres and give pain. This type of pain will continue for as long as the nociceptor irritation continues. With rest, irritation will settle and healing progress. Part of this healing process is scar formation, so the type of pain will change from a constant chemical pain to a mechanical pain developed through adaptive shortening of the affected tissues. Non-mechanical conditions also include those which refer pain to the spine, such as vascular or visceral damage and carcinoma. Clearly, it is essential to differentiate between mechanical and non-mechanical pain in the lower back. When no movement can be found which reduces the patient's symptoms and if a period of rest does not allow the symptoms to subside, the patient requires medical investigation.

| Posture score sheet | Name _____ | | | Scoring dates | | | |
|---|---|---|---|---|---|---|---|
| | Good − 10 | Fair − 5 | Poor − 0 | | | | |
| Head Left Right 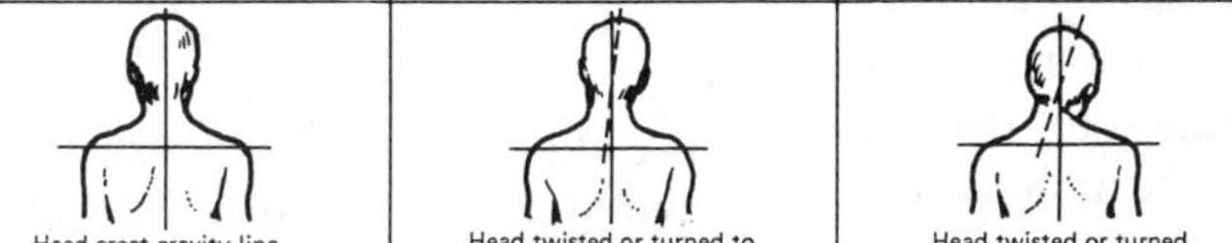 | Head erect gravity line passes directly through centre | Head twisted or turned to one side slightly | Head twisted or turned to one side markedly | | | | |
| Shoulders Left Right 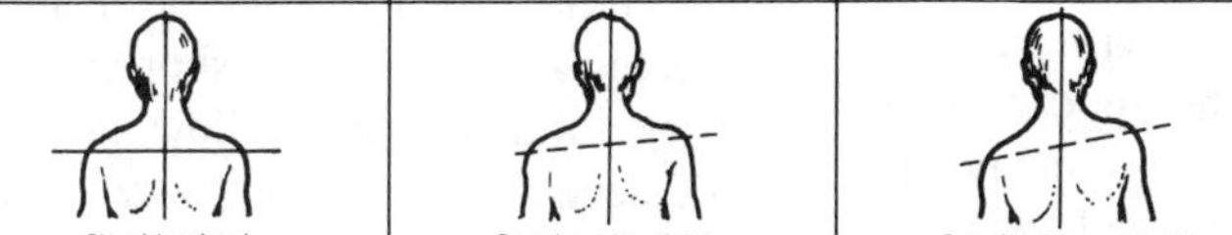 | Shoulders level (horizontally) | One shoulder slightly higher than other | One shoulder markedly higher than other | | | | |
| Spine Left Right 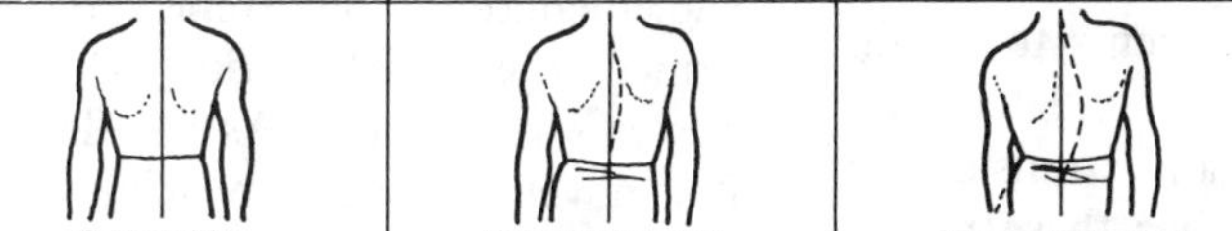 | Spine straight | Spine slightly curved laterally | Spine markedly curved laterally | | | | |
| Hips Left Right 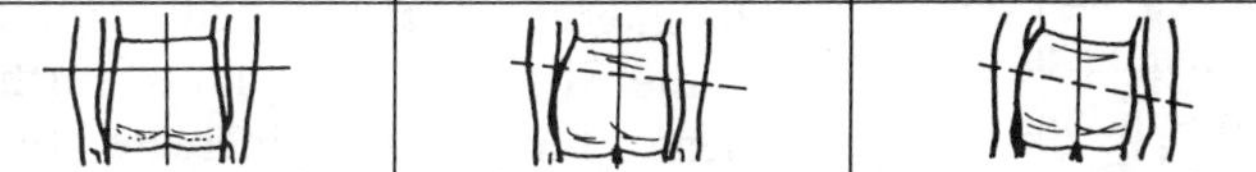 | Hips level (horizontally) | One hip slightly higher | One hip markedly higher | | | | |
| Ankles 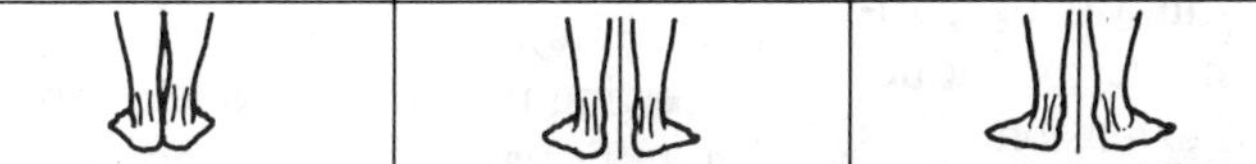 | Feet pointed straight ahead | Feet pointed out | Feet pointed out markedly ankles sag in (pronation) | | | | |
| Neck 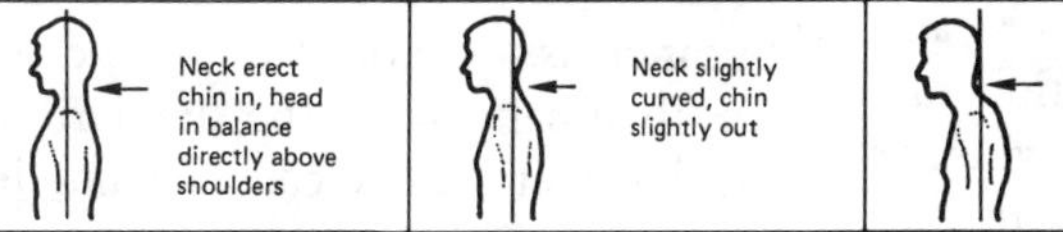 | Neck erect chin in, head in balance directly above shoulders | Neck slightly curved, chin slightly out | Neck markedly forward, chin markedly out | | | | |
| Upper back 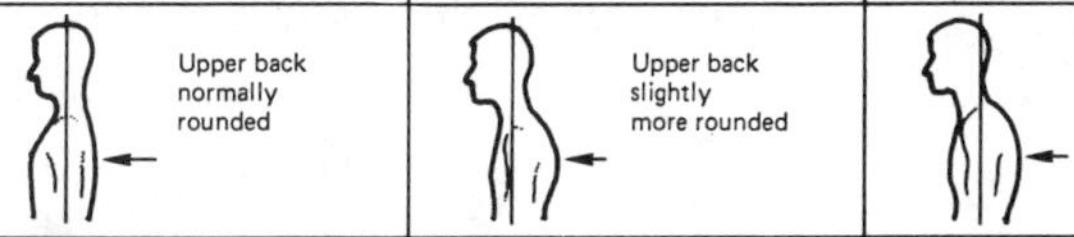 | Upper back normally rounded | Upper back slightly more rounded | Upper back markedly rounded | | | | |
| Trunk 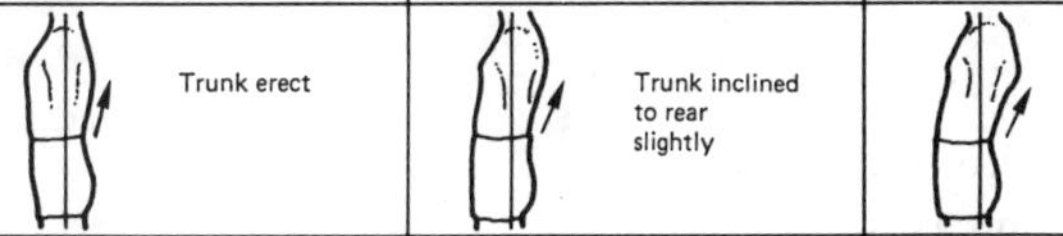 | Trunk erect | Trunk inclined to rear slightly | Trunk inclined to rear markedly | | | | |
| Abdomen 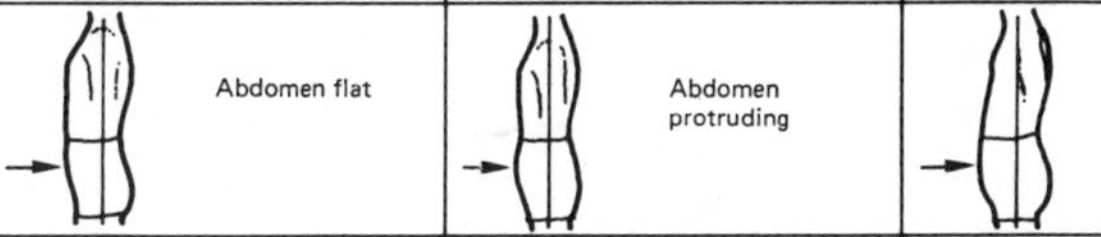 | Abdomen flat | Abdomen protruding | Abdomen protruding and sagging | | | | |
| Lower back 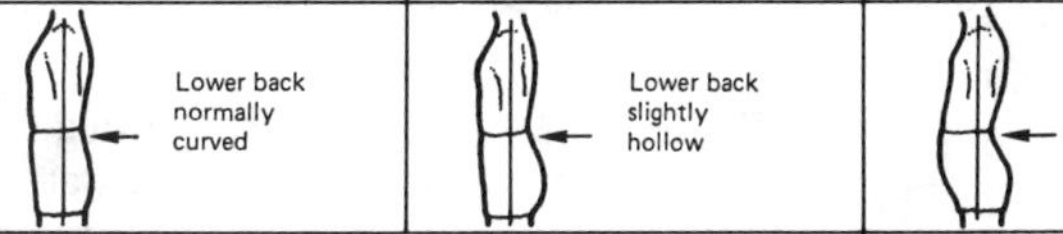 | Lower back normally curved | Lower back slightly hollow | Lower back markedly hollow | | | | |
| | | | Total scores | | | | |

**Figure 15.5**  Posture score sheet.

## Screening examination

Examination of the lumbar spine can be very complex or relatively simple, depending on the approach taken. Initially, the approaches taken by Cyriax (1982) and McKenzie (1981) are extremely useful and provide enough information to treat the majority of patients, or provide the practitioner with an indication that further investigation is necessary.

Observation deals particularly with posture while standing and sitting, and the appearance of the spine at rest. Scoliosis and loss of normal lordosis are of particular note, as is the level of the iliac crests. Flexion, extension and lateral flexion are tested initially as single movements to obtain information about range of motion, end feel and presence of a painful arc. Flexion and extension are then repeated to determine whether these movements change the intensity or site of pain, bearing in mind the centralization phenomenon and dysfunction stretch (see p. 235). Side-gliding movements are also tested to repetition. Flexion and extension may be further assessed in a lying position to obtain information about nerve root adhesion (flexion) and greater range of extension. This initial examination then indicates whether neurological testing of sensation, power, reflexes and further nerve stretch is required. In addition, the history, signs and symptoms will indicate whether the pelvis and sacro-iliac joints warrant further attention, or if resisted tests should be included.

## The straight leg raise

The straight leg raise (SLR) or Laseague's sign is a widely used test to assess the sciatic nerve in cases of back pain. The test also places stretch on the hamstrings, buttock tissues, sacro-iliac joint, posterior lumbar ligaments, and facet joints, in addition to lengthening the spinal canal (Urban, 1986). Confirmation that the nerve root is the source of pain may be made by raising the leg to the point of pain and then lowering it a few degrees. The neuromeningeal structures are then further stretched either from below by dorsiflexing the foot, or applying firm pressure to the popliteal fossa over the posterior tibial nerve. Pressure from above is produced by flexing the cervical spine. In addition, the slump test (see p. 164) is useful. When performing the SLR, as the leg is raised, the knee should not be allowed to bend and the pelvis should stay on the couch.

The dura within the spinal canal is firmly attached to the foramen magnum above and the filum terminale below. Trunk flexion causes the spinal canal to lengthen and therefore stretches the dura, whereas extension, by shortening the canal, induces dural relaxation allowing the sheath to fold. The neuromeningeal pathway is elastic, so tension imparted at one point will spread throughout the whole length of the spine. As the SLR is performed, the initial motion is of the nerve at the greater sciatic notch. As hip flexion goes through 35°, movement occurs proximally to the ala of the sacrum, and during the next 35° the movement is at the intervertebral foramen itself. The last degrees of the SLR do not produce further nerve movement, but simply increase the tension over the whole course of the nerve (Grieve, 1970) (Fig. 15.6).

Testing the unaffected leg (crossed SLR or 'well leg' test) may also give symptoms. This manoeuvre pulls the nerve root and dura distally and medially, but increases the pressure on the nerve complex by less than half that of the standard SLR test. When the ipsilateral SLR causes pain, it simply means that one of the tissues connected to the nerve

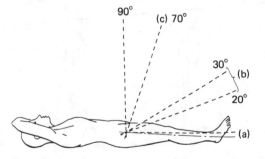

**Figure 15.6**  Effects of straight-leg raising (a) Movement of sciatic nerve begins at the greater sciatic notch. (b) Movement of roots begins at the intervertebral foramen. (c) Minimal movement only, but increase in tension. From Oliver and Middleditch (1991), with permission.

pathway is sensitized. Because the crossed SLR stretches the neural structures less, the resting tension of these tissues must be higher to cause pain. The crossed SLR may therefore be a more reliable predictor of large disc protrusions than the ipsilateral SLR (Urban, 1986).

## Mechanical therapy

Three mechanical conditions are recognized in the lower back, the postural syndrome, dysfunction and derangement (McKenzie, 1981). The postural syndrome occurs when certain postures or body positions place soft tissues around the lumbar spine under prolonged stress. Pain is intermittent, and only occurs when the particular posture is taken up, and ceases when the offending posture is changed. This can be frustrating for the patient because they can find nothing wrong. There is no deformity, vigorous activity is frequently painless, as the stresses it imposes on the tissues are continually changing. The fault is usually poor sitting posture, which places the lumbar spine in flexion. After sport, the patient is warm and relaxed and so sits in a slumped position, perhaps in the bar after a game of squash. Discomfort occurs after some time and this gradually changes to pain. The patient often has the idea that sport makes the pain worse, but this is not the case. The poor sitting posture used when relaxing after sport is the true problem.

Pain may also occur in sport from extreme positions. Hyperflexion when lifting a weight from the ground or performing stretching exercises, hyperextension when pressing a weight overhead, or performing a back walkover in gymnastics are common examples.

The most important part of management of the postural syndrome is patient education. To this end, the slouch-overcorrect procedure for correcting sitting posture is useful (McKenzie, 1981). The patient sits on a stool, and is allowed to slouch into an incorrect sitting posture for some time until his or her back pain ensues. He or she is then taught a position of maximum lordosis, and learns how to change rapidly and at will, from the incorrect slouch to this overcorrect maximum lordosis. Once the patient has seen the relationship between poor

sitting posture and pain, he or she is taught a correct sitting posture mid-way between the two extreme movement ranges. The use of a lumbar pad or roll is helpful to maintain the lordosis in sitting.

If hyperflexion or hyperextension is the cause of postural pain, video is particularly useful in enabling the athlete to appreciate the strain he or she is placing on the lumbar spine. Re-education of movement, and skill training with emphasis on the position of the spine and hips, are helped by video-playback. Bony landmarks over the pelvis and spine are marked first using white adhesive dots (see p. 18). Biofeedback is also useful, especially when trying to correct hyperflexion. In its simplest form, strips of pre-stretched elastic tape are placed at either side of the lumbar spine. When the athlete flexes, the tape 'drags' on the skin and reminds him or her to avoid the flexed position. Various spinal motion monitors used in ergonomics and industrial physiotherapy are also useful in sport. These are attached over the sacrum and thoracic spine and record lumbar movement for feedback through a computer screen, and may be used to show angular displacement and angular velocity.

Dysfunction pain is caused by overstretching adaptively shortened structures within the lumbar spine. The previously damaged structures have shortened due to prolonged disuse, or scar tissue formation. When the normal range of motion is attempted at the affected segment, the shortened soft tissues are stretched prematurely. The essential feature with dysfunction is pain at the end of movement range which disappears as soon as the end range stretch is released. The position is self-perpetuating because the pain which occurs with stretching causes the patient to avoid the full range motion and so the adaptive shortening is compounded.

Dysfunction may occur secondary to trauma, or as a result of the postural syndrome. Typically, the patient is stiff first thing in the morning and his or her back 'works loose' through the day, so he or she is generally better with activity. Loss of extension leads to a reduced lordosis, and loss of flexion becomes apparent when the patient tries to touch his or her toes. Frequently, he or she will deviate to the side of the dysfunction. Once dysfunction has been detected, (static) stretching is required, and/or joint mobilization procedures. Although mobilizations at grades three and four are useful to help restore range of movement, this passive treatment must be coupled with active stretching procedures which the patient can practise at home to help regain lost physiological range. Accessory movements cannot usually be practised by the patient, and are perhaps a more appropriate form of manual therapy where physiological stretching causes excessive pain. It is important that stretching be practised little and often, to allow the patient to recover from the soreness which follows the lengthening of contracted tissues. The patient must be instructed to press gently into the painful end range point in an attempt to increase the range of motion. There is always a tendency to try to avoid the painful position with back pain, but with dysfunction this is precisely the position that should be worked in.

The most common dysfunction following low back pain is loss of extension (McKenzie, 1981). The extension loss may be regained by a combination of mobilization, manipulation and mechanical therapy. The classic mechanical therapy procedure is extension in lying (EIL), either with or without belt fixation. The patient lies prone on the treatment table, with his or her lumbar spine held by a webbing fixation belt. This is placed around both the lower spine and treatment table at a point just below the spinal segment which is blocked to extension. From this position, the patient performs a modified press-up exercise, trying to extend the arms fully while keeping the hips in contact with the couch surface. At home the patient should continue the exercise at regular intervals throughout the day. Various modifications may be used to apply the pressure—such as EIL with the patient lying on an ironing board using a thick belt, or positioning the spine under a low piece of furniture, or manual pressure from a spouse or the weight of a small child.

Loss of flexion may be similarly regained, but this time the mechanical therapy technique is flexion in lying (FIL), or flexion in standing (FIS). Initially, the patient uses FIL. The movement begins in a crook-lying position. From this position the patient pulls his or her knees to the chest. As maximum hip flexion is reached, further movement occurs initially by flexion of the lower lumbar and lumbo-sacral segments, and then the upper lumbar area. FIS is simply a toe-touching exercise performed very slowly. Gravitation effects place greater stress on the lumbar discs, so the exercise must proceed with caution. The differences between FIS and FIL are two-fold. First, with FIS the legs are straight, and so the nerve roots are stretched, a particularly useful effect when dealing with nerve root adhesion. Secondly, the sequence of flexion is reversed, with the upper lumbar areas moving before the lower lumbar and lumbo-sacral areas. Where there was a deviation in flexion at the initial examination, flexion in step standing may be used. Here, one leg is placed on a stool and the patient pulls his or her chest downwards onto the flexed knee. In so doing, flexion is combined with slight lateral bending. Other dysfunctions, such as loss of lateral flexion, side-gliding, or rotation may occur but they are less common. In addition, it must be remembered when assessing symmetry of bilateral movements that most people are slightly asymmetrical anyway. We must be certain that any asymmetry that exists is relevant to the patient's present symptoms before we spend time correcting it.

Derangement occurs when the nucleus or annulus of the disc is distorted or damaged, altering the normal resting position of two adjacent vertebrae. Pain is usually constant and movement loss is apparent, so much so in some cases that the condition is completely disabling. Derangement of the lumbar disc is a common cause of low back pain, and McKenzie (1981) described seven types, classified according to the site and behaviour of symptoms (Table 15.1), while Cyriax (1982) claimed that there are eight ways in which a damaged disc can move, and classified these according to discal position (Table 15.2).

Deformities of scoliosis and kyphosis are common, with local or referred pain over the lumbar and sacral dermatomes, depending on the severity of injury. Again, management may be by manual or mechanical therapy or a combination of the two. Mechanical therapy aims to centralize the pain, and reverse the sequence of pain development which

**Table 15.1 McKenzie classification of disc derangements**

*Derangement one*
Central or symmetrical pain across L4/5
Rarely buttock or thigh pain
No deformity

*Derangement two*
Central or symmetrical pain across L4/5
With or without buttock and/or thigh pain
With deformity of lumbar kyphosis

*Derangement three*
Unilateral or asymmetrical pain across L4/5
With or without buttock and/or thigh pain
No deformity

*Derangement four*
Unilateral or asymmetrical pain across L4/5
With or without buttock and/or thigh pain
With deformity of lumbar scoliosis

*Derangement five*
Unilateral or asymmetrical pain across L4/5
With or without buttock and/or thigh pain
With leg pain extending below the knee
No deformity

*Derangement six*
Unilateral or asymmetrical pain across L4/5
With or without buttock and/or thigh pain
With leg pain extending below the knee
With deformity of sciatic scoliosis

*Derangement seven*
Symmetrical or asymmetrical pain across L4/5
With or without buttock and/or thigh pain
With deformity of accentuated lumbar lordosis

From McKenzie (1981), with permission.

occurred as the disc lesion progressed. The aim is to transfer pain which is felt laterally in the spine or in the leg to a more central position. It is perfectly acceptable for the intensity of the pain to increase, providing its position is altered to a more central one.

The movements used are those which reduced the patient's symptoms in the initial examination. If a scoliosis exists, initially the most effective movement is usually side-gliding in standing (SGIS). The therapist stands at the side of the patient holding his or her hips. The therapist then presses the patient's shoulders gently towards the convexity of the scoliosis, aiming to obtain a sliding rather than laterally flexing, movement. The patient may continue this by placing his or her hand on a wall (with the arm abducted to 90°) and shifting his or her hips towards the wall. Once the pain moves into a more central position, the EIL exercise begins with the aim of centralizing the pain further. With most mechanical therapy procedures, the movement which centralizes or reduces the pain is chosen as the technique for the patient to practise. The patient's response to a particular movement must, therefore, be assessed throughout a treatment session to give continuous feedback about the effectiveness of a procedure.

## Manual therapy of the lumbar spine

The point at which manual therapy is used will vary depending on both the condition and the practitioner using the therapy. Some practitioners rarely use manual therapy, claiming that to do so could make a patient dependent upon this type of care, while others use only mobilization and manipulation, claiming that it gives a more rapid response. The true picture probably lies somewhere between the two extremes. There are certainly patients for whom mechanical therapy is initially too painful. These patients usually respond to mobilization to relieve pain and then to increase mobility, and this treatment may be followed by mechanical and exercise therapy at a later date. Equally, there are patients who look upon manual treatment as a panacea which will always cure them, and so they feel they have no need to care for their own spine. For these, clearly mechanical therapy must be emphasized.

The differences between the various grades of mobilization, and between mobilization and manipulation were discussed on pp. 139–140. For the lumbar spine, there are two techniques (out of literally thousands) which are especially valuable and will be described briefly here. The first is the rotation movement. This is performed in a side-lying starting position, with the painful side uppermost, so that the pelvis is rotated away from the painful side. In the side-lying position both knees and hips are bent (crook side-lying) with the upper

**Table 15.2  Cyriax classification of disc lesions**

*Gradual small posterior displacement*
Pain brought on by stooping or lifting and relieved by standing or resting. Articular signs only, sometimes with painful arc, SLR is full

*Swift large posterior displacement*
Severe low back pain of traumatic origin, or from overuse following prolonged stooping. Constant ache with intermittent twinges. Articular signs of flexion deformity, dural signs of limited SLR and lumbar pain in full neck flexion

*Massive posterior protrusion*
Posterior longitudinal ligaments may rupture, compressing sciatic nerve roots and giving sympathetic signs. Perineal pain and bilateral symptoms, limited SLR with root palsy. Saddle analgesia with bladder weakness

*Posterolateral protrusion*
Previous history of general backache, changing to unilateral pain, pins and needles or numbness, aggravated by coughing. Limitation of trunk flexion and SLR. Pain often increased by neck flexion

*Anterior protrusion in the elderly*
Backache and or unilateral pain with pins and needles in the feet, often mimicking claudication. Symptoms are present only when the patient has been upright for some time and relieved by sitting or lying. Flexion reduces symptoms. SLR full, no neurological deficit

*Anterior protrusion in adolescents*
Osteochondrosis giving pressure erosion of the vertebral body, and kyphotic posture. Associated with excessive weightbearing

*Vertical protrusion*
Schmorl's node formation. No pain, but radiographic appearance confirms abnormality. T10 most commonly effected. Alternatively, biconcave disc phenomenon with osteoporosis

*Circular protrusion*
Compression causes uniform discal bulging, with traction to the periosteum and subsequent osteophyte formation. Limited spinal mobility

Adapted from Cyriax (1982).

leg bending slightly more than the lower. The therapist stands behind the patient and imparts a grade one or two mobilization by pushing rhythmically on the patient's pelvis, allowing the thorax to rock freely. With grades three and four, the patient's underneath arm is pulled through to rotate the thorax, so that the chest faces more towards the ceiling. The upper leg bends slightly further, so that the knee clears the couch side, and the lower leg is straighter to act as a pivot (increasing the flexion of the lower leg will flex the lumbar spine further). Therapist pressure is now over the pelvis and humeral head. This movement may be taken further to apply a manipulation. A lower couch position is used, and the end range point of spinal rotation is maintained by the therapist pushing down on the patient's pelvis and shoulder through straight arms, and in so doing applying slight traction. As the patient exhales, a high velocity, low amplitude thrust is applied. A tremendous number of variations exist to allow for alterations in range of motion, direction of rotation, and combined movements. These procedures are described in detail by Maitland (1986) and Cyriax and Cyriax (1983).

Extension movements in their simplest form may be produced by using postero-anterior pressures and derivatives of this technique. Postero-anterior central vertebral pressure (Maitland, 1986) may be performed with the patient prone. The pressure may be imparted with the pads of the thumbs, or the ulnar border of the hand (pisiform/

hamate) pressing over the spinous processes. Movement is gradually taken up as the therapist moves his or her weight directly over the patient's spine and an oscillation is begun. Variations include combined movements, unilateral pressures, bilateral pressure over the transverse processes, and the addition of hip extension among others.

## The facet joint

The zygapophyseal or facet joints are synovial plane joints. The joint surfaces are covered by hyaline cartilage and each joint has a loose capsule, especially in the cervical region where gliding movements are free. The orientation of the joint surfaces varies depending on the spinal level, so that in the cervical region the joints are angled at 45° in the antero-posterior direction and permit movement in all directions. In the thoracic region the facets face mainly backwards, allowing free lateral flexion and rotation but limiting flexion and extension. In the lumbar spine however, the facets are positioned in the sagittal plane and rotation is the most limited movement, the others being largely free.

The major function of the lumbar facets is the limitation and control of torsion. Normally, the facets take about 20% of axial loading on the spine, but this is increased substantially as the spine is extended. In later life, facet degeneration may occur, and this can be completely independent of any damage to the lumbar discs. The facet joint capsule is a lax structure, enabling the joint to hold about 2 ml of fluid. The loose capsule may actually move into the joint cavity when the joint surfaces are parted with extreme movement or manipulation. Following injury, adhesions can form between the capsule and the joint itself, giving pain to end range motion. The facet has an overlapping neural supply, with ascending, local and descending facet branches coming from the posterior primary ramus. The nerve endings in the facet joint capsules are similar to those in the annulus of the disc, and although the disc is more sensitive, the facet joints can be a source of referred pain to the lower limb (Hirsch, Ingelmark and Miller, 1963),

but not neurological deficit (Mooney and Robertson, 1976).

Relief from facet joint pain has been attempted by both denervation and desensitization as well as manual therapy. Denervation not only destroys the sensation to the facet, but also the motor supply to the spinal extensor muscles as these also receive their supply from the posterior primary ramus. Desensitization with local anaesthesia and hydrocortisone can be useful diagnostically, but persistent pain relief with this technique is rare.

As the facets are synovial joints it seems logical to assume that they will be subject to inflammation and adhesions in the same fashion as any other diarthrodial joint. Manual therapy, especially rotation mobilizations and manipulation to gap the facets, and mechanical therapy to correct any flexion dysfunction caused by capsular adhesions is useful.

## Nags and snags

Many patients who have disc lesions seem to respond well to techniques aimed at the facet joints. The connection between these seemingly dissociate conditions is a biomechanical one. As the disc bulges posteriorly, it causes the vertebrae to flex with a loss of lordosis. For this to happen, the facet joints must be mobile enough to open fully. However, in many cases, these joints are far from mobile, and the soft tissue surrounding them is placed on stretch, giving pain, which can be reduced using mobilization procedures.

Mulligan (1989) described a number of procedures which combine manual and mechanical therapy, taking into account the planes of movement at the facet joints. In the lumbar spine, movement may be assisted (snag procedure) by applying therapist pressure over the spinous processes or particular pillars of the lumbar spine as the patient moves. Flexion, extension or lateral flexion may be used either in sitting or standing. Either pisiform or thumb contact is used, and the direction of pressure is vertical in an attempt to separate, or at least assist separation of, the facets.

The direction of motion and level of pressure application are decided both by the movement which is limited, and the action which relieves the patient's symptoms. As the patient moves, the vertical pressure is applied until end range is obtained. Pressure is continued until the patient resumes the neutral position once more. Nag procedures for the cervical spine are described on p. 264.

## The sacro-iliac joint

The three bones of the pelvis, the two innominates and the sacrum, form a closed ring. Anteriorly, the innominates join together at the pubic symphysis and posteriorly they join the sacrum via the sacro-iliac joints (SIJ). Disorders of the pubic symphysis will often have repercussions on the SIJ, so examination should take in both joints.

The sacral articular surface is shaped like a letter 'L' lying on its side, and is covered by hyaline cartilage, while the corresponding surface on the ilium is covered by fibrocartilage. The SIJ is a synovial joint, but its posterior surface is firmly secured by the interosseous ligament and so the joint may be considered as fibrous. There is great variation between individuals, in terms of the size, shape and number of articular surfaces, with 30% of subjects having accessory articulations between the sacrum and ilium (Grieve, 1976). With increasing age the joint becomes fibrosed and may eventually show partial bony fusion.

The sacrum is inserted like the keystone of an arch, but seemingly the wrong way round, tending to be displaced rather than forced inwards with pressure. However, as the bodyweight is taken, the tension developed in the interosseous sacro-iliac ligaments pulls the two halves of the pelvic ring together (Fig. 15.7). The normal SIJ does move. As the trunk is flexed, the sacral base moves forwards between the ilia, and with trunk extension in standing, the sacrum moves back again. The range of movement is usually only about 5 mm, but ranges of up to 26 mm have been recorded (Frigerio, Stowe and Howe, 1974).

Postural asymmetry of the pelvis is common, and is evident when there is torsion of one ilium in relation to the other. On examination, one anterior superior iliac spine may be higher and one posterior superior iliac spine may be lower, for example.

Unequal leg lengths, although normally asymptomatic, may cause the SIJ to become 'blocked', with a consequent alteration in gluteal muscle tone (Grieve, 1976). When the shortening is more than 1–2 cm, torsion of the pelvis occurs, with the ilium and sacral base on the side of the longer leg moving backwards and the pubis moving upwards. The degree of postural compensation between individuals will differ and so the pelvic position in reaction to altered leg length is variable.

Hormonal changes in pregnancy and, to a lesser extent, menstruation and menopause will also influence the SIJ. The general softening and relaxation of the pelvic ligaments leads to an increased range of motion which may remain for up to 12 weeks following child birth. Local irritation of the SIJ leads to pain on gapping tests and limited hip abduction on the painful side. In addition, the lower PSIS is usually on the painful side.

Subjective examination usually reveals a unilateral distribution of symptoms, perhaps spreading to the buttock, lower abdomen, groin, or thigh, although pain may be referred to the foot. The traumatic history is frequently one of a fall, landing on the ischial tuberosity with patients unable to walk distances without marked pain. The footballer in a mistimed sliding tackle, or the youngster who falls while ice-skating are prime examples. In any sports where the range of motion required at the hip is great, or repetitive unilateral leg movements are performed, SIJ irritation may be encountered. Tensile forces are increased with jumping activities on to both legs, while shear forces are raised with single leg activities, such as running and hopping. Dancers, gymnasts and high-jumpers are particularly prone to SIJ involvement, but any athlete may suffer trauma to the joint leading to local inflammation or mechanical disturbance.

Objective examination of the pelvis and SIJ is made initially with the patient standing. The general bony alignment and muscle contour is noted. The patient may be reluctant to take weight through the affected leg, and might walk with a limp. Loss of gluteal and abdominal muscle bulk has also been reported (Wells, 1986). The level of the gluteal folds and gluteal cleft is noted, as is that of the iliac crests and iliac spines. Movement of the SIJ is assessed both in standing and sitting posi-

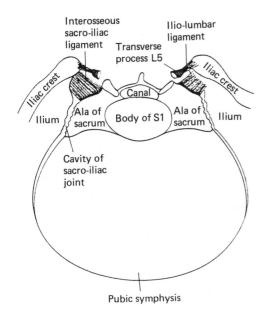

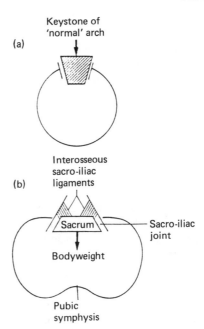

**Figure 15.7** The sacro-iliac joint. (a) Normal keystone of arch principle (not used by body). (b) Diagram of principle found. The bodyweight is transmitted by the interosseous sacro-iliac ligaments and joints.

tions (to eliminate leg length discrepancy). The examiner places his or her thumbs over S2/3 and the PSIS. From the standing position, the patient flexes one hip, and movement of the PSIS is noted. Normally with hip flexion the PSIS moves caudally and as the leg is brought back to the ground it moves cephalically (Wells, 1986). Both PSISs are palpated as the patient flexes his or her spine. If one joint is markedly restricted, the joint which is lower and more prominent in standing moves higher up as the patient flexes (Piedallu's sign).

Flexibility and power of the hip muscles is tested, and passive movements of the hip joint assessed. Range and end feel are noted, with particular attention being paid to passive flexion adduction (SI ligaments) and flexion/abduction/external rotation of the hip with the knee flexed, and lateral malleolus resting above the opposite knee (FABERE, or Patrick's test). Pain produced in the groin or anterior thigh with this test indicates hip involvement, while SIJ pain is localized to the joint. Baer's point, one third of the way down a line joining the umbilicus to the ASIS, is often tender. Iliac gapping and approximation tests will often reproduce SIJ pain, and the apex test is most useful. With the patient in a prone position, the pelvis rests on the ASIS and the pubis. Firm pressure over the sacrum will shear the SIJs and may reproduce unilateral pain if positive.

With persistent bilateral SIJ pain, the possibility of ankylosing spondylitis should be considered. The range of motion, especially lateral flexion, of the lumbar spine is limited, and muscle spasm may be evident. Where costo-vertebral involvement is present, chest expansion will be affected—often an early sign. The use of radiographs, erythrocyte sedimentation rate (ESR), and the presence of the antigen HLA B27 aid the diagnosis.

Treatment of SIJ conditions will obviously depend on the findings at examination, and may include correction of leg length discrepancy, muscle stretching or strengthening, support, modalities or manual therapy. A useful mobilization procedure when unilateral pain is the only symptom is approximation of the ASIS in crook side-lying, with pressure directed to the opposite trochanter. In half crook side-lying (upper hip and knee flexed to 90°) pressure may be imparted to the ischial tuberosity and ASIS to place a rotatory strain on the SIJ, especially helpful when pain is associated with a lower PSIS. As with other mobilization techniques, the movement which reproduces the patient's pain on test is used as a technique, at a grade which produces only minimal discomfort (Maitland, 1986).

## Spondylolysis

Spondylolysis is a defect in the neural arch (pars interarticularis) between the lamina and pedicle of the fifth lumbar vertebra (Fig. 15.8). Occasionally, L4 is also affected. It is a fracture of the pars without slippage. Where symptoms are present but no deformity is detectable on X-ray or bone scan, a pars interarticularis stress reaction has occurred (Weber and Woodall, 1991). At one stage a congenital defect was thought to be present. However, the condition is not present from birth and increases in incidence with age. Furthermore, the

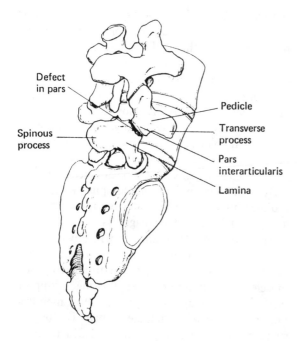

Defect in pars

Spinous process

Pedicle

Transverse process

Pars interarticularis

Lamina

**Figure 15.8** Site of defect in spondylolysis. From Gould (1990), with permission.

ossification centres of the vertebrae do not correspond to the position of the defect. Familial tendencies do exist, and racial differences have been described (Coucher and Hursh, 1952).

The most important consideration from the point of view of sport is that of trauma. Direct trauma may result in a non-union of the area or, more likely, a stress fracture forms over a prolonged period, especially as a result of repeated flexion overload, hyperextension, or shearing stress to the lumbar spine. Athletes with hypolordosis in the lumbar spine are at risk from flexion overload, whereas those demonstrating hyperlordosis may suffer the condition as a result of forced rotation causing torsion overload (Farfan, Osteria and Lamy, 1976). The pars interarticularis is positioned as a pivot between the disc and facet joints, and so subjected to considerable stress. The condition has been described in weight-lifters and oarsmen (Kotanis et al., 1971), hockey players (Letts et al., 1985), gymnasts (Jackson et al., 1981; Weber and Woodall, 1991), and fast bowlers (Williams and Sperryn, 1976). The incidence of spondylolysis in young athletes has been reported to be as high as almost 20% (Hoshina, 1980).

Repeated stress can lead to microfractures, especially if overtraining has occurred. As these heal they produce an elongated appearance of the bone. Lumbar pain is apparent, which may be unilateral or bilateral, but this is rarely associated with nerve root compression. Pain is experienced first with hyperextension, such as walk-over movements in gymnastics, and increases in intensity. Pain is aggravated by hyperextension or rotation, and may present with paraspinal muscle spasm. Unilateral pain may be reproduced if the athlete performs hyperextension in single-leg standing. It is thought that this movement causes compression on the pars interarticularis (Weber and Woodall, 1991). Flexion is normally painless, although pain may occur as the athlete returns to standing. Oblique X-rays give the classic 'terrier dog' appearance (Fig. 15.9) with the dog's collar represented by the pars interarticularis defect, which is bridged by fibrous tissue rather than bone. A negative X-ray does not rule out spondylogenic conditions, and bone scan may be required (Ciullo and Jackson, 1985).

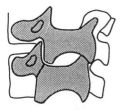

**Figure 15.9** An oblique X-ray of the lumbar spine, which has the appearance of a terrier dog. In the lower segment a spondylolysis through the pars interarticularis appears as a collar around the dog's neck. From Corrigan and Maitland (1983), with permission.

## Spondylolisthesis

Spondylolisthesis is an anterior shift of one vertebra on another, usually L5 on S1. In sport, the condition is usually a progression from spondylolysis, but it may also occur in the elderly as a result of degeneration, or congenitally in association with spina bifida. The first degree injury involves slippage to a distance of one quarter the vertebral diameter, but further movement may occur up to a fourth degree injury which involves a full diameter displacement (Corrigan and Maitland, 1983). The major symptom is of back pain referred to the buttocks, which is aggravated by exercise. Sciatica may be present, as the condition is associated with disc protrusion in 5% of cases (Williams and Sperryn, 1976). The alteration in spinal alignment causes dimpling of the skin and extra skin folds above the level of injury. A step deformity to the spinous process at the lower level is normally apparent to palpation. The lordosis is usually increased, and severe spasm of the erector spinae may be present. Lumbar extension is often severely limited, and passive intervertebral pressure over the spinous process at the affected level is painful.

## Management of spondylogenic disorders

Treatment aims mainly to eliminate the symptoms of the condition rather than to obtain bony union. Initially, rest is required. This varies from 'active rest' by avoiding painful movements with mild conditions, to total bed rest with very severe les-

ions. Occasionally, braces and casts are used to protect the spine until the acute pain subsides, but the most important component of management is closely supervised exercise therapy. Thorough functional assessment is carried out to investigate strength and flexibility In addition to absolute values in comparison to norms for a particular athlete population, muscle imbalance is important. Transmission of ground forces to the spine is governed to a large extent by hip and spine musculature, and weakness or asymmetry here must be corrected. Anterior shear forces are compensated

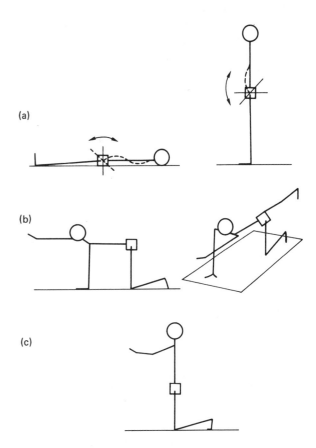

**Figure 15.10** Lumbar stabilization exercises. (a) Pelvic tilting in a lying position to establish a neutral spinal position, and pelvic tilting followed by spinal bracing in a standing position. (b) Prone kneeling leg–arm raising. The spine and pelvis should remain level. Placing a stick across the spine is helpful, the stick will fall if the pelvis tilts. (c) High kneeling activities maintaining neutral spinal position. After Saal and Saal (1989).

by an extension moment created by the abdominal muscles (especially the internal obliques and transversus) and the latissimus dorsi pulling on the thoracolumbar fascia. In addition, the paraspinal muscles counteract shear forces in the lumbar spine (Farfan, Osteria and Lamy, 1976).

The athlete is therefore required to follow an exercise programme to emphasize lumbar stabilization, and re-educate pelvic positioning. The programme (Saal and Saal, 1989; Weber and Woodall, 1991) begins by teaching the neutral spinal position, and then maintaining this by co-contraction of the trunk muscles. This is performed in positions of supine lying, prone kneeling, high kneeling, sitting, standing, and finally during athletic training. The lumbar stabilization is maintained as the athlete performs overhead arm raising in a supine position, single arm lifting and single leg lifting in prone kneeling, and arm actions in high kneeling (Fig. 15.10). Video playback is a valuable tool in this re-education process, especially when athletic activity is resumed.

# References

Adams, M.A. and Hutton, W.C. (1982) Prolapsed intervertebral disc. A hyperflexion injury. *Spine*, **8**, (3) 327

Adams, M.A. and Hutton, W.C. (1985) The effect of fatigue on the lumbar intervertebral disc. *Journal of Bone and Joint Surgery*, **65B**, (2) 199

Cappozzo, A., Felici, F., Figura, F. and Gazzani, F. (1985) Lumbar spine loading during half-squat exercises. *Medicine and Science in Sports and Exercise*, **17**, (5) 613–620

Ciullo, J.V. and Jackson, D.W. (1985) Pars interarticularis stress reaction, spondylolysis, and spondylolisthesis in gymnasts. *Clinics in Sports Medicine*, **4**, 95–110

Colcher, A.E. and Hursh, A.M.W. (1952) Pre-employment low back X-ray survey: A review of 1500 cases. *Industrial Medicine and Surgery*, **21**, 319

Corrigan, B. and Maitland, G.D (1983) *Practical Orthopaedic Medicine*, Butterworth, London

Cyriax, J. (1982) *Textbook of Orthopaedic Medicine*, Vol. one, 8th edn, Baillière Tindall, London

Cyriax, J.H. and Cyriax, P.J. (1983) *Illustrated Manual of Orthopaedic Medicine*, Butterworth, London

Farfan, H.F., Osteria, V. and Lamy, C. (1976) The mechanical etiology of spondylolysis and spondylolisthesis. *Clinical Orthopaedics and Related Research*, 117, 40–55

Frigerio, N.A., Stowe, R.R. and Howe, J.W. (1974) Movement of the sacro-iliac joint. *Clinical Orthopaedics and Related Research*, **100**, 370

Gould, J.A. (1990) *Orthopaedic and Sports Physical Therapy* (2nd edn), C.V. Mosby, St Louis

Grieve, G.P. (1970) Sciatica and the straight leg raising test in manipulative treatment. *Physiotherapy*, **56**, 337

Grieve, G.P. (1976) The sacro-iliac joint. *Physiotherapy*, **62**, (12) 384–400

Harman, E.A., Rosenstein, R.M., Frykman, P.N. and Nigro, G.A. (1989) Effects of a belt on intra-abdominal pressure during weight lifting. *Medicine and Science in Sports and Exercise*, **21**, 186–190

Hirsch, C., Ingelmark, V.E. and Miller, N. (1963) The anatomic basis for low back pain: studies on the presence of sensory endings in ligamentous capsular and intervertebral disc structures in the human lumbar spine. *Acta Orthopaedica Scandinavica*, **33**, 1–17

Holm, S., Maroudas, A., Urban, J.P.G., Selstam, G. and Nachemson, A. (1981) Nutrition of the intervertebral disc: solute transport and metabolism. *Connective Tissue Research*, **8**, 101–119

Hoshina, H (1980) Spondylolysis in young athletes. *Physician and Sportsmedicine*, **8**, 75–79

Hukins, D.W.L. (1987) Properties of spinal materials. In *The Lumbar Spine and Back Pain*, (ed. M.I.V. Jayson), Churchill Livingstone, London

Hunter, G.R., McGuirk, J., Mitrano, N., Pearman, P., Thomas, B. and Arrington, R. (1989) The effects of a weight training belt on blood pressure during exercise. *Journal of Applied Sports Science Research*, **3**, 13–18

Jackson, D.W. et al. (1981) Stress reactions involving the pars interarticularis in young athletes. *American Journal of Sports Medicine*, **9**, 304–312

Johnson, C. and Reid, J.G. (1991) Lumbar compressive and shear forces during various trunk curl-up exercises. *Clinical Biomechanics*, **6**, 97–104

Kapandji, I. (1974) *The Physiology of Joints, Vol. 3, The Spine*, Churchill Livingstone, London

Kisner, C. and Colby, L.A. (1990) *Therapeutic Exercise. Foundations and Techniques*, Davis, Philadelphia

Klein, J.A. and Hukins, D.W.L. (1983) Relocation of the bending axis during flexion-extension of the lumbar intervertebral discs and its implications for prolapse. *Spine*, **8**, 659–664

Kotanis, P.T., Ichikawa, N., Wakabayashi, W., Yoshii, T. and Koshimune, M (1971) Studies of spondylolysis found among weight lifters. *British Journal of Sports Medicine*, **6**, 4

Leatt, P., Reilly, T. and Troupe, J.G.D. (1986) Spinal loading during circuit weight-training and running. *British Journal of Sports Medicine*, **20**, 119–124

Letts, M., Smallman, T., Afanasiev, R. and Gouw, G. (1985) Fracture of the pars interarticularis in adolescent athletes: A clinical-biomechanical analysis.

*Journal of Pediatric Orthopaedics*, **6**, 40–46

Maitland, G.D. (1986) *Vertebral Manipulation*, 5th edn, Butterworths, London

McKenzie, R.A. (1981) *The Lumbar Spine. Mechanical Diagnosis and Therapy*, Spinal Publications, Lower Hutt, New Zealand

McKenzie, R.A. (1990) *The Cervical and Thoracic Spine. Mechanical Diagnosis and Therapy*, Spinal Publications, Waikanae, New Zealand

Mooney, V. and Robertson, J. (1976) The facet syndrome. *Clinical Orthopaedics*, **115**, 149–156

Mulligan, B.R. (1989) *Manual Therapy — Nags, Snags, and PRP's etc*, Plane View Services, Wellington, New Zealand

Nachemson, A. (1976) The lumbar spine: an orthopaedic challenge. *Spine*, **1**, 59–71

Nachemson, A. (1987) Lumbar intradiscal pressure. In *The Lumbar Spine and Back Pain*, (ed. M.I.V. Jayson), Churchill Livingstone, London

Nachemson, A. and Evans, J. (1968) Some mechanical properties of the third lumbar inter-laminar ligament (ligamentum flavum). *Journal of Biomechanics*, **1**, 211

Nachemson, A. and Elfstrom, G. (1970) Intravital dynamic pressure measurements in lumbar discs. *Scandinavian Journal of Rehabilitation Medicine*, Suppl. 1

Oliver, J. and Middleditch, A. (1991) *Functional Anatomy of the Spine*, Butterworth–Heinemann, Oxford

Palastanga, N., Field, D. and Soames, R. (1989) *Anatomy and Human Movement*, Heinemann Medical, Oxford

Panjabi, M.M., Jorneus, L. and Greenstein, G. (1984) *Lumbar Spine Ligaments: an in vitro Biomechanical Study*, ORS Transactions

Panjabi, M.M., Hult, J.E. and White, A.A. (1987) Biomechanical studies in cadaveric spines. In *The Lumbar Spine and Back Pain*, (ed. M.I.V. Jayson), Churchill Livingstone, London

Reilly, T., Tyrrell, A.R. and Troup, J.D.G. (1984) Circadian variation in human stature. *Chronobiology International*, **1**, 121–126

Russell, P.J., and Phillips, S.J. (1989) A preliminary comparison of front and back squat exercises. *Research Quarterly for Exercise and Sport*, **60**, (3) 201–208

Saal, J.A. and Saal, J.S. (1989) Nonoperative treatment of herniated lumbar intervertebral disc with radiculopathy. *Spine*, **14**, 431–437

Sullivan, S.M. (1989) Back support mechanisms during manual lifting. *Physical Therapy*, **69**, (1) 38–44

Tkaczuk, H. (1968) Tensile properties of human lumbar longitudinal ligaments. *Acta Orthopaedica Scandinavica*, **115** (Suppl).

Tyrrell, A.R., Reilly, T. and Troup, J.D.G. (1985) Circadian variation in stature and the effects of spinal loading. *Spine*, **10**, 161–164

Urban, L.M. (1986) The straight-leg raising test: a review. In *Modern Manual Therapy of the Vertebral Column*, (ed. G. P. Grieve), Churchill Livingstone, London

Vernon-Roberts, B. (1987) Pathology of intervertebral discs and apophyseal joints. In *The Lumbar Spine and Back Pain*, (ed. M.I.V. Jayson), Churchill Livingstone, London

Weber, M.D. and Woodall, W.R. (1991) Spondylogenic disorders in gymnasts. *Journal of Orthopaedics and Sports Physical Therapy*, **14**, (1) 6–13

Wells, P. (1986) The examination of the pelvic joints. In *Modern Manual Therapy of the Vertebral Column*, (ed. G.P. Grieve), Churchill Livingstone, London

Williams, J.G.P. and Sperryn, P.N. (1976) *Sports Medicine*, Edward Arnold, London

# 16 The thorax

## Thoracic spine

The unique feature of the vertebrae in the thoracic region is the presence of facets, both on the sides of the vertebral bodies, and on the transverse processes. These are for articulation with the ribs, forming the costo-vertebral and costo-transverse joints. Most of the ribs articulate with two adjacent vertebral bodies and one transverse process. The facets on the head of the ribs articulate in turn with demi-facets on the upper and lower borders of the vertebrae, and the crest on the rib head butts onto the intervertebral disc. The joint capsule is loose and strengthened anteriorly to form the radiate ligament. The costo-vertebral joint cavity is divided into two by the intra-articular ligament, except for ribs one, ten, eleven and twelve which articulate with a single vertebra and have a single joint cavity.

The costo-transverse joints are formed only with the upper ten ribs. The joint is made between the articular facet of the transverse process and the oval facet on the rib tubercle. The thin joint capsule is strengthened by the costo-transverse ligaments.

## Sternal articulations

The sternocostal joints are formed between the medial end of the costal cartilages of ribs one to seven. The joint between the first rib and the sternum is cartilaginous, but all the others are synovial. Each is surrounded by a capsule and supported by radiate ligaments. The fibres of these ligaments fan out and intertwine with those of the ligaments above and below, and also with those of the opposite sternocostal joints. In addition, the radiate ligament fibres fuse with the tendinous fibres of the pectoralis major. The eighth, ninth

and tenth ribs form interchondral joints between their costal cartilages.

The costo-chondral joints are formed between the end of the rib and the lateral edge of the costal cartilage. The joint formed is cartilaginous, its perichondrium being continuous with the periosteum of the rib itself. Only slight bending and twisting actions are possible at this joint. The manubriosternal articulation is that between the upper part of the sternum and the manubrium. The joint is cartilaginous, with a hollow disc in its centre, and is strengthened by the sternocostal ligaments and longitudinal fibrous bands. About 7° of movement occurs at the joint in association with breathing.

## Rib movements

Movement of the diaphragm, ribs and sternum increases the volume within the thorax with inspiration. Each rib acts as a lever, with one axis travelling through the costo-vertebral and sternocostal joints, and another through the costo-vertebral and costo-transverse joints (Fig. 16.1). The two axes permit two types of motion, known as 'pump handle' and 'bucket handle'. In the pump handle action the upper ribs and sternum are raised, increasing the antero-posterior diameter of the thorax. With bucket handle motion the lower ribs move both up and out, widening the infrasternal angle and increasing the transverse diameter of the thorax. The variation in movement between the upper and lower ribs accounts for the different structure of their respective costo-transverse joints. The upper joints are cup shaped, permitting mainly rotation (pump handle), while those lower down are flat, permitting both rotation and gliding movements (bucket handle).

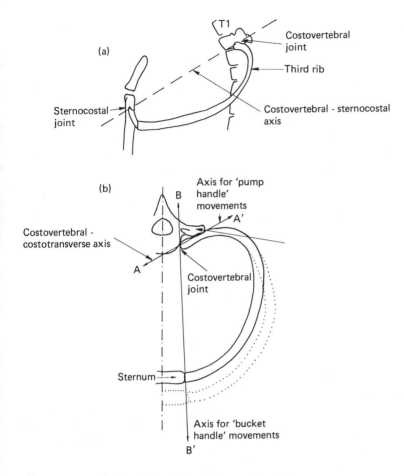

**Figure 16.1** (a) The relationship of the anterior and posterior ends of a rib. (b) The axes of movement of the ribs during respiration. From Palastanga (1989).

In addition to respiratory motion, the ribs also move in association with the thoracic spine. With flexion of the spine the ribs move closer together and with extension they are pulled further apart. Lateral flexion causes the ribs on the concave side to move together and those on the convex side to move apart. Rotation gives horizontal gliding of one rib relative to another.

## Movement of the thoracic spine

The relative thinness of the discs in the thoracic region, coupled with the presence of the ribs, makes movement here more limited than in other spinal areas. Extension is limited to about 30°, with slightly more flexion being possible—roughly 40°. Flexion is freer in the lower thoracic region but is still restricted by the ribs. Extension is limited by approximation of the facets and spinous processes as well as tissue tension, and causes the thoracic cage to become flatter. Lateral flexion is limited to roughly 25° to each side, a greater range being available in the lower region. Lateral flexion is accompanied by the same amount of rotation, which occurs contralaterally. For example, right lateral flexion is accompanied by right axial rotation, causing the tip of the spinous process to rest to the left of the midline. Rib movements accompany lateral flexion, with the ribs on the concave side compressing and those on the side of the convexity being pulled apart.

The range of rotation is larger than other movements with 35° being possible to either side. However, when the spine is extended, both lateral flexion and rotation are dramatically reduced. As rotation occurs, the inferior facets of the upper vertebrae slide laterally with respect to the lower vertebrae, towards the direction of the rotation. The transition from thoracic to lumbar movement may occur at any level between T10 and L1 (Grieve, 1988). Movement of the vertebrae is accompanied by distortion of the ribs. The rib cage becomes more rounded on the side to which the rotation is occurring, and flattens on the opposite side.

Rotation of the thoracic spine is an important constituent of locomotion. In walking, when the right leg swings forward the lower trunk and the pelvis rotate to the left about the fixed left leg. To keep the head facing forwards the upper spine must rotate to the right, pulling the shoulders back into a forward facing direction. As the upper and lower parts of the spine are rotating in opposite directions, there is a point at which the two movements cancel each other out. This point is the intervertebral disc between T7 and T8 which is not subjected to any rotation, while those vertebrae immediately above and below rotate maximally, but in opposite directions.

## Examination

The screening examination is essentially similar to that of the lumbar spine, except that rotation is the movement most likely to be revealing, as this normally has the greatest range. Rotation is performed in a sitting position, with overpressure being given through the shoulders. Resisted flexion and extension may be performed in a lying or a sitting position. Resisted lateral flexion is tested in a standing position with the therapist initially at the patient's side. The patient's near wrist of his or her straight arm is gripped, as is the far shoulder. Stability is improved if the therapist widens his or her base of support by placing his or her near foot between those of the patient.

As rotation and lateral flexion accompany each other in the thoracic spine it is often revealing to combine these movements at examination. Thoracic rotation is performed, and is followed by lateral flexion, firstly in one direction and then the other.

Palpation takes in the vertebrae, rib joints and ribs themselves, and is carried out with the patient in a prone position with his or her arms over the couch side to move the scapulae apart. In a prone-lying position the spinous processes of the thoracic vertebrae are angled downwards like the 'scales of a fish'. The thoracic verebrae may be considered in threes, with the transverse processes being found relative to the spinous processes as follows (Grieve, 1991):

T1, 2, 3 — At the same level as spinous process.
T4, 5, 6 — Between two successive levels.
T7, 8, 9 — Level with spinous process of vertebra below.
T10 — Level with vertebra below.
T11 — Between two successive levels.
T12 — At same level.

As an approximate guide to levels, the AC joint is normally aligned with the C7–T1 interspace, the spine of the scapula at T3 and the inferior scapular angle at T7.

The rib angles gradually spread out from the spine with the eighth rib being furthest (about 6 cm) from the mid-line. The rib angles can be palpated at the same levels as the transverse processes down to the T8/T9, by pushing the soft tissue to one side. The apophyseal joints lie in the paravertebral sulci, and the transverse processes, which overlie the costotransverse, are found 3–4 cm from the mid-line.

## Injury to the rib cage

Direct trauma to the rib cage can result in damage to the ribs, intercostal muscles or, indirectly, to the rib joints. Deep breathing will usually reproduce the pain of rib or intercostal injury, and palpation can be used to reveal the exact site of injury as these structures are superficial. Trunk extension will open the rib cage and cause pain, and intercostal muscle tearing will generally give pain to resisted trunk flexion. Rib springing at a distance from the point of injury usually produces pain from a rib fracture.

With rib fracture, it is the tearing of the intercostal muscles which causes the pain, rather than the fracture itself (Cyriax, 1982). The acute pain may be relieved by local strapping. Pre-stretched elastic adhesive strapping is applied across the area to restrict rib cage expansion and give the athlete a feeling of support. In the sub-acute phase active mobilization is required. If scar tissue formation is excessive and the source of pain, transverse frictions to the intercostal muscles along the line of the ribs are helpful. In addition, holding the rib down with the fingertips and practising deep inspiration will help to stretch the injured area. Exercises to expand the rib cage, such as deep inspiration and overhead reaching, or trunk lateral flexion to the contralateral side with or without rotation is also helpful to stretch the area.

The sternocostal joints may be sprained, causing local swelling and tenderness, as may the costochondral joints (Tietze's syndrome). Pressure on the sternum, or applied to the lateral aspect of the thorax, reproduces the pain and palpation localizes the lesion. The injury can occur when performing exercises which force the arms into extension and abduction. Weight training movements, such as bench pressing, and gymnastic exercises, such as dips on parallel bars, may both cause problems. Both the costo-vertebral and costo-transverse joints may be subject to sprain, with pain occurring to rib movements and local palpation.

## First rib

The first is the shortest and roundest of the ribs. It slopes downwards and forwards, from its attachment to the first thoracic vertebra. It forms attachment for the scalene muscles, serratus anterior, and subclavius. Its superior surface bears a deep groove for the subclavian artery (posterior) and the subclavian vein (anterior). The arterial groove is the weakest part of the rib (Gurtler, Pavlov and Torg, 1985).

Fractures of the first rib may either be traumatic or the result of overuse. Overuse injuries have been reported as a result of repeated arm movements, such as heavy lifting and pitching (Bailey, 1985; Lankenner and Micheli, 1985; Gurtler, Pavlov and Torg, 1985). Symptoms are of pain associated with deep breathing, tenderness in the root of the neck, posterior aspect of the shoulder, or axilla. Often the patient hears or feels a snap in the shoulder as he or she performs a sudden violent movement. Range of shoulder movement will usually be full but painful, especially to extension. Accurate diagnosis by radiographs in traumatic lesions is essential because of the proximity of the major vessels, nerves and the lung. Bailey (1985) recommended serial radiographs for up to 6 months after stress fracture

Management is by rest from the causal action, with shoulder support in a sling if pain is limiting. Gentle isometric shoulder exercises are used, and the condition usually resolves within 4–6 weeks.

## Manual therapy

### Joint mobilization

Postero-anterior central vertebral pressure is the technique normally used first in the thoracic spine, for both unilateral and bilateral symptoms (Maitland, 1986). The technique is essentially the same as that described for the cervical spine. In the thoracic spine, however, the spinous processes are larger, and so the therapist may use his or her thumbs side by side or one in front of the other. For the upper thoracic spine the therapist stands at the patient's head, and for the lower regions at the patient's side. The oscillatory motion is given as described for the cervical spine, with the range of movement being particularly great in the middle and lower thoracic areas, but somewhat limited between T1 and T2.

The costo-vertebral and costo-transverse joints are mobilized by springing the rib. The therapist places the thumbs, or the ulnar border of the hand and little finger, along the line of the rib to be mobilized to give a broad (and more comfortable) area of contact. The mobilization must take the patient's respiratory movements into account, pressure for higher grade movements coinciding with expiration.

Antero-posterior movements may be performed on any of the costal joints (costo-chondral, interchondral or sterno-costal). The therapist's thumbs are placed over the joint to be mobilized with the fingers fanning out over the patient's chest. The movement may be directed towards the patient's head or feet to reproduce the symptoms, and then continued in this direction at a lesser grade.

Intervertebral rotations may be applied both locally and generally. Local rotation may be carried out using pressure over the transverse processes. The thenar eminence of one hand is placed on the transverse process of one vertebra with the fingers pointing towards the patient's head. The hypothenar eminence of the other hand is placed on the transverse process on the opposing side of the spine either of the same vertebra or that of the vertebra below, with the fingers towards the patient's feet. A number of techniques are used. Rotation may be applied by using alternating pressure from one hand and then the other with the hands over the same spinal level (McKenzie, 1990). Or a high velocity, low amplitude thrust may be applied as the patient breathes out, with the hands over the transverse processes of two levels (Bourdillon, 1982).

General rotation may be performed with the patient seated over the couch end, with his or her arms folded, with the hands gripping the shoulders, the therapist stands to the side of the patient. The patient rotates as far as is possible away from the therapist, who reaches across the patient's chest and grasps the patient's far shoulder. Overpressure is applied as the therapist pulls the far shoulder towards him or herself and presses the far scapula away with the flat of his or her hand. Slight traction may be applied by gripping the far elbow rather than the shoulder. The therapist bends his or her knees before applying the grip and then straightens them as he or she pulls up and round. This technique may be used for mobilization or contract-relax stretching (Fig. 16.2).

The close proximity of structures within this area makes it difficult to assess precisely whether a patient's symptoms are coming from the interver-

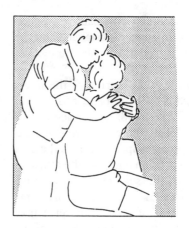

**Figure 16.2** Thoracic rotation mobilization. From Maitland (1986), with permission.

tebral joint, the costo-transverse joint, the costo-vertebral joints or a combination of all three. For this reason many of the mobilizations affect all of these joints.

## Trunk muscles

The trunk muscles are open to injury in the same way as any other muscle in the body, but muscle conditions are often overlooked in the search for signs of more complex injuries involving the intervertebral joints. Injury to the intercostal muscles has already been mentioned, but the abdominal muscles and erector spinae may also give pain from injury or muscle soreness.

The abdominal muscles are tested isometrically to eliminate involvement of the spine. A crook-lying position is preferred, as this partially relaxes the ilio-psoas. Straight flexion taxes the rectus abdominis while flexion-rotation works the oblique abdominals. Pure rotation is tested in a sitting position, while lateral flexion is tested either in a sitting or standing position.

The upper (supra-umbilical) portion of the rectus abdominis is assessed from a sit-up position, while the lower (infra-umbilical) portion is assessed by lowering the straight legs from 90° hip flexion to work the muscle in a reverse origin to insertion fashion. Comparison is made between the right and left sides of the rectus by palpation, and watching the displacement of the umbilicus which will be pulled to the side of the stronger muscle (Lacote et al., 1987). The oblique abdominals are worked by performing a sit-up motion with rotation, for example reaching the right arm towards the left knee. Rotation to the left works the right external oblique and left internal oblique and vice versa. The transversus abdominis acts to support the viscera and is active in forced expiration. It may be tested with the patient in a prone kneeling position. From this position the subject breathes out against a resistance (balloon or spirometer) and pulls the abdominal wall in.

The erector spinae are tested in a prone lying position, the subject being asked to extend his or her trunk and lift his or her chest from the couch. Isometric contraction is assessed by having the patient (in a prone lying position) maintain a horizontal position of the trunk with only the legs supported. Alternatively, the patient should rest his or her chest over the couch end and attempt to straighten the legs to a horizontal position. The quadratus lumborum is tested with the subject prone, leg extended and slightly abducted, to elevate the pelvis laterally. Traction is placed through the elevated leg to oppose the pull of quadratus lumborum (Kendall and McCreary, 1983).

## Exercise in the treatment of spinal pain

The use of exercise in the management of back pain is the subject of considerable debate. Some authors favour flexion exercises, arguing that this will allow more room for the posteriorly bulging disc (Williams, 1955). Others recommend passive extension to compress the posterior aspect of the disc and move it forwards away from the compressing force (McKenzie, 1981). Controversy also exists between the use of passive or active exercise. Passive exercise (mechanical therapy) avoids muscle contraction and therefore longitudinal compression of the lumbar spine, but will not lead to increases in muscle strength. Active exercise will strengthen muscle, but may also considerably raise lumbar intradiscal pressure.

Part of the confusion comes from a failure to assess each patient individually and a desire to find a common exercise regime for a condition which has a multifactorial aetiology. If assessment reveals a reduction in mobility in one direction, then this is the direction that will ultimately require an increase in mobility. Muscle weakness, if identified, will require re-strengthening. The time at which these two procedures is used will depend on the stage of pathology, and the behaviour of the patient's symptoms. The aim is always a centralization or reduction of the patient's symptoms, and a restoration of normal function.

In addition to treatment, exercise may help to prevent the onset of back pain. An increase in general physical fitness has been associated with a reduction in the risk of developing back pain in firefighters (Cody et al., 1979), and reduced isometric strength of the erector spinae was cited as an important risk factor in occupational back pain (Biering-Sorenson, 1984). Isometric strength of the cervical musculature has been proposed as a mechanism to control stability of the neck in football tackling (Franco and Herzog, 1987).

While the physically active sportsperson is no less likely to suffer from a traumatic disc lesion than his or her inactive counterpart, quality and quantity of exercise is important. Postural back pain in a sedentary office worker will usually respond well to correctly applied exercise therapy (Sarno, 1984), and maintenance exercises for back health should include mobility, abdominal/dorsal muscle strengthening, stretching to the psoas and hamstrings (if restricted), re-education of pelvic tilt and general cardiopulmonary endurance (Grieve, 1988).

## Muscle imbalance

Imbalance of both strength and flexibility in the trunk muscles is common. In the normal (pain-free) subject, spinal extensor strength usually exceeds that of the flexors by a ratio of 5:3 (Suzuki and Endo, 1983). Favouring certain muscles in daily living and through training faults can accentuate the imbalance already present. Similarly, an imbalance frequently exists in the flexibility of the trunk and hip muscles, again as the result of a daily living or training effect. This is important because tight muscles have been shown to have an inhibitory effect on their antagonists (Janda, 1986). Attempts to strengthen a weakened muscle without restoring adequate flexibility to its antagonist usually leads to poor results. However, stretching will produce a dis-inhibition and a consequent improvement in muscle activity without the requirement for resistance exercise (Janda, 1978).

An important distinction must be made between postural and phasic muscles. The muscles with mainly dynamic (phasic) function are listed below. (Janda, 1983).

Scaleni
Pectoralis major (abdominal part)
Subscapularis
Extensors of the upper extremity
Trapezius (lower part)
Rhomboidei
Serratus anterior
Rectus abdominis
Obliquus abdominis externus, obliquus abdominis internus
Gluteus minimus, gluteus medius, gluteus maximus
Vastus medialis and lateralis
Tibalis anterior
Peronei

The muscles involved in the standing posture, especially single leg-standing, show a tendency to shorten. These are thought to be genetically older, and demonstrate less reaction to injury (Janda, 1982a). Conversely, phasic muscles have been shown to weaken through inhibition. The muscles commonly found to be short around the lower spine include the iliopsoas, tensor fascia lata, piriformis, adductors, hamstrings, quadratus lumborum and spinal extensors, while the gluteals, quadriceps and abdominals are frequently weak. In the upper spine, tightness is usual in the upper trapezius, sternomastoid, levator scapulae and the upper limb flexors, while weakness may be found in the middle and lower trapezius, rhomboids, prevertebral muscles and upper limb extensors (Janda, 1983).

During the rehabilitation of sports injury, we must be concerned not simply with the morphological damage to a particular tissue but, perhaps more importantly, with the functional consequences of this damage. Phasic muscles have been shown to atrophy more quickly than postural muscles (Janda, 1982b), and so the imbalance in favour of the postural muscles is compounded after injury. An evaluation must always be made of this postural-phasic muscle balance before a stretching or strengthening programme is begun.

Assessment of the flexibility and strength of the limb muscles is made by comparing both sides of the body. Strength evaluation of the spinal and abdominal muscles may be made using a strain gauge or dynamometer. Comparisons between abdominal and spinal extensor strength and endurance can be made, but the results can be confusing. Differences in trunk strength between normal subjects and back pain sufferers are usually only apparent when the condition is chronic (Karvonen et al., 1980; Smidt et al., 1983), and are more noticeable in the back extensors (McNeil et al., 1980).

Various flexibility exercises are presented in Fig. 6.2, and the reader is referred to Evjenth and Hamberg (1991) and Bower (1986) for a more detailed description of spinal and peripheral flexibility programmes.

## Therapeutic muscle strengthening

In cases of chronic back pain where muscle weakness is found, isometric exercise is useful initially. Isometric spinal flexion is performed with the knees and hips flexed to 90° (see below) or in a crook-lying position. Extension is performed in a prone position, with a pillow under the abdomen. Alternatively, the legs may be unsupported over the end of a couch and held in the horizontal position (prone double straight leg raise). The oblique abdominal muscles are taxed by combining flexion and rotation, while the lateral flexor muscles are worked from a side-lying position.

In addition to strength and flexibility of the spine, muscular endurance is important, especially with respect to manual handling. The erector spinae muscles show little activity in normal standing. However, when an object is carried in front of the body the muscles contract vigorously, and when heavy objects are held in one hand, the contralateral muscles are active. As the spine is flexed from the standing position, the erector spinae work eccentrically to lower the body weight. A critical point occurs when the fingertips are reached below the patellae. At this point erector spinae activity ceases, and the body weight is supported by tension in the posterior spinal ligaments.

Muscle endurance of the erector spine is increased by using high repetitions of resistance exercise, and by prolonged static contractions. Contraction of the muscles from a standing flexed position is to be avoided because of the large increase in intradiscal pressure.

Contraction of the abdominals or erector spinae will cause longitudinal compression of the lumbar spine and so raise intradiscal pressure. In the acute phase of discal injury strength exercises may therefore be contraindicated, and mechanical therapy using passive spinal extension is to be preferred.

A rehabilitation programme which concentrates initially on pain relief using mechanical therapy (EIL) and modalities, and later on exercise therapy to improve the stabilization of the spine has been shown to be effective in the treatment of a herniated lumbar disc (Saal and Saal, 1989), and in the rehabilitation of football players with back injury (Saal, 1988a, b). The programme used stretching exercises to the hamstrings, quadriceps, iliopsoas, hip rotators and gastroc-soleus complex, mobilization procedures and strengthening exercises.

The strengthening exercises were designed to obtain adequate dynamic control of the lumbar spine, and were prescribed at two levels of intensity. Level one aimed to establish postural control initially in prone and supine positions, later progressing to kneeling and standing. The aim was to use co-contraction of the abdominal muscles to stabilize the lumbar spine in a neutral position. Advanced level exercises involved other activities such as weight training, running, swimming and cycling, while maintaining the stabilized lumbar posture. Finally, sport specific actions were used again with the athlete maintaining lumbar stabilization.

## Abdominal muscle training in sport

A flat stomach has become synonymous with a visually appealing physique, making abdominal strengthening exercises tremendously popular during sport and fitness training. Although adequate tone is important, abdominal strengthening exercises can be dangerous to the spine if performed incorrectly. The traditional sit-up exercise performed from supine lying has been shown to place an intradiscal pressure of 1200 N on the third lumbar disc of a 70 kg subject, while the same exercise performed isometrically resulted in a load of 600 N, and a bilateral straight leg raise produced an 800 N load (Nachemson, 1987). In addition, we have seen (p. 228) that lumbar shear forces are significantly reduced when a bench-curl exercise is used instead of the normal sit-up (Johnson and Reid, 1991).

The action of the iliopsoas muscle on the spine is of particular importance during abdominal exercise. The iliopsoas muscle is a hip flexor, but when the leg is fixed, it can move the trunk on the hip, by reverse origin-insertion action (the psoas paradox). The standard sit-up action therefore is an exercise which taxes the iliopsoas muscle as much as, and in some cases more than, the rectus abdominis muscle. With inactive individuals the iliopsoas muscle, because of its intense use in everyday activities, is generally the stronger of the two muscles. When a full range sit-up is performed from the supine position the iliopsoas muscle will tend to pull the lumbar spine into hyperextension as the movement commences. This movement is normally resisted by the rectus abdominis muscle, but if weakness of this muscle is present, the spine will suffer. Exercises such as the bilateral straight leg raise place an intense demand on the iliopsoas muscle, and the abdominal muscles are unable to successfully act as fixators of the lumbar spine, and so hyperextension occurs once more.

To reduce the stress on the lumbar spine and increase the work of the rectus abdominis muscle, full range abdominal flexion exercises if they are to be performed should be carried out with the iliopsoas muscle shortened, and without the feet fixed (Lipetz and Gutin, 1970; Ricci, Marchetti, and Figura, 1981; Silvermetz, 1990). This will reduce the ability of the muscle to produce force through the length–tension relationship (see p. 14). The full sit-up movement is therefore better performed in a crook-lying position, or with the hips flexed to 90°. It must be emphasized that the flexed hip position will not eliminate the work of the iliopsoas muscle, nor reduce it substantially, so long as hip flexion remains part of the motion. The hip flexion action is only reduced if the lower spine remains in contact with the supporting surface.

As the sit-up is performed slowly from a supine lying position, the rib cage is depressed anteriorly. The ribs themselves flare outwards, increasing the infrasternal angle. The attachment of the rectus abdominis will tend to tilt the pelvis upwards, but in an individual with weakness of this muscle the reverse may occur. Now the stronger ilio-psoas tilts the pelvis downwards through its iliacus attachment to the iliac fossa. With a straight knee sit-up, a weaker subject is unlikely to be able to perform the exercise keeping the spine neutral. As the spine is flexed however, the body's centre of gravity moves downwards from the upper sacral level to the hip, and the exercise is performed more easily, providing the trunk curl portion of the exercise precedes the hip flexion (Kendall and McCreary, 1983).

As we have seen, in many subjects, the iliopsoas muscle is shortened as a result of prolonged sitting and inactivity. In the supine lying starting position the shortened muscle pulls the lumbar spine into hyperextension. This factor in combination with weak abdominal muscles means that the lumbar spine will further hyperextend as the exercise progresses, placing strain on the lower spine. For these subjects the answer is not to continue sit-up exercises which maintain (or increase) the lack of flexibility of the hip flexors, but to perform a slow trunk curl-up action without hip movement and with the feet unsupported, and to separately stretch the hip flexors. The trunk curl-up is simply the first portion of the straight leg sit-up, involving lumbar flexion but no hip motion. This maintains the length of the hip flexors, involves little hip flexor work and reduces lumbar intradiscal pressure (Nachemson and Elfstrom, 1970; Kendall and McCreary, 1983)

Most forms of sit-up exercise emphasize the supra-umbilical portion of the rectus abdominis (Lipetz and Gutin, 1970). To increase the work on the infra-umbilical portion, lumbar flexion must be performed from below upwards. With the hips and knees at 90°, the lumbar spine is flexed to bring the knees towards the head without increasing hip joint movement. Alternatively, hip and trunk flexion may be performed from a hanging position.

The need to exercise the spinal rotators and lateral flexors must be emphasized to athletes, as these muscles are often neglected in favour of sit-ups alone. In all sit-up type movements, adding trunk rotation will place a greater emphasis on the oblique abdominal muscles (see muscle testing above). The spinal lateral flexor muscles (in combination with the hip abductor muscles) may be exercised from the side-lying position with the legs fixed.

## Hernia

A hernia is a protrusion of the contents of a cavity through the cavity wall. Most usually an organ or peritoneum is forced through the muscular layer of the abdominal wall, at sites of natural weakness where nerves and blood vessels leave the abdomen. The most common types are femoral, inguinal and incisional. Less common types include umbilical, epigastric and hiatus herniae.

Inguinal herniae may be either direct or indirect, and are more common in men. As the testis descends during fetal life, it drags with it a tube-like covering of peritoneum, the processus vaginalis, which is usually obliterated. If this tube remains, it constitutes a weakness which may lead to an indirect inguinal hernia. This usually occurs in males and on the right side of the body. Direct inguinal herniae are more common in older men, and rupture occurs through the weak abdominal wall. They are precipitated by obesity, persistent coughing and straining.

Symptoms of an inguinal hernia are of a dragging sensation in the groin, especially when straining. A swelling may be noticeable over the external ring of the inguinal canal above and medial to the pubic tubercle, the point of attachment of adductor longus. In the case of an indirect hernia, the bulge may be in the upper scrotum. A bulge may be palpated over the hernia when the patient coughs.

It is sometimes possible to pass the little finger through the skin of the upper scrotum to the external ring of the inguinal canal, following the line of the spermatic cord. The patient is supine, and the examining finger is directed upwards, backwards and laterally. Again, coughing will produce a bulge when hernia is present.

A femoral hernia is a protrusion of the abdominal contents through the femoral ring, the point below the inguinal ligament where the blood vessels enter the leg. The condition is more common in women. The features are essentially similar to that of the inguinal hernia, except that the femoral hernia is generally smaller and more difficult to detect. An epigastric hernia travels through the linea alba. A small bulge (usually of fat) is found between the two recti above the umbilicus. An umbilical hernia is due to failure of the umbilical ring to close completely. Later in life this may dilate as a result of a rapid increase in intra-abdominal pressure. These hernias may be very large. Incisional hernias occur after abdominal surgery through the weak area created by the incision. A hiatus hernia is a rupture of a portion of the stomach through the oesophageal hiatus in the diaphragm. This type of hernia generally gives no symptoms in itself, but may in turn cause reflux and oesophagitis giving heartburn. In addition, reflux of bitter irritating fluid into the pharynx and mouth may occur. Antacids are used to neutralize gastric contents, and weight loss and dietary modification (small frequent meals, avoidance of foods that induce symptoms) are used initially.

Initial management of hernia is conservative, and involves instruction on actions to avoid an increase in intra-abdominal pressure. When symptoms persist, surgery is required.

## Thoracic outlet syndrome

Thoracic outlet syndrome is a compression of the brachial plexus rather than the nerve roots, and so symptoms appear in the arm instead of the neck. The lower trunk (C8/T1) is most commonly affected, with bilateral tingling appearing over the median or ulnar distributions into the forearm and hand. The anatomy of the region favours compression. The nervous structures travel through the costoclavicular space, formed by the inner clavicle, first rib and insertions of the scalene muscles. The lower trunk of the brachial plexus and the subclavian artery travel through the outlet formed between the scalenus anterior and scalenus medius to rest on the first rib. The more oblique slope of the first rib in the female changes the costoscalene angle (Grieve, 1986) and may account for the increased incidence of the condition in females.

Middle-aged women are more commonly affected, with the typical clinical picture consisting of a round-shouldered posture displaying a 'dowager's hump' between C7 and T1. The thoracic kyphosis is usually stiff, showing tight pectoral tissues and limited shoulder movements. The thoracic segments and rib angles are often exquisitely tender. The pectoral girdle muscles may have weakened through prolonged disuse, and a 'poking chin' head position is common. This postural complex is summarized in the following list (Grieve, 1986).

1 Descended scapulae, compressing the subclavian artery and lower trunk of the brachial plexus over the first rib.
2 Possible complication of cervical rib seen on X-ray.
3 Soft tissue contracture limiting range of motion at shoulder joint and girdle.
4 Reduced movement in upper/mid-thoracic region (dowager's hump).
5 Tenderness to palpation of upper/mid-thoracic segments and costal joints.
6 Head protraction.

Carrying heavy objects or wearing a heavy coat exacerbates the problem, and simply allowing the arm to hang freely by the side can cause aching. The condition is seen commonly as an occupational injury, with the subject often noticing increased pain when he or she reaches overhead. Typically this pattern also occurs when a middle-aged female takes up exercise in a keep-fit class. When severe, vascular signs such as coldness, blueing or whiteness of the skin may occur if the subclavian artery is affected. Equally, the patient may be woken at night with pain, or can experience numbness first thing in the morning.

Various provocative tests are available which aim to reproduce the patient's symptoms. Sustained scapular elevation, or simply holding the arms overhead may increase the signs. The Adson test examines the radial pulse while the patient breathes in deeply and holds her breath, at the same time extending the neck and rotating it towards the affected side (Halbach and Tank, 1990). Abduction of the shoulder to 90° with full external rotation, combined with vigorous hand movements may give rise to symptoms if compression is significant. In addition, exaggerating the military posture and at the same time placing longitudinal traction through the arms may limit the costoclavicular space and reproduce symptoms (Grieve, 1986). Examination of the thoracic spine should also be made to differentiate the condition from T4 syndrome (see below).

Conservative management is to elevate the scapulae in the first instance. Simply strengthening the trapezius may have little effect. First, because the trapezius, as an antigravity muscle, is usually very strong, and secondly because the stronger muscle may still not be used correctly. Postural re-education is more successful (Cyriax, 1982), teaching a less depressed shoulder girdle resting position. Muscle and non-contractile structures should be stretched using PNF techniques and autotherapy respectively. Postural strengthening exercises using shoulder retraction and elevation are combined with stretching of the pectoral tissues to restore a more normal alignment of the shoulder/ thoracic region. Klapp's crawling position is useful. The patient starts in a prone kneeling position with his or her arms reaching forwards to grasp the couch end. The motion is then to lean back pressing the buttocks towards the heels, and at the same time stretching the shoulders. Retraction strength may be increased with exercises such as supine lying shoulder bracing.

## T4 syndrome

The T4 syndrome (Maitland, 1986; McGuckin, 1986) produces vague widespread symptoms of pain and paraesthesia in the upper limbs and head, possibly with autonomic involvement. Any region between T2 and T7 may be affected, but the focus is normally around T4. The distribution of symp-toms in the hand is glove-like, in contrast to that of thoracic outlet syndrome, but many subjects have sensations extending from the wrist and forearm. Head symptoms appear in a 'skull cap' distribution, and the patient is commonly woken by the pain. Onset may be due to unaccustomed activities or trauma (road traffic accident), but in many cases there is no specific history of injury. As with thoracic outlet syndrome, a predisposing factor is postural. Head protraction, shoulder girdle protraction and accentuated thoracic kyphosis are common, and place a stretch on the thoracic tissues.

On examination, movements can be localized by performing rotations and flexion/extension from a slumped sitting starting position. Palpation is carried out with the patient prone, head in midposition, with the therapist standing at the patient's head. The patient's forearms hang over the couch side and his or her upper arms are abducted to 90° to widen the interscapular space. Signs of joint localization include pain, resistance to passive movement and guarding muscle spasm. Common findings include alteration of the alignment of one spinous process in comparison with its neighbours, with local pain to palpation. Examination must take in the cervical spine and first rib. The first rib is palpated through the trapezius muscle, with the direction of pressure aimed towards the patient's feet, as well as postero-anteriorly.

Mobilization is used for any joints which exhibited signs at examination, and may be carried out with the patient in a supine position, arms folded across his or her chest, and hands placed over the anterior aspect of the shoulders. The therapist places one hand beneath the patient's thoracic spine, with the side of his or her thumb or hand in contact with the area to be mobilized. Downward pressure is exerted through the patient's arms onto the therapist's hand. Postural correction may be carried out as with thoracic outlet syndrome.

## Scheuermann's disease

Scheuermann's disease is a condition predominantly affecting the thoracic spine around T9, although the lumbar levels may be involved

(Greene, Hensinger and Hunter, 1985). The condition is more common in males, and occurs in about 6% of the adolescent population in the age group 12–18 years (Corrigan and Maitland, 1983). There is a disturbance of the normal ossification of the vertebrae. The vertebrae ossify from three centres, one at the centre of the vertebral body, and two secondary centres (the ring epiphyses) in the cartilage end plates. In Scheuermann's disease there is an alteration of the normal development of the ring epiphyses, but a vascular necrosis does not occur (Garland, 1987) in contrast to true osteochondrosis. Penetration of discal material is often seen through the cartilage end plate of the disc and into the vertebral body (Schmorl's nodes). The changes are largely developmental, but trauma may play a part in exacerbating the condition. In contrast, when the central bony nucleus is affected Calvé's vertebral osteochondritis is present, a much less common condition affecting a single vertebra.

The changes in Scheuermann's disease are primarily to the anterior margins of the thoracic vertebra as these bear greater weight. The disc narrows anteriorly, and deficient growth of the vertebral body occurs as a result of epiphyseal malformation. The vertebra gradually takes on a wedged formation. Normally, several vertebrae are affected in the thoracic spine. The athlete is usually a skeletally immature adolescent, with a 'rounded back' posture. In the active stage of the condition there may be localized pain, often provoked by repeated thoracic flexion as occurs in certain swimming strokes (butterflier's back) and aerobic dance classes. Deep notches are visible over the anterior corners of the vertebrae on X-ray, and these appear sclerotic rather than rarefied. The ring epiphyses are irregular, but the erythrocyte sedimentation rate is normal.

The condition is self-limiting, but in the active stage rest is required. In more severe cases, especially those affecting a number of thoracic segments where kyphosis exceeds 30°, a spinal brace (Milwaukee brace) may be required to prevent gross deformity. An exercise programme to prevent further deformity is essential. This normally involves strengthening in extension, and patient education to avoid repeated flexion during activities and prolonged flexion in sitting and lying.

In addition, increasing the lumbar lordosis and stretching the hamstrings has been recommended (Corrigan and Maitland, 1983).

## References

Bailey, P. (1985) Surfer's rib: isolated first rib fracture secondary to indirect trauma. *Annals of Emergency Medicine*, **14**, 346–349

Biering-Sorenson, R. (1984) Physical measurement as risk indicators for low back trouble over a one year period. *Spine*, **9**, 106–119

Bourdillon, J.F. (1982) *Spinal Manipulation*, Butterworth–Heinemann, Oxford

Bower, K.D. (1986) The role of exercises in the management of low back pain. In *Modern Manual Therapy of the Vertebral Column*, (ed. G.R. Grieve), Churchill Livingstone, London

Cady, L.D., Bischoff, D.P., O'Connell, E.R., Thomas, P.C., and Allan, J.K. (1979). Strength and fitness and subsequent back injuries in firefighters. *Journal of Occupational Medicine*, **21**, 269–272

Corrigan, B. and Maitland, G.D (1983). *Practical Orthopaedic Medicine*, Butterworth, London

Cyriax, J. (1982) *Textbook of Orthopaedic Medicine*, Vol. one, 8th edn, Baillière Tindall, London

Evjenth, O. and Hamberg, J. (1991) *Autostretching*. Alfta Rehab Forlag, Sweden

Franco, J.L. and Herzog, A. (1987) A comparative assessment of neck muscle strength and vertebral stability. *Journal of Orthopaedic and Sports Physical Therapy*, **8**, (7) 351–356

Gartland, J.J. (1987) *Fundamentals of Orthopaedics*, 4th edn, W.B. Saunders, Philadelphia

Greene, T.L., Hensinger, R.N. and Hunter, L.Y. (1985) Back pain and vertebral changes simulating Scheuermann's disease. *Journal of Pediatric Orthopaedics*, **5**, 1–7

Grieve, G.P. (1986) *Modern Manual Therapy of the Vertebral Column*, Churchill Livingstone, Edinburgh

Grieve, G.P. (1988). *Common Vertebral Joint Problems*, 2nd edn, Churchill Livingstone, Edinburgh

Grieve G.P. (1991) *Mobilisation of the Spine*, 5th edn, Churchill Livingstone, Edinburgh, p. 5

Gurtler, R., Pavlov, H. and Torg, J.S. (1985) Stress fracture of the ipsilateral first rib in a pitcher. *American Journal of Sports Medicine*, **13**, 277–279

Halbach, J.W. and Tank, R.T. (1990) The shoulder. In *Orthopaedic and Sports Physical Therapy*, (ed. J.A. Gould), 2nd edn, Mosby

Humphrey, D. (1988) Abdominal muscle strength and endurance. *Physician and Sportsmedicine*, **16**, (2) 201–202

Janda, V. (1986) Muscle weakness and inhibition (pseudoparesis) in back pain syndromes. In *Modern Manual*

*Therapy of the Vertebral Column*, (ed. G.P. Grieve), Churchill Livingstone, London

Janda, V. (1978) Muscles, motor regulation and back problems. In *Neurological Mechanisms of Manipulative Therapy*, (ed. I.M. Korr), Plenum, New York

Janda, V. (1982a) Introduction to functional pathology of the motor system. In *Proceedings of the VII Commonwealth and International Conference on Sport, Physical Education, Recreation and Dance*, (ed. M.L. Howell and M.I. Bulloch), Department of human movement studies, University of Queensland

Janda, V. (1982b) Prevention of injuries and their late sequelae. In *Proceedings of the VII Commonwealth and International Conference on Sport, Physical Education, Recreation and Dance*, (ed. M.L. Howell and M.I. Bulloch), Department of human movement studies, University of Queensland

Janda, V. (1983) *Muscle Function Testing*, Butterworth–Heinemann, Oxford

Johnson, C. and Reid, J.G. (1991) Lumbar compressive and shear forces during various trunk curl-up exercises. *Clinical Biomechanics*, **6**, (2) 97–104

Karvonen, M.J., Viltasalo, J.T., Komi, P.V., Nummi, J. and Jarvinen, T. (1980) Back and leg complaints in relation to muscle strength in young men. *Scandinavian Journal of Rehabilitation Medicine*, **12**, 53–59

Kendall, F.P. and McCreary, E.K. (1983) *Muscles Testing and Function*, 3rd edn, Williams and Wilkins, Baltimore

Lacote, M., Chevalier, A.M., Miranda, A., Bleton, J.P. and Stevenin, P. (1987) *Clinical Evaluation of Muscle Function*, Churchill Livingstone, London

Lankenner, P.A. and Micheli, L.J. (1985) Stress fracture of the first rib: a case report. *Journal of Bone and Joint Surgery*, **67A**, 159–160

Lipetz, S. and Gutin, B. (1970) An electromyographic study of four abdominal exercises. *Medicine and Science in Sports*, **2**, (1) 35–38

Maitland, G.D. (1986) *Vertebral Manipulation*, 5th edn, Butterworth, London

McGuckin, N. (1986) The T4 syndrome. In *Modern Manual Therapy of the Vertebral Column*, (ed. G.P. Grieve), Churchill Livingstone, London

McKenzie, R.A. (1981) *The Lumbar Spine. Mechanical Diagnosis and Therapy*, Spinal Publications, Lower Hutt, New Zealand

McKenzie, R.A. (1990) *The Cervical and Thoracic Spine. Mechanical Diagnosis and Therapy*, Spinal Publications, Waikanae, New Zealand

McNeil, T., Warwick, D., Andersson, G. and Schultz, A. (1980) Trunk strength in attempted flexion, extension and lateral bending in healthy subjects and patients with low back disorder. *Spine*, **5**, 529–538

Nachemson, A. (1987) Lumbar intradiscal pressure. In *The Lumbar Spine and Backpain*, (ed. M.I.V. Jayson), Churchill Livingstone, London

Nachemson, A. and Elfstrom, G. (1970) Intravital dynamic pressure measurements in lumbar discs. *Scandinavian Journal of Rehabilitation Medicine*, Suppl. 1

Palastanga, N., Field, D. and Soames, R. (1989) *Anatomy and Human Movement: Structure and Function*, Butterworth–Heinemann, Oxford

Ricci, B., Marchetti, M. and Figura, F. (1981) Biomechanics of sit-up exercises. *Medicine and Science in Sports and Exercise*, **13**, (1) 54–59

Saal, J.A. (1988a) Rehabilitation of football players with lumbar spine injury (Part 1 of 2) *Physician and Sportsmedicine*, **16**, (9) 61–67

Saal, J.A. (1988b) Rehabilitation of football players with lumbar spine injury (Part 2 of 2) *Physician and Sportsmedicine*, **16**,(10) 117–125

Saal, J.A. and Saal, J.S. (1989) Nonoperative treatment of herniated lumbar intervertebral disc with radiculopathy. *Spine*, **14**, (4) 431–437

Sarno, J.E. (1984) Therapeutic exercise for back pain. In *Therapeutic Exercise*, (ed. J.V. Basmajian), 4th edn, Williams and Wilkins

Silvermetz, M. A. (1990) Pathokinesiology of supine double leg lifts as an abdominal strengthener and suggested alternative exercises. *Athletic Training*, **25**, (1) 17–22

Smidt, G., Herring, T., Amundsen, L., Rogers, M., Russell, A. and Lehmann, T. (1983) Assessment of abdominal and back extensor function: a quantitative approach and results for chronic low back patients. *Spine*, **8**, 211–219

Suzuki, N. and Endo, S. (1983) A quantitative study of trunk muscle strength and fatigability in the low back pain syndrome. *Spine*, **8**, 69

Williams, D.C. (1955) Examination and conservative treatment for disc lesions of the lumbo-sacral spine. *Clinical Orthopaedics*, **5**, 28–35

# 17 The cervical spine

The cervical spine consists of eight mobile segments made up of seven cervical vertabrae and the occipital region of the skull. These are generally categorized into two functional units. The first comprises the occiput, C1 and C2 (the sub-occipital region) and the second the segments from C2 to T1 (the lower cervical region).

Within the sub-occipital region, an important distinction is made between the atlanto-occipital and atlanto-axial joints. The atlanto-occipital joint, formed between the occipital condyles and lateral masses of Cl allows no rotation, but free flexion/extension and some lateral flexion. There are three atlanto-axial joints. The median joint is formed between the odontoid peg of the axis and the anterior arch and transverse ligament of the atlas. The lateral two joints are between the lateral articular processes of the atlas and axis. The atlanto-axial joint allows free rotation to about 35°, and only minimal flexion/extension. As rotation occurs, the head is depressed vertically by about 1 mm, causing ligamentous slackening and increasing the available range of motion.

The discs of the lower cervical region are fairly thick, allowing free movement in all planes. Flexion and extension combined has a range of about 110°, with only 25° being flexion, and the least amount of movement occurring between C7 and T1. With flexion, the upper vertebra of a pair slides anteriorly, pulling its inferior facet up and forwards, thus widening the facet joint space posteriorly. With extension, the situation is reversed, the upper vertebra tilting and sliding posteriorly, gapping the facet joint anteriorly but narrowing the intervertebral foramen. Lateral flexion has a range of about 40° to each side. This is not a pure movement, but is combined with rotation and slight extension. Rotation occurs in the lower cervical region in either direction to about 50°, and is limited by grinding of the facets, and torsion stress on the discs and facet capsules. The functional size of the intervertebral foramen is increased on the opposite side to the rotation, but reduced on the same side. Thus, manual therapy to the cervical spine for unilateral pain often involves contralateral rotation to relieve root pressure.

The lateral edge of each vertebra in the cervical region is lipped to form an uncovertebral joint, lying anteriorly to the intervertebral foramen. Each joint is surrounded by a capsule which blends medially with the disc. The joints help to stabilize the neck and control its movements.

Within the total range of any cervical movement some regions move more than others. The upper cervical segments allow more rotation than the lower, but less lateral flexion. With head retraction the upper segments flex while the lower ones extend. In fact, with this movement a greater range of upper cervical flexion is obtained than with neck flexion itself (McKenzie, 1990). As flexion occurs, the spinal canal lengthens, stretching the spinal cord and nerve roots. Extension reverses this effect, relaxing the spinal structures.

## Vertebral arteries

One important difference between the cervical and other spinal areas is the presence of the vertebral arteries. These branch from the subclavian artery and pass through the foramina transversaria of each cervical vertebra from C6 and above (Fig. 17.1). When the artery reaches the atlas, it runs almost horizontally and then enters the foramen magnum to join with its neighbour and form the basilar artery. Variations in the diameter of the vertebral arteries are common, and in some cases the basilar artery is supplied almost entirely by one dominant

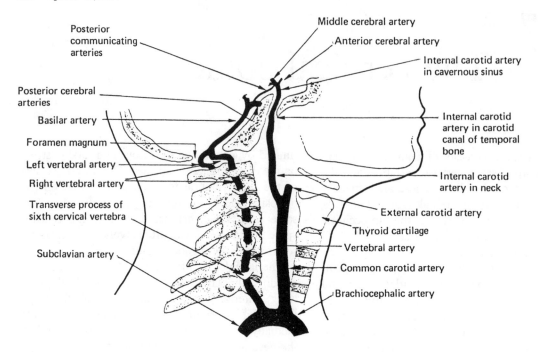

**Figure 17.1**   The vertebral arteries and their connections. From Palastanga, Field and Soames (1989), with permission.

vertebral artery (Bogduk, 1986). During its course, the artery is in close relation to a number of structures, including the scalenus anterior and longus colli muscles, the uncinate processes, the superior surface of the facet joint, and of course the transverse process itself.

If the artery is occluded the predominant symptom is dizziness. Occlusion may be either intrinsic or extrinsic. Intrinsic causes include atherosclerosis blocking the artery causing either focal narrowing, or more extensive constriction over the whole length of the artery Extrinsic causes of occlusion occur by compression to the vessel wall. This is most commonly caused during rotation of the neck if an anomaly of the artery exists. Three such anomalies have been described in the lower part of the artery (Bogduk, 1986). First, an irregularity in the origin of the artery from the subclavian, secondly, bands of deep cervical fascia crossing the artery which tighten on rotation, and thirdly squeezing of the artery within the fascicles of either longus colli or scalenus anterior.

The major portion of the artery is most commonly affected by osteophytes and adhesive scar tissue, with neck rotation compromising the ipsilateral vessel. In the upper region, the artery may be occluded should the atlas move on the axis, through trauma, rheumatoid arthritis or abnormalities of the odontoid. Passive rotation of the neck can shut the contralateral artery by stretching it (Brown and Tatlow, 1963).

Occlusion of the vertebral arteries is a potential danger in any manual therapy to the neck, particularly rotation; in one study some 60 cases of stroke were reported following neck manipulation (Bogduk, 1986). For this reason a basilar test should be performed for any patient who is to receive rotation movements. The test is to combine cervical extension and rotation, maintain this position for 10 seconds and then repeat the movement to the opposite side. In addition, any position described in the patient's history as causing dizziness is tested. To eliminate the possibility of dizziness being vestibular in origin, the patient may be being vestibular in origin, the patient may be assessed in a sitting position as well. The therapist holds the patient's head (but does not cover the ears) and body rotation is performed (for example in a swivel chair) to both sides and held for 10 seconds. The test may then be repeated as a continuous swinging action (Magarey, 1986). As the head itself is not moving, any symptoms are due to cervical rotation rather than vestibular disturbance. For further details of cervical spine testing prior to manipulation, the reader is referred to the Australian Physiotherapy Association (APA) testing protocol (1989).

The production of dizziness, nausea or nystagmus from vertebral artery occlusion is an obvious bar to full range rotation manual therapy. However, even if the test is negative, a small risk still remains so the patient should be continually questioned about dizziness throughout any treatment involving rotation techniques.

## Nature of cervical injury in sport

The most common mechanism of severe cervical injury is axial loading (Torg et al., 1985). This may be caused if a player hits another using his or her head as a battering ram (spearing), or if the athlete falls on to his or her head or runs into an object head-first. In this situation the neck is slightly flexed, flattening the cervical lordosis. Now, the cervical spine absorbs considerably less energy than it would in its normal state as a flexible column. Initially, maximal discal compression occurs, and then the spine rapidly buckles and fails in flexion, resulting in fracture, subluxation or dislocation.

An illustration of the importance of this mechanism and its preventive possibilities is found in American football. The incidence of cervical quadriplegia in this sport dropped dramatically from a peak of 34 cases per year to 5 since head-first tackling and blocking were forbidden (Torg et al., 1985).

A similar mechanism has been described in rugby football. Spinal cord injuries have occurred in scrum, ruck, and maul situations when a player was attempting to pick the ball up from the ground (Silver and Gill, 1988), and as two forwards engage (Taylor and Coolican, 1987). The vertex of the head is restrained, either against another player or against the ground, and the trunk continues to move forwards forcing the cervical spine into flexion and dislocation (McCoy et al., 1984).

In ice hockey, axial loading is again the culprit, when a player hits the boards or an opponent with his or her helmeted head while the neck is slightly flexed (Tator and Edmonds, 1986). In all full-body contact sports such as rugby, American football and ice hockey, it is essential that players are taught that the initial point of contact in a tackle or block should be the shoulders or chest and not the head. In addition, strengthening the neck musculature may reduce the intensity of potential injury (Torg, 1982).

Less severe trauma may occur to the neck with indirect impact or a sudden mis-timed movement. A type of whiplash injury may occur in a rear impact where one player runs into another. Hyperextension of the neck can result in varying degrees of tissue damage.

Diving into a shallow swimming pool or lake is also a common cause of injury, with fracture dislocation occurring as the neck is forced into flexion (or extension in some cases) when the head strikes the pool bottom. The condition may occur if a swimming pool is too shallow, especially if it is left unsupervised or without depth markings. In addition, this tragic injury is common in lakes and rivers with youngsters under the influence of alcohol or drugs.

In gymnastics the most usual mechanism of injury is flexion of the cervical spine, with injury occurring most commonly at C4 and C7 levels (Silver, Silver and Godfrey, 1986). Again, there is an axial loading, with the gymnast landing on his or her head. Of note is the potential for abuse of the trampette by young athletes. This piece of equipment enables the young athlete to gain both height and speed in an inverted body position — a potentially lethal combination.

## Screening examination

The subjective assessment will give the practitioner an indication of the depth of examination required objectively. A great number of tests and procedures exist, but not all will be used with every patient. Following the subjective assessment, a screening examination is used to indicate where further tests, including palpation, should concentrate.

Initial objective examination includes posture and head position in both sitting and standing. Muscle tension and both active and passive motions are examined. Flexion/extension, rotation and lateral flexion are examined for range and end feel. Movements are isolated by eliminating unwanted shoulder elevation or trunk rotation. Resisted movements may be similarly tested, and the shoulder range to abduction and flexion/abduction assessed to determine if there is an associated shoulder or arm pathology. Pain referral and any sensation loss is mapped, and upper limb muscle power and reflexes assessed if the history suggests neurological involvement.

Two further movements and their adaptations are important with reference to mechanical therapy, these are head protrusion and retraction. As with other tests, the location and intensity of symptoms is established prior to testing. Head protrusion is performed in sitting, with the patient instructed to slide the head forwards horizontally as far as possible by 'poking the chin out'. This is performed singly and to repetition. Head retraction is the opposite action, sliding the head back and 'pulling the chin in'. Again overpressure may be used to assess end feel and symptoms. If postural pain is suspected, the movements are performed statically and maintained to load the structures and cause tissue deformation. The capsular pattern of the cervical spine is an equal limitation of all movements, except flexion which is usually of greater range. Asymmetrical limitation of movement suggests a non-capsular lesion such as disc displacement (Cyriax and Cyriax, 1983).

Classification of disc displacement by pain pattern and presence of deformity is similar to that of the lumbar spine (McKenzie, 1990). Derangements one and two give pain travelling as far as the shoulder, three and four give pain referred into the arm but no further than the elbow. Derangements five and six can refer pain down to the wrist. Derangements one, three, and five do not show deformity, whereas derangement two may show cervical kyphosis, and derangements four and six may show torticollis.

### Special tests

Further detail in cervical examination is gained by palpation to test accessory movements, and special tests such as the quadrant position and the upper limb tension test (ULTT). These two latter procedures are useful if the clinical picture is not clear, and to confirm or refute involvement of the cervical spine. The quadrant test combines extension, lateral flexion and rotation to the same side. For the lower cervical spine the neck is taken back into extension and lateral flexion towards the painful side, and then rotated, again towards the pain. The upper cervical spine is tested by extension with pressure to localize the movement to the upper cervical segments. When full extension has been gained, rotation is added towards the pain, followed by lateral flexion. Various sequences of combined movements may produce the patient's symptoms, and it is important that the same sequence of movements be used when comparing both sides or assessing prior to and following treatment.

The ULTT may be thought of as the 'straight leg raise of the upper limb'. It develops tension in the cervical nerve roots and their sheaths and dura, and places greatest stress on the C5 and C6 structures. The movement may be performed in a supine lying position, and combines glenohumeral abduction and external rotation, with elbow, wrist and finger extension and forearm supination. At the same time, the shoulder girdle is depressed and the neck laterally flexed to the painless side. Pain from two-joint muscle stretch over the shoulder is eliminated by altering the head or finger position (which will not affect the shoulder muscles but will alter the nerve tension) to establish if this affects the pain.

In normal subjects an ache is usually felt in the cubital fossa, and some sensation on the radial side of the forearm and hand is common. The test is only positive if symptoms other than these, and similar to the patient's complaint are produced. The ULTT is useful in patients with shoulder girdle or upper limb involvement where the origin of the symptoms is unclear, or where other tests do not reproduce the symptoms (Magarey, 1986).

In sport, traction injury of the brachial plexus can occur, in a position similar to that of the ULTT. With blocking or tackling in rugby or American football, the shoulder may be forcibly depressed while the cervical spine is simultaneously laterally flexed to the contralateral side. The upper trunk of the brachial plexus may suffer a neurapraxia as a result. Nerve function is temporarily disturbed and a burning sensation is felt in the upper limb. The condition is often referred to as a 'stinger' or 'burner' by players, and recovery is usually full in a matter of minutes.

## Manual therapy for the cervical spine

### Joint mobilization

One of the most useful mobilization techniques for the cervical spine in the presence of unilateral symptoms is rotation, usually performed in a direction away from the patient's pain (Maitland, 1986). The patient lies supine on the treatment couch with his or her head extending over the couch end. The therapist grasps the patient's occiput and chin, and rotates the head away from the painful side. The upper cervical (sub-occipital) spine is better mobilized with the head and neck in line. With the lower cervical area the neck is flexed further the lower down the spine the lesion is. Rotation procedures should be stopped if dizziness ensues.

If pain is intense, or if the patient is particularly nervous, longitudinal oscillations are useful. The same grip may be used as with rotation movements, and the longitudinal motion is imparted by the therapist pulling through his or her arms. Stronger manual traction is also of use (Cyriax, 1980). To apply strong traction, the patient's shoulders should be stabilized to avoid the patient being pulled up the couch as the traction force is applied. An assistant can apply pressure onto the patient's shoulder as the therapist increases the traction

force. Alternatively, padded bars (horns) may be used. These are fixed to the couch and jut out vertically from the couch top. In the case of a heavier patient, the patient's bodyweight alone may be sufficient to provide counter-traction and stop the patient sliding on the couch surface.

Traction is applied through straight arms by the therapist leaning back. The use of a belt or harness can reduce the strain on the therapist considerably, and the use of isometric traction is also helpful (Lewit, 1991). Here, the patient is instructed to 'look up' (eyes moving only) and breathe in as his head is held. As the traction force is applied, the patient breathes out and looks down, helping the muscles around the neck to relax. Rotational mobilizations and manipulations may also be applied during traction. Some authors claim that this procedure makes cervical manipulation safe by ensuring that any displaced fragment will move centrally (Cyriax and Cyriax, 1983), while others dispute this claim (Grieve, 1986).

Accessory intervertebral movements are normally performed with the patient in a prone lying position with his or her hands beneath the forehead. The chin is tucked in slightly to reduce the cervical lordosis. The tips or pads of the therapist's thumbs are used to impart the mobilization. Power for the movement comes from the shoulders and is transmitted through the arms and hands, so that the thumbs deliver rather than create the force.

Postero-anterior central vertebral pressures are performed with the therapist's thumbs in contact with the patient's spinous process. More pressure is required to feel movement in the mid-cervical region than in the sub-occipital or lower cervical areas. The atlas has no spinous process, but rather a posterior tubercle, and pressure here is through the overlying muscles and ligaments. The spinous process of C2 overhangs that of C3, so palpation is aided in this region by asking the patient to tuck the chin in further and so increase cervical flexion. The oscillation is repeated two or three times each second, and the direction of travel may be angled towards the patient's head or feet depending on comfort. Postero-anterior central pressures are very useful where symptoms are central, or evenly distributed to either side.

Postero-anterior unilateral pressures are similarly performed, but this time the therapist's thumbs are in contact with the patient's articular processes, and angled towards the mid-line. The technique is used for unilateral symptoms over the painful side. Transverse vertebral pressures are given against the side of a single spinous process with one thumb reinforcing the other. This technique is used mostly where there are unilateral symptoms which are well localized to the vertebrae. The movement is usually performed from the painless side, pressing towards the pain.

## Mechanical therapy

The same rules apply for the assessment of mechanical lesions as for the lumbar spine (p. 235). The postural syndrome is managed largely by correcting sitting posture with the slouch overcorrect exercise. This time, however, the elimination of head protrusion is an important aim.

Extension dysfunction occurs more commonly in the lower cervical spine, making it impossible for the patient to sit correctly. Retraction is performed initially in sitting or standing, followed by extension. Overpressure is most easily given with the patient in a prone lying position. From this position the patient props him or herself on to the elbows, and places the fingers beneath the chin, pushing the head into further extension. Alternatively, a supine lying position may be used with the head over the couch end. The patient allows his or her head to move slowly back into full extension (traction being applied by the weight of the head). Small rotation movements may be used at end range to complete the movement. This latter procedure is really only suitable for younger patients, and even then caution should be exercised with consideration to the vertebral arteries.

Rotation and flexion movements may also be performed with overpressure. The patient gently presses on the chin or pulls the back of the head down respectively.

## Nags and snags

Nags are mid-range oscillatory mobilizations applied to the facet joints between C2 and T3, in an antero-superior direction (Mulligan, 1989). They are used with the patient seated, placing the cervical spine in a functional weight-bearing position.

Assuming the therapist is using the right hand, he or she stands to the right of the patient, blocking any unwanted shoulder movement with his or her own lower trunk. The patient's head is held in the therapist's cupped right hand, with the little finger hooked below the spinous process at the level to be treated. The therapist's left thenar eminence reinforces the pressure of his or her right little finger. The mobilization is applied through the hand and little finger at an angle of 45° to the cervical spine, and repeated 6–10 times.

Varying degrees of flexion and traction may be applied, until a movement is found which reduces the patient's symptoms. The cradled head position is particularly useful in that it gives confidence to the especially nervous patient.

Snags are sustained motions applied at end range. The therapist places the side of his or her thumb over the level to be treated, and presses upwards along the plane of the facet joint as the patient rotates or laterally flexes his or her head. His or her thumb follows the motion as the neck moves. Similar snags may be used if flexion or extension is limited, and to C2 in the case of headaches. In this case the direction of movement is horizontal, again in line with the facet joint plane.

## Soft tissue techniques

Additional soft tissue techniques involve massage and muscle stretching, which are particularly effective when used in combination with other forms of manual therapy. Stretching of the sternomastoid and upper fibres of the trapezius is useful if the neck has been held to one side for any time, or if the athlete (usually a child) wakes with an acute torticollis. The technique is used initially as a passive stretch in a supine lying position and continued as an autostretch technique in a sitting position. In a supine position, the neck is straightened as far as possible. For tightness on the left side, the therapist places his or her left hand against the left side of the patient's head, and his or her right hand over the antero-lateral aspect of the left shoulder, so that the forearms cross. The movement is left shoulder depression combined with right cervical lateral flexion and rotation where this increases the stretch of tight structures. A gentle continuous pressure is used initially, followed by PNF stretching techniques or spray stretch procedures. The autotherapy stretch is applied with the patient sitting on a dining chair. The head is laterally flexed to the right, and the patient grips the chair seat with the left hand to stabilize the shoulder. The patient's right hand reaches over the head and he or she grips the left side of the head and gently pulls the neck into right lateral flexion and right or left rotation, depending on which is the tighter movement (Fig. 17.2).

If the pain is initially too intense for stretching, positional traction is used. Here the patient is supine and the head is straightened as far as possible and held in this position with a rolled towel until the pain starts to subside. The neck is then taken to a new end-range position limited by the pain. This procedure is continued over a 30 minute period, until full lateral flexion (with or without rotation) to the contralateral side is achieved.

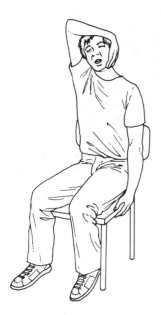

**Figure 17.2** Autotherapy neck stretch. Right hand pulls neck into right lateral flexion. Left hand holds shoulder down by gripping chair seat.

The suboccipital muscles may be massaged and stretched in the supine lying position. The therapist places his or her supinated forearms beneath the patient's head, and grips the suboccipital structures with the pads of his or her flexed fingers. Gently gripping and relaxing the fingers imparts the massage. The muscles are stretched by retracting and flexing the neck, and then applying gentle overpressure. Transverse frictions may be given in prone lying or lean support sitting, using the thumb and forefinger or forefinger supported by the middle finger.

## The temporomandibular joint

The temporomandibular joint (TMJ) can give rise to facial pain of various types, and although this is not strictly a sporting injury, it will be briefly considered. TMJ pain may be the result of alterations in the way the teeth come together (occlusion), and this in turn is affected by mouth guards used in contact sports (see p. 269).

### Structure and function

The TMJ is a synovial condyloid joint found between the mandibular fossa of the temporal bone, and the condyle of the mandible. The two bony surfaces are covered with fibrocartilage, and separated by an articular disc. Movements of the jaw include protraction, retraction, elevation, depression,and lateral gliding, all of which are used to some extent when chewing. The three main muscles contributing to TMJ motion are the temporalis, masseter, and the pterygoids. The temporalis fans out from the temporal fossa to insert into the coronoid process of mandible. The masseter has both deep and superficial portions, and attaches from the zygomatic arch and maxillary process to the angle of the mandible. The medial pterygoid is similar in position to the masseter, but the lateral pterygoid arises from the sphenoid bone and inserts into the mandibular condyle and articular disc, playing a large part in stabilization of the TMJ.

In the occluded position, the upper teeth are normally in front of the lower ones. As the mouth is opened, the lower incisors move downwards and forwards, a movement encompassing forward gliding and rotation at the TMJ. Depression of the mandible is controlled by eccentric action of the temporalis but, if resisted, the geniohyoid, mylohyoid and digastric muscles contract. The jaw is closed powerfully by the masseter, temporalis and the medial pterygoid. The lateral pterygoid pulls the mandible forwards (protraction), while the temporalis is the main effector of retraction.

## Pathology

Dysfunction of the TMJ may present as local muscle tenderness, limited motion and a general dull ache over the side of the face. Clicking may be present, and patients often protrude the mandible as the jaw is opened, or sublux the joint. When chronic, the condition may show reduced range of motion, with contracture of the masticatory muscles. Pain and muscle spasm are common, with the lateral pterygoids most usually affected (Hertling and Kessler, 1990). Emotional stress which presents as teeth clenching is a common factor, as is an alteration in bite pattern and chewing action.

Trauma to the area is common in contact sports, and soft tissue damage and subluxation/dislocation may occur. Whiplash injuries can also give rise to the condition. As the head tips back rapidly, the jaw flies open, stretching the masseter and joint structures. Immediately after this the jaw snaps shut, which may in turn compromise the articular meniscus.

## Management

Limited mandibular movement can be corrected by a number of autotherapy techniques. Initially, the patient starts by simply opening and closing the mouth, gradually increasing the range until a yawning motion is used. Prolonged static stretch is used by placing a number of tongue depressors (about ten to begin with) between the teeth. The stretched position is maintained for 5–10 minutes until the muscles relax. Ice is useful for cryostretch. As the range of motion increases, the number of tongue depressors is increased. Alternatively, a tapered cork may be used to hold the teeth apart. This is inserted thin side first and gradually moved inwards as movement range increases. Translation movements occur when the mouth is opened further than about 1 cm. From this position the patient is instructed to protrude and retract the chin, and to use lateral gliding movements.

Mobilization procedures include caudal traction, in which the therapist presses down on the patient's lower jaw, and medial-lateral gliding and protrusion. In each case the hold is over the chin using the web of the therapist's hand, or over the inner aspect of the lower molars. Direct mobilization may be used with the patient in a side lying position, with the head supported on a pillow. Contact is made with the therapist's thumbs over the posterior surface of the head of the mandible.

In persistent cases referral to a dental practitioner is recommended. Bite patterns may be corrected with the use of a dental appliance, but the precise value of mandibular orthopaedic repositioning appliances (MORA) is still largely uncertain. Some authors (Laskin and Greene, 1972; Gelb, 1977) have used these devices to optimize the positioning of the condyles and fossa of the TMJ to restore neuromotor function to the joint. It has been suggested (Gelb, 1977) that in addition to TMJ pain, cervical and spinal problems may also benefit, and muscle strength may be enhanced in other parts of the body (Schwartz and Novich, 1980). The use of a MORA has however been criticized. Burkett and Berstein (1982), and McArdle et al. (1984) found no increase in strength with subjects using a MORA, and Kerr (1986) concluded that physiological improvement by the use of a MORA had not been scientifically proven.

In all cases of TMJ pain, the cervical and thoracic spines must be examined and excluded as a cause or contributory factor of the patient's complaint.

## References

Australian Physiotherapy Association (APA) (1989). Testing of the cervical spine prior to manipulation. *Physiotherapy Practice*, 5, 207–211

Bogduk, N. (1986) Cervical causes of headache and dizziness. In *Modern Manual Therapy of the Vertebral Column*, (ed. G.P. Grieve), Churchill Livingstone, Edinburgh

Bourdillon, J.F. (1982) *Spinal Manipulation*, Butterworth–Heinemann, Oxford

Brown, B. St J. and Tatlow, W.F.T. (1963) Radiographic studies of the vertebral arteries in cadavers. *Radiology*, **81**, 80–88

Burkett, L.N. and Berstein, A.K. (1982) Strength testing after jaw repositioning with a mandibular orthopaedic appliance. *Physician and Sportsmedicine*, **10**, (2) 101–107

Cyriax, J (1980) *Textbook of Orthopaedic Medicine*, Vol. 2, 10th edn, Treatment by manipulation massage and injection, Baillière Tindall, London

Cyriax, J.H. and Cyriax, P.J. (1983) *Illustrated Manual of Orthopaedic Medicine*, Butterworth, London

Gelb, H. (1977) *Clinical Management of Head, Neck and Temporomandibular Joint Pain and Dysfunction*, W.B. Saunders, Philadelphia

Grieve, G.P. (1986) *Modern Manual Therapy of the Vertebral Column*, Churchill Livingstone, Edinburgh

Hertling, D. and Kessler, R.M. (1990) *Management of Common Musculoskeletal Disorders*, J.B. Lippincott, Philadelphia

Kerr, I.L. (1986) Mouth guards for the prevention of injuries in contact sports. *Sports Medicine*, 415–427

Laskin, D.M. and Greene, G.S. (1972) Splint therapy for the myofacial pain dysfunction (MPD) syndrome in a comparative study. *Journal of the American Dental Association*, **84**, 624–628

Lewit, K. (1991) *Manipulative Therapy in Rehabilitation of the Locomotor System*, 2nd edn, Butterworth-Heinemann, Oxford

Magarey, M.E. (1986) Examination and assessment in spinal joint dysfunction. In *Modern Manual Therapy of the Vertebral Column*, (ed. G.P. Grieve), Churchill Livingstone, Edinburgh

Maitland, G.D. (1986) *Vertebral Manipulation*, 5th edn, Butterworth, London

McArdle, W.D., Goldstein, L.B., Last, F.C., Spena, R. and Lechtman, S. (1984) Temporomandibular joint repositioning and exercise performance: a double blind study. *Medicine and Science in Sports and Exercise*, **16**, (3) 228–233

McCoy, G.F. et al. (1984) Injuries of the cervical spine in schoolboy rugby football. *Journal of Bone and Joint Surgery*, **66B**, 500–503

McKenzie, R.A. (1990) *The Cervical and Thoracic Spine. Mechanical Diagnosis and Therapy*, Spinal Publications, Waikanae, New Zealand

Mulligan, B.R. (1989) *Manual Therapy Nags, Snags, and PRP's etc*, Plane View Services, Wellington, New Zealand

Palastanga, N., Field, D. and Soames, R. (1989) *Anatomy and Human Movement*, Heinemann Medical, Oxford

Schwartz, R. and Novich, M.M. (1980) The athlete's mouthpiece. *American Journal of Sports Medicine*, **8**, (5) 357–359

Silver, J.R., Silver, D.D. and Godfrey, J.J. (1986). Injuries of the spine sustained during gymnastic activities. *British Medical Journal*, **293**, 861–863

Silver, J.R. and Gill, S. (1988) Injuries of the spine sustained during rugby. *Sports Medicine*, **5**, 328–334

Tator, C.H. and Edmonds, V.E. (1986) Sports and recreation are a rising cause of spinal-cord injury. *Physician and Sportsmedicine*, **14**, 157–167

Taylor, T.K.F. and Coolican, M.R.J. (1987) Spinal-cord injuries in Australian footballers, 1960–1985. *Medical Journal of Australia*, **147**, 112–118

Torg, J.S., Vegso, J.J., Sennett, B. and Das, M (1985) The national football head and neck injury registry: 14-year report on cervical quadriplegia, 1971 through 1984. *Journal of the American Medical Association*, **254**, 3439–3443

Torg, J.S. (1982) *Athletic Injuries to the Head, Neck, and Face*, Lea and Febiger, Philadelphia

Verban, E.M., Groppel, J.L., Pfautsch, M.S. and Ramsmeyer, G.C. (1984) The effects of a mandibular orthopaedic repositioning appliance on shoulder strength. *Journal of Craniomandibular Practice*, **2**, (3) 232–237

# 18 Facial injury

## Ocular injury

Eye injuries may arise from collisions in which a finger or elbow goes into the eye. Small balls (especially squash balls) may damage the eye, and mud, grit or stone chips can enter the eye.

If there is a foreign body in the eye, quantities of water should be used to irrigate the eye and wash the object out (a squeeze bottle is particularly useful). No attempt should be made to probe the eye, as this may cause the object to scratch the cornea. In some instances, particularly if the foreign body is an eyelash, the eyelid may be rolled back on itself. This procedure is carried out by first asking the athlete to look downwards. The practitioner then grasps the lashes of the upper lid, pulling them down and out, away from the eye. A cotton swab is placed on the outside of the lid, level with the lid crease. The lashes are then folded upwards over the swab to reveal the inside of the eyelid, and the foreign body is washed away. The eyelid returns to its normal position when the athlete looks upwards and blinks.

A foreign body is one of the most common eye problems on the sports field. The reaction is usually pain and tear production. If the object is not removed, blinking may cause corneal abrasion and extreme pain for about 48 hours.

Contact lenses can cause problems. Hard lenses may break or become scratched or roughened, causing corneal damage. Soft lenses are easily torn. If the eye has been injured or infected, a contact lens should never be re-inserted until the eye has healed completely for at least 24 hours.

When contact lenses become dislodged, the wearer, with the aid of a mirror, is often the person most capable of removing them. Hard lenses may be removed using a small suction cup, which is available from an optician, and persistent soft lenses may be dislodged by water from a squeeze bottle, or by gently wiping with a cotton swab.

Following injury, basic vision assessment should be carried out and if any abnormalities are detected the athlete should be referred to an ophthalmologist. A distance chart (placed 6 metres from the subject) and a near vision chart (35 cm from the eyes) should be used. Failure to read the 20/40 line on either chart is a reason for referral (Ellis, 1987). The visual field is tested in all four quadrants. One eye is covered, and the athlete should look into the examiner's eyes. The examiner moves his or her finger to the edge of the visual field in both horizontal and vertical directions until the athlete loses sight of it. Decreased visual acuity or loss of the visual field in one area warrants referral (Ellis, 1987).

The reaction of the pupils may be tested with a small pen torch. Pupil size, shape and speed of reaction is noted. Pupil dilation in reaction to illumination requires immediate referral, as does any irregularity in pupil shape and an inability to clear blurring of vision by blinking.

## Eye protection

Sports trauma accounts for 25% of all serious ocular injuries (Jones, 1989), an even more tragic statistic when we realize that 90% of sports injuries to the eye could be prevented by wearing eye protection (Pashby, 1989). Prevention of ocular trauma comes from two sources, sports practice and eye protection.

Changes in sports practice include rule modification and increasing player awareness. For example, rule changes in Canadian ice hockey to prevent high sticking have greatly reduced eye injury. Injury in badminton is more frequent at the net, so teaching young players to cover their face with the racquet when receiving a smash at the net would seem sensible.

Individual athletes should also protect themselves. The eye protectors worn must be capable of dissipating force, but should not restrict the field of vision or the players comfort. In addition if they are to be acceptable to a player they must be cosmetically attractive and inexpensive.

Each sport will have its own specific requirements. If potential blows are of great intensity, the eye protector must be incorporated into a helmet, and if there is danger of irritation (for example, due to chlorine in a swimming pool) the material used must be chemically resistant. Goggles for skiing must filter out ultraviolet light, while those for shooting may have to be suitable for low light conditions or capable of screening out glare.

For general protection in racquet sports polycarbonate lenses mounted in plastic, rather than wire, frames are the choice. The nasal bridge and sides of such a protector should be broad and strong to deflect or absorb force.

## Dental injury

The simplest form of tooth injury is a concussion in which the anterior teeth are knocked against something. This may occur from a head butt, a punch, or someone running into a piece of apparatus. There is only minor soft tissue damage and the teeth and mouth are sore. The front teeth may be painful when the athlete eats, so he or she should avoid eating hard foods until the pain subsides.

Tooth subluxation occurs when a tooth becomes mobile after a direct injury, but is not displaced. On examination the tooth may be loose and tender, and there may be some gum damage. It is usual for the teeth to tighten up and heal within a week, but the athlete should see his or her dentist.

Displacement of a tooth is more common when a gum shield is not worn. The displaced tooth should be washed in tepid water and replaced in the socket, taking care to put the tooth back the right way round. The athlete may hold the tooth in place by biting on a cloth or handkerchief, until specialist advice can be sought. In children, a displaced tooth may be soaked in whole milk (Mackie and Warren, 1988) until help is available. The tooth should be handled by the crown to avoid further damage to the cells at its root. Good results may be expected if reimplantation is carried out within 30 minutes of trauma, but after 2 hours the prognosis is poor.

## Mouth guards

Custom-made mouth guards (gum shields) have been shown to reduce the incidence of dental injuries by as much as 90% (Jennings, 1990). In addition, they stop the teeth from cutting into the lips and cheeks. When the jaw is hit from below, the bottom teeth will impact into the guard, absorbing some of the impact force. A mouth guard will also modify the transmission of force through the temporo-mandibular joints. The combination of altered force transmission and shock absorption can reduce the likelihood of concussion and mandibular fracture (Chapman, 1990). Any guard must cover the surfaces of the upper teeth, be comfortable to wear, and allow unhindered breathing and speech. Furthermore, they must show good properties of retention in the mouth, and give proper inter-maxillary positioning.

Mouth guards were originally worn in boxing, and they were simply curved pieces of rubber gripped between the teeth. Progress has been made in their design, and nowadays three types are available, custom-made, mouth-formed and ready-moulded. Most protection is given to the upper front teeth, as these are the ones most susceptible to injury.

For custom-made gum shields the first step is to take an impression of the upper teeth using a material such as alginate. Dental stone is poured into the impression to create a positive model of the teeth. Polyvinyl acetate-polyethelene (PVAc-PE) is vacuum-formed over the model, and the mouth guard is trimmed and smoothed off (Kerr, 1986).

Self-moulded guards come in two types. The first type is soaked in hot water to soften it and then moulded over the upper teeth ('boil and bite'). The second type consists of a pre-formed outer shell into which a plasticized acrylic gel or silicone rubber is added. The outer shell and fluid gel are placed over the teeth and pressed into position until the gel sets.

The dentally fitted type of mouth protector is better in terms of both safety and effectiveness. The model made from the impression of the athlete's mouth can be re-used to form a number of mouth shields.

The ready-moulded kind are available off the shelf in many sports shops. They do not fit well, and have to be held in place by gritting the teeth. They should not be recommended to athletes as they are easily dislodged and may block the airway.

## Auricular injury

### Cauliflower ear

Auricular haematoma (cauliflower ear) is normally caused by a direct blow to the ear. Blood and serum accumulate between the perichondrium and external ear cartilage, and secondary infection may arise. First aid involves the use of ice and compression. As soon as possible the haematoma should be aspirated or drained through an incision, and the ear compressed to prevent further fluid accumulation. The injury occurs particularly in contact sports, such as wrestling, boxing and rugby, and is very common. Schuller et al. (1989) found that 39% of high school and collegiate wrestlers from a group of 537 had one or both of the auricles permanently deformed by injury. Some degree of prevention may be achieved by wearing protective headgear.

### Underwater diving injury

The air on either side of the tympanic membrane should be at equal pressure. Externally, the air is at atmospheric pressure, and internally the Eustachian tube leads to the nasopharynx. Pressure changes, such as those which occur in an aeroplane, are equalized by swallowing or yawning, through the Eustachian tube mechanism. If the free exchange of air is impaired, barotrauma may occur. If the outside air pressure rises, such as may occur in diving, and the Eustachian tube mechanism is unable to equalize pressure, pain will result, a condition referred to as 'the squeeze'. Small haemorrhages may occur in the middle ear, and the tympanic membrane may burst in depths below 3 m (Sperryn, 1985). With a severe cold, the Eustachian tube may be blocked, so an athlete should not dive (or fly if the condition is severe).

Barotrauma to the inner ear secondary to decompression is less common, but considerably more serious. This type of trauma usually occurs at depths below 35 m. Symptoms may be caused by the formation of gas bubbles in the blood vessels supplying the inner ear (Renon et al., 1986).

The reduction in air volume at increasing depths is responsible for another danger in diving and underwater swimming, the phenomenon of 'mask squeeze'. A relative vacuum is created in a diving mask or swimming goggles, as the diver descends. With a mask, this is equalized by breathing out through the nose into the mask, but with swimming goggles this is not possible. A swimming pool may be as deep as 3 or 4 m. Children who dive for objects at this depth, face the very real danger of conjunctival haemorrhage and oedema (Craig, 1984). As the air space within the goggles is not connected to a body cavity, the air pressure will not be equalized. The pressure within the goggles will drop lower than that inside the body, causing the ocular vascular system to over-distend and fluid to accumulate in the tissues covered by the goggles.

Diving with ear plugs in, or with an upper respiratory tract infection, should also be avoided because of danger to the eardrum (tympanic membrane). The water pressure will press an ear plug further in, compressing the air between the plug and eardrum. This can cause severe pain and may even rupture the eardrum. During any change in air pressure, the pressure inside the eardrum is equalized through the Eustachian tube mechanism when swallowing or yawning. With upper respiratory tract infections, this tube can become blocked, causing severe pain (middle-ear squeeze) as the eardrum is stretched inwards.

## Maxillofacial injuries

Sport accounts for about 12% of maxillofacial injuries (Handler, 1991), with fractures of the maxilla and zygomatic bones being more common in contact sports. If the upper jaw has been subjected to a blow, injury should be suspected if the teeth are out of alignment or if one half of the cheek feels numb. Direct palpation of these fractures is painful, and pain may be elicited as far back as the temporomandibular joint if the athlete is asked to bite on a folded cloth. Chewing will be painful and local swelling may be apparent. Bony deformity is often better assessed by looking at both cheekbones from the top of the patient's head.

Mandibular fracture may occur with a direct blow to the chin, with pain being experienced as the mouth is opened or closed, in an area in front of the ear. There is malocclusion and abnormal mobility of the mandible. Most of these fractures extend through the intraoral mucosa and so bleeding from the mouth is often noticed. The primary aim is to ensure a clear airway. Blood, bone and tooth fragments and saliva must be cleared from the mouth. The mobile jaw fragment may be secured temporarily with a bandage around the head and chin.

The local application of ice will ease pain, and direct pressure by the athlete supports the area until hospitalization is achieved.

## Nasal injury

Nasal injuries require treatment mainly for haemorrhage (nose bleed). Direct pressure should be applied to the distal part of the nose with the head held forward. The athlete is able to breathe through his or her mouth. In cases in which bleeding is severe a cotton-wool ball or compress may be placed inside the nostril, providing the pad is large enough not to be inhaled. If bleeding continues, hospitalization may be required to cauterize the ruptured vessels or apply vessel-constricting agents.

Nasal fracture is one of the most common maxillofacial injuries in sport. Often the nasal bones are obviously deviated to one side or depressed. Running the finger gently down the edge or bridge of nose may reveal a step deformity, but this can easily be disguised when oedema is excessive (which is frequently the case). Radiographs are useful, but not definitive, as many nasal fractures cannot be identified on X-ray (Handler, 1991). The nasal septum and orbit must be examined at the same time as the nose, as concurrent injuries here can often go unnoticed.

Reduction of a displaced fracture should be performed within 7 days, because, after this, fibrosis makes accurate realignment of the bony fragments difficult.

## References

Chapman, P.J. (1990) Orofacial injuries and international rugby players' attitudes to mouthguards. *British Journal of Sports Medicine*, **24**, 3

Craig, A.B. (1984) Physics and physiology of swimming goggles. *Physician and Sportsmedicine*, **12**, (12) 107

Ellis, G.S. (1987) Sports eye injuires: first aid and prevention. In *Sports Ophthalmology*, (ed. L.D. Pizzarello and B.G. Haik), Charles C. Thomas, Springfield, Illinois

Handler, S.D. (1991) Diagnosis and management of maxillofacial injuries. In *Athletic Injuries to the Head, Neck, and Face*, 2nd edn, (ed. J.S. Torg), Mosby Year Book, St Louis

Jennings, D.C. (1990) Injuries sustained by users and non-users of gum shields in local rugby union. *British Journal of Sports Medicine*, **24**, 3

Jones, N.P. (1989) Eye injury in sport. *Sports Medicine*, **7**, 163–181

Kerr, I.L. (1986). Mouth guards for the prevention of injuries in contact sports. *Sports Medicine*, 415–427

Mackie, I.C. and Warren V.N. (1988) Dental trauma: 4. Avulsion of immature incisor teeth. *Dental Update*, December, 406–407

Pashby, T. (1989) *Journal of Ophthalmic Nursing and Technology*, **8**, (3) 99–101

Renon, P., Lory, R., Belliato, R. and Casanova, M. (1986) Inner ear trauma caused by decompression accidents following deep sea diving. *Annals of Otolaryngology (Paris)*, **103**, 259–264

Schuller, D.E., Dankle, S.K., Martin, M. and Strauss, R.H. (1989) Auricular injury and the use of headgear in wrestlers. *Archives of Otolaryngology: Head and Neck Surgery*, **115**, 714–717

Sperryn, P.N. (1985) *Sport and Medicine*, Butterworth, London

# 19 The shoulder girdle

The upper limb attaches to the trunk via the shoulder (pectoral) girdle, which consists of the scapula and clavicle. The girdle articulates with the axial skeleton through the sternoclavicular joints, while the scapula itself rests only on muscle tissue. The clavicle forms a strut for the shoulder, holding the arm away from the side of the body, and allowing a greater range of unencumbered movement.

The arm has little function in locomotion. Instead, it has developed for power and manipulation. The various articulations and levers which make up the arm enable the hand to be taken to a point in space with exceptional accuracy, and held there with great stability.

Injury to the shoulder girdle is common in sport. Clavicular fracture and disruption of the sternoclavicular or acromioclavicular joints are injuries frequently encountered following a fall. When this happens, both the stability and mobility of the whole shoulder region is affected.

## Sternoclavicular joint

The sternoclavicular (SC) joint performs functionally as a ball and socket. The medial end of the clavicle articulates with the clavicular notch of the sternum, and the adjacent edge of the first costal cartilage. The congruity of the joint is enhanced by the presence of an interarticular fibrocartilage disc, which divides the joint cavity into two. In addition to improving the congruity of the joint, the disc also provides cushioning between the two bone ends. Furthermore, it holds the medial end of the clavicle against the sternum, preventing it moving upwards and medially when pushing actions are performed.

The joint is strengthened by a capsule attached to the articular margins, and four ligaments. The anterior SC ligament strengthens the superior aspect of the joint and is reinforced by the origin of the sternomastoid. The posterior SC ligament, which is weaker than its anterior counterpart, runs downwards and laterally and is strengthened by the sternohyoid muscle. The interclavicular ligament attaches between the two clavicles, passing across the jugular notch. The costoclavicular ligament is a short dense band running from the first costal cartilage to the rhomboid impression on the undersurface of the clavicle. This ligament strengthens the inferior part of the joint capsule and limits elevation of the clavicle.

The joint has three degrees of movement, displaying elevation-depression, protraction-retraction, and axial rotation. The axis of rotation for the first two movements (not rotation) is lateral to the joint itself, passing through the costoclavicular ligament. Consequently, when the lateral end of the clavicle moves in one direction, its medial end moves in the opposite direction (Fig. 19.1), an important consideration with clavicular joint dislocation.

A total of about 60° of elevation and depression is available, elevation being limited by tension in the costoclavicular ligament, and depression by the interclavicular ligament and articular disc. When the lateral end of the clavicle is protracted, the medial end moves backwards, the opposite movement occurring with retraction. The total range of motion here is about 35°. Axial rotation is purely a passive action accompanying scapular movements. The range of rotation is small (20–40°), but increases slightly as the lateral end of the clavicle is pulled back.

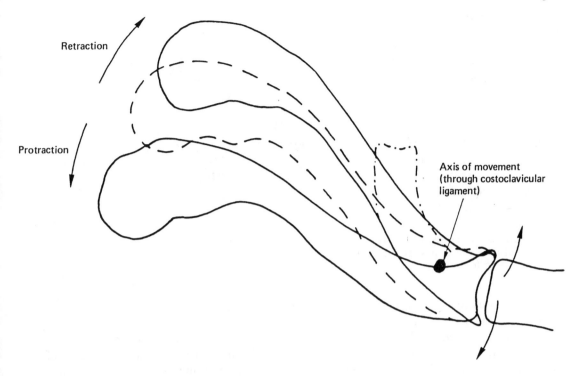

Retraction

Protraction

Axis of movement
(through costoclavicular
ligament)

**Figure 19.1** Movement of the clavicle. After
Palastanga, Field and Soames (1989).

## Injury

Injury to the SC joint is unusual. Normally, the
clavicle will fracture, or the acromioclavicular joint
will give way, before the SC joint is seriously
injured. However, when damage does occur, it is
frequently the result of direct lateral compression
of the shoulder, such as occurs when falling onto
the side of the body. The injury is more common in
horse-riding and cycling where sufficient force is
produced, but is seen in rugby and wrestling. The
SC joint will dislocate in the opposite direction to
the applied force (Fig. 19.2), thus an anterior force
(falling on to the back) will dislocate the joint
backwards. Several important structures lie in close
proximity to the joint, including the oesophagus,
trachea, lungs, pleurae, brachial plexus and major
arteries and veins. Posterior dislocation therefore,
if it is severe, may be potentially life threatening.
In contrast, anterior dislocation can occur in the
absence of trauma, and frequently results only
in slight discomfort.

Initial examination (of posterior dislocation) on
the field must obviously aim to rule out life-
threatening injury. The presence of stridor, dyspnoea, cyanosis, difficulty with speech, pulsating
vessels and neurological signs may all necessitate
immediate hospitalization.

If these are not present, joint examination may
continue. Pain is generally well localized, and may
become progressively more limiting over time.
Anterior dislocation leaves a visible step deformity,
and with posterior dislocation the usual prominence over the medial clavicle is lost. Local swelling is sometimes present, with crepitus and pain to
motion, especially horizontal flexion. The shoulder
is frequently held in a protracted position.

Radiographic investigation will rule out clavicular fracture, and may enable differentiation between fracture and epiphyseal injury in athletes

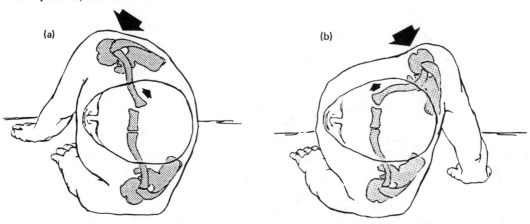

(a)   (b)

**Figure 19.2** Sternoclavicular dislocation. (a) Anteriorly directed force causes posterior dislocation. (b) Posteriorly directed force causes anterior dislocation. From Garrick and Webb (1990), with permission.

below 25 years. Closed reduction is often possible immediately after injury if pain is not too severe and before muscle spasm sets in. Both anterior and posterior dislocations may be reduced by placing a knee between the scapulae of the seated athlete and gently pulling the shoulders back. The joint often reduces with an audible thud. After reduction, the joint is immobilized with a figure-of-eight bandage and ice is used to reduce local swelling. Posterior dislocations, even if successfully reduced, will still require hospital referral and observation. Posterior dislocations usually remain reduced, but anterior dislocations are apt to recur. Surgical fixation of anterior dislocation is possible, but the number of complications makes the procedure undesirable. Migration of a Steinmann pin or Kirchner wire into the heart or major vessels has been reported (Garrick and Webb, 1990). Rockwood and Odor (1989) reported excellent results following conservative management of atraumatic anterior displacement 8 years after initial treatment. Patients treated surgically (not by these authors) in the same study had complications including scarring, instability, pain and limitation of activity.

Even though the joint is frequently hypermobile, joint mobilizations may be used to relieve pain (Maitland, 1991). Antero-posterior gliding may be performed with the therapist placing his or her thumbs over the sternal end of the clavicle.

## Acromioclavicular joint

The acromioclavicular (AC) joint is formed between the oval facet on the lateral end of the clavicle and the similarly shaped area on the acromion process. The lateral end of the clavicle overrides the acromion, slightly. The AC joint capsule is fairly loose and strengthened above by fibres from the trapezius, and by capsular thickenings, the superior and inferior AC ligaments. As with the SC joint there is an intra-articular disc, but this time it does not divide the cavity into two. The joint is further stabilized by the coracoclavicular ligament, running from the lateral end of the clavicle to the coracoid process. This ligament is in two parts, known as the conoid and trapezoid ligaments. The conoid ligament is fan-shaped and resists forward movement of the scapula, while the stronger trapezoid ligament is flat and restricts backward movements. As with the SC joints, the AC joint moves only in association with the scapula. Three types of movement are again present; protraction–retraction, elevation–depression and axial rotation.

### Injury

The most common conditions affecting the AC joint are sprains and degeneration. AC joint sprains vary in intensity between minor grade I injuries to grade III ruptures representing complete disruption of the coracoclavicular ligament and AC joint dislocation (sprung shoulder) (Fig. 19.3). The injury may be further classified using weight-lifting radiographs. Here, the anterior deltoid is contracted by having the patient hold a weight with the elbow flexed and the arm next to the body. If the clavicular attachment of the deltoid is intact, the joint may reduce as weight is taken (IIIa), or there may be no change in the joint appearance (IIIb). However, if the lateral end of the clavicle becomes more prominent, the clavicular attachment of the deltoid may have been stripped off (Dias and Gregg, 1991). Radiographs are also used to differentiate the condition from fractures of the distal clavicle where this is suspected.

Injury is usually the result of a superiorly directed force as occurs with a fall on to the point of the shoulder or being struck from above. The force drives the scapula downwards, an action resisted by the coracoclavicular ligament. Examination reveals local tenderness over the AC joint, sometimes with a noticeable step deformity. The deformity may occur later, if initial muscle spasm reduces acromioclavicular separation.

Initial treatment aims to reduce the symptoms. Ice and a sling support to take the weight of the arm are recommended. The joint is immobilized in the sling for 2–3 weeks, and then gradually mobilized within pain-free limits. With grade I injuries, some relief may be provided by two strips of elastic

adhesive strapping placed (pre-stretched) over the joint from the sternum to the scapula. As inflammation subsides, exercise therapy is commenced to restore function, although a permanent step deformity is usual, and joint degeneration may occur in later years. When returning to sport, the player participating in contact sports may need a felt doughnut pad placed over the joint to limit the effects of direct trauma.

There is some controversy concerning the treatment of this condition. Both conservative and surgical approaches restore function to a similar degree (Larsen, Berg-Nielsen and Christensen, 1986; Dias et al., 1987; Bannister et al., 1989), and some surgical methods have been shown to lead to long-term functional detriment. Certainly, removal of the distal end of the clavicle will disrupt the AC ligament, a main stabilizer of the joint (Fukuda et al., 1986). In the literature the main argument for surgery has been the development of degenerative changes in the joint as a result of non-operative management. However, degeneration does not occur in all patients, and when it does occur, it is not necessarily a limitation (Dias et al., 1987). In addition, surgery is often as effective if done in the acute or chronic condition, so there is normally no advantage in operating immediately. Importantly, surgery carries with it a high risk of complications (Ejeskar, 1974; Lancaster, Horowitz and Alonso, 1987; Taft, Wilson and Oglesby, 1987).

In a literature review of 11 papers detailing the long-term results of both surgical and conservative management of this injury, Dias and Gregg (1991) found poor results to have occurred in 13 out of 247 patients treated conservatively (5.3%), and 22 out of 233 managed surgically (9.4%). These authors argued that as comparable results were obtained regardless of the method used, conservative management was the treatment of choice for most AC joint injuries.

### AC joint degeneration

Joint degeneration is common in later years following injury, regardless of the grade of damage which occurred, and particularly after repeated trauma. In addition, some sports, such as weight-lifting,

Classification

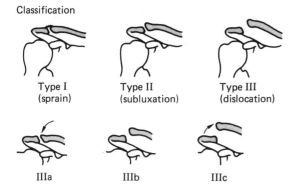

| Type I | Type II | Type III |
| (sprain) | (subluxation) | (dislocation) |

| IIIa | IIIb | IIIc |

**Figure 19.3**  Acromioclavicular joint injuries.

lead to a higher incidence of degenerative changes in the AC joint, even where no incidents of trauma have occurred. Cahill (1982) reported 46 cases of osteolysis of the distal clavicle, all but one occurring in weight-lifters. He argued that degeneration occurred as a result of sub-chondral stress fractures resulting from repeated microtrauma. The condition presents as pain, which is usually dull and aching in nature, brought on by activities such as lifting and throwing. To examination there is point tenderness over the joint, with pain and crepitus to passive horizontal flexion.

Where the diagnosis is uncertain, radiographs will frequently reveal degeneration, and injection of local anaesthetic into the joint is helpful to establish whether the degeneration is the cause of the patient's symptoms.

Movements which stress the joint (for example, press-ups, weight training or throwing) should be avoided. Initially, immobilization in a sling may be required in the very acute lesion. Later, joint mobilization provides good results. Antero-posterior gliding may be performed with the patient in a sitting position. The therapist grasps the distal end of the clavicle with his or her thumb and the forefingers of one hand, and the acromion process in a similar fashion with the other hand. The hands are worked against each other to glide the joint. Injection of corticosteroid may give many months of relief, a technique made easier if the shoulder is laterally rotated to distract the AC joint.

# Fractures of the clavicle

The most common mechanism of injury is a fall onto the outstretched arm, and occasionally direct trauma to the shoulder. Although common, these injuries should not be taken too lightly, as it must be remembered that the subclavian vessels and brachial plexus lie in close proximity, as does the upper lobe of the lung. There is usually a cracking sensation at the time of injury, with immediate pain over the fracture site, and rapid swelling. Signs of injury to vital structures are rare, but include dyspnoea and paraesthesia and obviously warrant immediate hospitalization. Laceration of the subclavian artery presents as a readily expanding pulsating haematoma. Deformity is common, as is crepitus.

Fractures of the proximal and middle thirds of the clavicle make up the largest proportion (80%) of such injuries. If not displaced these should be immobilized with the shoulders retracted in a figure-of-eight bandage for 6 weeks. With young athletes the risk of non-union may make it necessary to curtail activity for up to 3 months after injury. Figure-of-eight bandages must not be applied so tightly as to constrict the blood or nerve supply to the arm. Some step deformity usually occurs as complete immobilization of athletes (other than in a cast) is difficult. This type of deformity is usually cosmetic rather than functional.

Distal fractures tend to be displaced by retraction immobilization, and are better wired. Internal fixation of the proximal clavicle carries with it similar complications to that of the SC joint.

# Shoulder girdle movements

Motion of the shoulder girdle as a whole changes the position of the glenoid fossa, placing it in the most favourable location for the maximum range of humeral movement. When the glenoid cavity moves, it does so in an arc, the diameter of which is the length of the clavicle (Palastanga, Field and Soames, 1989). The medial border of the scapula moves in a similar, but smaller, arc and as a consequence the positions of the shoulder girdle structures change in relation to each other.

As the scapula moves medially and laterally towards and away from the vertebral column, the curvature of the rib cage forces the scapula to change from a frontal to a more sagittal position. This, in turn, alters the direction in which the glenoid cavity faces. With elevation, the scapula is accompanied by some rotation, the glenoid cavity gradually pointing further upwards as the scapula gets higher (Fig. 19.4).

In both shoulder abduction and flexion, the clavicle axially rotates. As the scapula twists, the coracoclavicular ligament 'winds up' and tightens, causing the clavicle itself to rotate. For this reason a diminished range of movement at either the AC or

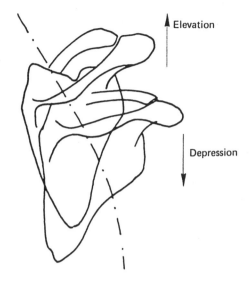

Elevation

Depression

**Figure 19.4** Elevation of the scapula. Elevation is accompanied by rotation. As the scapula gets higher, the glenoid cavity points further upwards.

SC joints, which reduces clavicular rotation will also impair scapular and therefore glenohumeral motion.

### Muscle actions

Shoulder retraction is carried out by the rhomboids and trapezius, while protraction occurs as a result of contraction of the serratus anterior and the pectoralis major. The shoulder girdle is elevated by the upper fibres of the trapezius and the levator scapulae.

Scapular rotation is most important in scapulo-humeral rhythm accompanying shoulder joint flexion and abduction. Abduction of the shoulder above 30% requires scapular rotation, movement of the scapula and humerus occurring in a ratio of about 1:2. Scapular rotation occurs as a result of force-couples between the various muscles attached to the scapula. Lateral rotation, accompanying shoulder joint abduction or flexion, is brought about by contraction of the upper and lower fibres of the trapezius and serratus anterior. The serratus anterior is probably the most important of the group, pulling powerfully on the inferior border of the scapula as the trapezius lifts the lateral end of

the clavicle and the acromion process. Medial rotation frequently occurs as a result of eccentric action of the above muscles. However, in activities such as hanging and chinning a beam, active scapular rotation is accomplished by the levator scapulae and the rhomboids pulling upwards on the medial side of the scapula, together with the pectoralis minor pulling the coracoid process down (Fig. 19.5).

Contracting the muscles which attach to the clavicle and acromion will stress the clavicle bone. When the trapezius and pectoralis major contract, a compression stress is transmitted to the clavicle, and when the deltoid is active, a tension stress similarly occurs.

### Winged scapula

During normal scapulo-humeral rhythm, the scapula slides over the rib cage, and is held in place by the serratus anterior. If weakness or paralysis of the serratus anterior occurs, the scapula will stand prominent from the rib cage when the arm is protracted against resistance. In addition to muscular weakness, there are a number of causes, including damage to the long thoracic nerve, brachial plexus injury, conditions affecting the fifth, sixth and seventh cervical nerve roots, and certain types of muscular dystrophy (Apley and Solomon, 1989).

If weakness is due to nerve palsy, spontaneous recovery is to be expected. Re-education of scapulohumeral movement is required, as habitual alteration of scapulo-humeral rhythm is often seen. Strengthening the shoulder musculature in general and especially the serratus anterior, is also useful.

Occasionally, a congenitally undescended scapula (Sprengel's shoulder) is seen, sometimes associated with marked thoracic kyphosis. The scapulae normally descend completely by the third month of fetal life. However, if undescended, the scapula appears slightly smaller, higher, and more prominent. Scapulo-humeral rhythm is affected and abduction is limited as a consequence. Minor cases respond to rehabilitation, although marked deformity may require surgery.

Scapular conditions such as these are not strictly 'sports injuries', but are included because they are

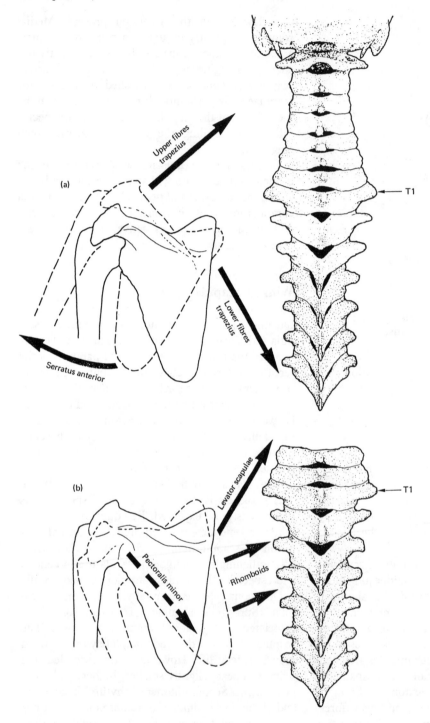

**Figure 19.5**    Muscle-force couples which create
scapular rotation. (a) Lateral rotation. (b) Medial
rotation. From Palastanga, Field and Soames (1989),
with permission.

often noticed first by the club physiotherapist when treating young athletes.

# References

Apley, A.G. and Solomon, L. (1989) *Concise System of Orthopaedics and Fractures*, Butterworth, London

Bannister, G.C., Wallace, W.A., Stableforth, P.G. and Hutson, M.A. (1989) The management of acute acromioclavicular dislocation: a randomised prospective controlled trial. *Journal of Bone and Joint Surgery*, **71B**, 848–850

Cahill, B.R. (1982) Osteolysis of distal part of clavicle in male athletes. *Journal of Bone and Joint Surgery*, **64A**, 1053–1058

Dias, J.J., Steingold, R.F., Richardson, R.A., Tesfayohannes, B. and Gregg, P.J. (1987) The conservative treatment of acromioclavicular dislocation: review after five years. *Journal of Bone and Joint Surgery*, **69B**, 719–722

Dias, J.J. and Gregg, P.J. (1991) Acromioclavicular joint injuries in sport. *Sports Medicine*, **11**, (2) 125–132

Ejeskar, A. (1974) Coracoclavicular wiring for acromioclavicular joint dislocation: a ten year follow-up study. *Acta Orthopaedica Scandinavica*, **45**, 652–661

Fukuda, K., Craig, E.V., An, K. Cofield, R.H. and Chao, E.Y.S. (1986) Biomechanical study of the ligamentous system of the acromioclavicular joint. *Journal of Bone and Joint Surgery*, **68A**, 434–439

Garrick, J.G. and Webb, D.R. (1990). *Sports injuries: Diagnosis and Management*, W.B. Saunders, London

Lancaster, S., Horowitz, M. and Alonso, J. (1987) Complete acromioclavicular separations: a comparison of operative methods. *Clinical Orthopaedics*, **216**, 80–88

Larsen, E., Bjerg-Nielsen, A., and Christensen, P. (1986) Conservative or surgical treatment of acromioclavicular dislocation: a prospective controlled randomised study. *Journal of Bone and Joint Surgery (Am)*, **68A**, 552–555

Maitland, G.D. (1991) *Peripheral Manipulation*, 3rd edn, Butterworth–Heinemann, London

Palastanga, N., Field, D. and Soames, R. (1989) *Anatomy and Human Movement*, Heinemann Medical, Oxford

Rockwood, C.A. and Odor, J.M. (1989) Spontaneous atraumatic subluxation of the sternoclavicular joint. *Journal of Bone and Joint Surgery*, **71A**, 1280–1288

Taft, T.N., Wilson, F.C. and Oglesby, J.W. (1987) Dislocation of the acromioclavicular joint: an end-result study. *Journal of Bone and Joint Surgery*, **69A**, 1045–1051

# 20 The shoulder joint

The shoulder (glenohumeral) joint is the articulation between the head of the humerus and the shallow glenoid fossa of the scapula. The glenoid fossa is only one third the size of the humeral head, but it is extended by the glenoid labrum attached to its periphery. This fibrocartilage rim is about 4 mm deep, with its inner surface lined by, and continuous with, the joint cartilage. The joint itself is surrounded by a loose capsule with a volume twice as large as the humeral head. The anterior capsule is strengthened by the three glenohumeral ligaments. The lower portion of the capsule is lax in the anatomical position, and hangs down in folds. It has two openings, one for the passage of the long head of the biceps, and the other between the superior and middle glenohumeral ligaments which communicates with the subscapular bursa (between the subscapularis and the joint capsule). The capsule is further strengthened by the rotator cuff muscles which act as 'active ligaments' and blend with the lateral capsule. The 'roof' of the joint is formed by the bony coracoid and acromion processes and the coracoacromial ligament which runs between them, the three structures together forming an arch.

Most joints have a high degree of passive stability provided by their capsules and ligaments. The shoulder, however, depends more on the active stability provided by its muscles to maintain joint integrity. In the anatomical position, the weight of the arm is largely supported by the coracohumeral ligament and superior capsule. When the arm moves away from the side of the body, tension in the superior capsule is immediately lost. Now joint stability is provided only by the rotator cuff muscles. Athletes with a pronounced kyphosis will move the shoulder joint forward, leaving the arm hanging in a slightly abducted position This position tenses the rotator cuff and may in turn give shoulder pain.

The fibres of the joint capsule are angled forwards and slightly medially when the arm is hanging by the side of the body. As abduction progresses, tension within these fibres causes the shoulder to rotate passively and externally. This movement prevents the humeral head from being pulled closer to the glenoid and facilitates a greater range of movement. Importantly, the external rotation also allows the greater tuberosity to clear the acromion process.

Abduction of the humerus is accomplished by the supraspinatus and deltoid muscles. With the arm dependent, contraction of the deltoid muscle (particularly the middle fibres) merely approximates the joint, because the medial muscle fibres run almost parallel with the humerus. The supraspinatus is better placed to produce a rotatory action and therefore initiates the movement, abducting the arm for the first 20°. After 30° of abduction the scapula starts to rotate to alter the glenoid position (see pp. 276–278).

## Screening examination

After a subjective history has been taken, a screening examination is performed to enable the examiner to focus more closely subsequently on the injured area. While the patient is undressing, his or her posture and actions are noted, and the area is then inspected for swelling, colour, and deformity. A combination of active, resisted and passive movements are used (Cyriax, 1982). The patient is viewed from behind, to note any alteration in scapulo-humeral rhythm. It is helpful to position the patient facing a full length mirror, so that the anterior aspect of the shoulder and the patient's facial expression may also be assessed. Active abduction, and flexion-abduction are performed with overpressure applied at end range, to assess end feel. Absence of correct scapulo-humeral rhythm, or winging of the scapula warrants closer inspection. Active rotations may be performed by asking the patient to place his or her hand behind the back (medial rotation) and then behind the head (lateral rotation). Passive lateral rotation is performed with the elbow flexed and upper arm held into the side. This is also the position for resisted lateral and medial rotations. Passive medial rotation is performed with the patient placing his or her hand into the small of the back. The examiner stabilizes the upper arm, and keeps the patient's elbow tucked into the side of the body. He or she then gently pulls the patient's forearm away from the body, increasing medial rotation. Any limitation of movement is noted, and the percentages of limitation relative to each other reveal whether a capsular pattern exists. The capsular pattern for the glenohumeral joint is gross limitation of abduction with some limitation of lateral rotation and little of medial rotation.

Resisted abduction and adduction are performed in mid range, the examiner stabilizing the patient's pelvis to prevent any lateral trunk flexion occurring at the same time as the shoulder moves. Elbow flexion, extension and forearm rotation may be assessed with the elbow flexed and the upper arm held close to the body. The patient's forearm rests on the examiner's when testing the triceps, and resistance is given from above when testing the biceps. Resisted shoulder shrugging tests the upper fibres of the trapezius. When a small physiotherapist is examining a large athlete, it is particularly important that resistance is applied from a position which gives maximum mechanical advantage to the therapist.

Referred pain from the neck must always be considered in cases of shoulder pain, and the neck screening examination (p. 262) is also carried out. This simple but methodical examination should take no more than 2–3 minutes and informs the examiner whether the shoulder is the cause of pain, whether a contractile or non-contractile structure is

affected, and reveals whether a capsular pattern exists to suggest an intracapsular lesion.

Should movement apparently be full, two further procedures are useful to reproduce the patient's symptoms, these are the locking test and the quadrant position (Maitland, 1991). The locking position combines internal rotation, extension and abduction of the shoulder with the scapula fixed. In this position the subacromial space is compressed and will give pain should an impingement syndrome be present. The quadrant position stresses the anterior capsule, and combines external rotation slight flexion and full abduction of the shoulder. Each test should be assessed for pain and end feel, and compared with the uninjured side.

To perform the tests, the patient is supine, and the practitioner stands by the patient's side towards his or her shoulders. To test the locking position, the therapist places the palmar aspect of his or her forearm beneath the patient's shoulder, and grips the trapezius muscle to stop the shoulder shrugging. The therapist holds the patient's elbow, slightly medially rotates the arm, and lifts it into abduction (Fig. 20.1). The movement is continued into the quadrant position (Fig. 20.2) by allowing the arm to rotate externally and flex, while the humerus is abducted to full range.

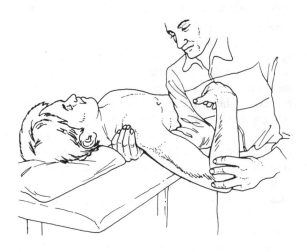

**Figure 20.1** Locking position.

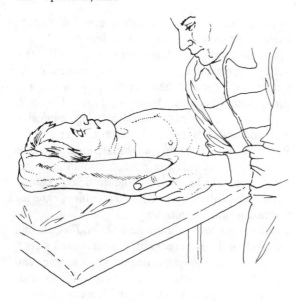

**Figure 20.2** Quadrant position.

## Impingement syndrome

The action of abduction is a complex series of movements involving many structures. At the point where the tuberosity comes close to the acromion (70–120° abduction), a number of structures may be pinched between the involved bones or the tuberosity and the coracoclavicular ligament. Normally the structures affected are the suprasinatus tendon, the long head of biceps, and the subacromial bursa.

In addition to a purely mechanical impingement, changes in the microvascular supply to the area have been noted. Pressure exerted by the humeral head on the supraspinatus tendon, and to a lesser extent on the intracapsular position of the biceps tendon, has the effect of 'wringing out' the tendon vessels and creating an avascular zone (Rathbun and Macnab, 1970). Furthermore, repeated microtrauma results in local oedema within the tendon and an increase in tissue volume. This, in turn, makes the structures more susceptible to impingement by reducing the subacromial space and so perpetuates the problem.

Impingement does not necessarily mean that there is a lack of subacromial space. Weakness in the rotator cuff can cause instability (see below)

and allow the humeral head to ride up through deltoid contraction, making examination of rotator cuff strength vital with this condition.

Three stages of impingement have been described (Neer, 1972). Stage I is a self-limiting overuse syndrome. It presents as a dull ache occurring after repeated overhead activity. The most significant sign is a painful arc of movement. Here, as abduction is commenced, no pain is felt. As the tuberosity moves closer to the glenoid, structures are compressed and pain occurs between 70 and 120°. As abduction goes further, the tuberosity moves away from the acromion and pain subsides as the arm is taken overhead (Fig. 20.3). In addition to a painful arc, palpable pain may be found over the anterior edge of the acromion in some cases. Resisted movements may or may not be painful, depending on whether a contractile structure is impinged. If the supraspinatus is affected, the painful arc exists in combination with pain to resisted lateral rotation and initiation of abduction. However, the situation is far from clear cut because pain is frequently caused when a

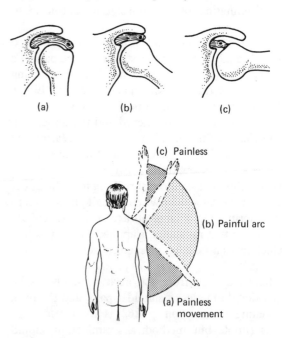

**Figure 20.3** The painful arc. (a) No impingements, painless. (b) Tuberosity pinches painful structure. (c) Tuberosity moves beneath acromion, pain disappears. From Crawford-Adams (1976), with permission.

resisted movement approximates the joint, pulling the humerus on to the acromion. In addition, pain in this condition may be so acute that resisted actions appear weak. However, the weakness is due to the pain itself rather than neurological involvement. Involvement of the biceps tendon gives pain along the intertubercular groove with resisted shoulder and elbow flexion in combination with resisted forearm supination. The stage I lesion is basically inflammatory in nature and so reversible. Treatment aims to reduce pain and swelling, and remove the cause of impingement by resting the impinged structures through training modification.

Stage II lesions involve the development of thickening and fibrosis. They generally give more intense pain, at night as well as with activity, and are not so readily reversed. Movement becomes increasingly limited as fibrosis and scarring occur in the subacromial space. Pain relief and reduction of inflammation are as for a stage I condition, but now stretching exercises become more important to limit loss of range through fibrosis. The stage III lesion involves chronic bony changes and is more usually seen in older athletes (Thein, 1989). Prolonged mechanical impingement gives rise to sclerosis and osteophyte formation of the acromion and tuberosity, and occasionally calcification of the supraspinatus tendon. Active movements are more limited than passive, with weakness and rotator cuff atrophy being commonly seen. Treatment aims essentially at restoring limited function, and frequently requires surgical intervention. Both decompression and anterior acromioplasty are used.

Internal rotation of the shoulder is one biomechanical factor which predisposes to impingement (Halbach and Tank, 1990), and should be limited in patients with this condition. While external rotation helps the greater tuberosity clear the acromion, internal rotation has the reverse effect, compressing the two structures.

The structures affected by impingement may also be injured in isolation. So, either the supraspinatus or biceps tendons may be subjected to tendinitis, and the subacromial bursa may be inflamed without muscular involvement.

## Tendinitis

Tendinitis of the rotator cuff muscles is common, both as a result of overuse and through trauma. Common examples of overuse include excessive repetitions on a single weight training exercise, while trauma may result from an ill-timed 'wrenching' action which combines rotation with abduction. The most commonly affected tendon in the shoulder is that of supraspinatus. Pain is elicited with resisted external rotation and initiation of abduction. Palpation to the muscle insertion is performed with the injured arm medially rotated (with the hand behind the back) to bring the greater tuberosity forwards and make the tendon more superficial (Fig. 20.4). This is also the most convenient position for transverse frictions, the area of scarring being found by palpating at about one finger width below the anterior tip of the acromion. The musculotendinous junction is more conveniently palpated with the injured arm abducted to 90° and supported (Cyriax and Cyriax, 1983). The palpating finger is directed at the space between the posterior aspect of the lateral clavicle and the scapular spine. Again, this is the most convenient starting position for transverse frictional massage (Fig. 20.5).

Pain on resisted lateral rotation but not abduction implicates the infraspinatus. Local pain may be found by palpation to the posterior aspect of the greater tuberosity, with the patient's shoulder flexed, slightly adducted and laterally rotated (elbow support prone lying). Should resisted medial rotation alone give pain, the subscapularis is most likely to be affected, at its insertion into the lesser tuberosity. Pain in combination with resisted adduction implicates the muscles attaching within the intertubercular sulcus (the pectoralis major, latissimus dorsi and teres major).

Tendinitis of the long head of the biceps presents as pain to resisted shoulder and elbow flexion and resisted forearm supination. The teno-osseous junction at the supraglenoid tubercle and adjacent glenoid labrum is difficult to palpate directly, but the tendon itself within the intertubercular groove is easier.

A painful arc is only present with these conditions if the inflamed area of tendon is within a

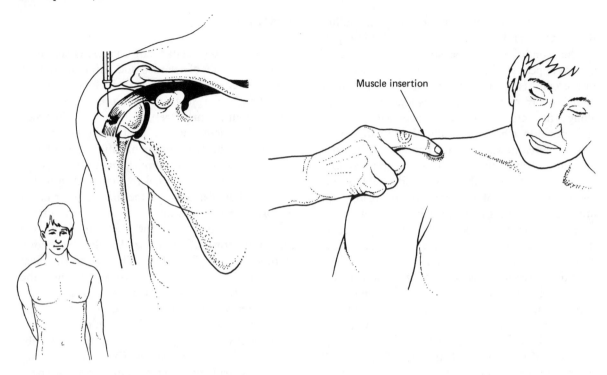

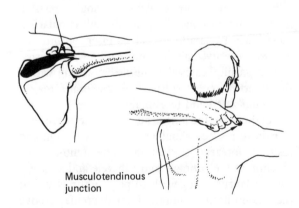

**Figure 20.4** Palpation and treatment of the supraspinatus tendon. From Cyriax and Cyriax (1983), with permission.

pinchable position in mid-range abduction. If the locking position and quadrant test reproduce pain, posteroanterior (PA) gliding should be assessed. If limited, PA pressures against the humeral head should be used (see below).

Musculotendinous junction

**Figure 20.5** Musculotendinous junction of the supraspinatus. From Cyriax and Cyriax (1983), with permission.

# Tendon rupture

## Pectoralis major

Rupture of the pectoralis major is unusual, but when it does occur, the muscle is usually already under tension when further force is imposed on it. The most common example of this phenomenon is the bench-press exercise in weight-training. The injury normally occurs during the eccentric phase of the exercise, as the bar is being lowered. When fatigued, the athlete may move his or her whole body in an attempt to lift the weight, and so bring accessory muscle groups into action enabling him or her to exceed the safe limit. When lowering this excessive weight, he or she loses control and the injury occurs.

A tearing sensation is felt, and a large haematoma is apparent over the anterior axilla. Weakness and pain to resisted adduction and medial rotation is noted on manual muscle testing. No defect may be seen at rest, but if the muscle is contracted isometrically by asking the athlete to press his or her hands together as if clapping, a defect may be apparent. Following injury, the muscle does not retract very far, perhaps due to its varied fibre direction and wide origin. The insertion into the humerus (just lateral to the intertubercular groove) of the non-dominant arm is more normally affected (Kretzler and Richardson, 1989).

Non-surgical treatment can be successful for partial tears (Roi, Respizzi and Dworzak, 1990), and in the non-athletic individual (Delport and Piper, 1982). However, surgical management is more generally recommended (Kretzler and Richardson, 1989; Reut, Bach and Johnson, 1991). At operation the deltoid is retracted and the tendon is re-attached, either via drill holes in the humerus, or by suturing the tendon to the remnant of tissue insertion.

The arm is immobilized in a sling and isometric contractions are started as soon as the pain stabilizes. Assisted movements are begun one week after surgery, and thereafter the rehabilitation programme aims to restore strength, mobility and function. As strength training progresses, eccentric movements must be used to prepare the muscle for its action of decelerating the bar in the bench-press exercise. In addition, pectoral muscle stretches, and retraction work must be used to avoid a protracted shoulder posture.

## Biceps

Rupture of the biceps brachii occurs more commonly at the insertion of the long head into the supraglenoid tubercle, but tears to the short head, distal attachment or belly may occur. The mechanism of injury for proximal tendon injuries is normally a forced extension while the muscle is contracting. This can result from an arm tackle or block where the arm is held abducted, and then pushed back behind trunk level. Distal tendon injuries may occur as a result of heavy lifting with the elbow flexed to 90°.

On examination, pain is elicited to resisted elbow flexion and supination (which may be combined with shoulder flexion), and passive end range extension. A visible defect may be noted in the muscle, with retraction of the tendon. In the case of the long head, the tendon may no longer be palpable in the intertubercular groove, and as the muscle is contracted the belly of the long head is seen to bunch up into a ball-shaped mass. Local swelling and bruising are noted, and lead to an increased arm girth measurement.

Both surgical and conservative management has been recommended in the literature (Friedman, 1963; Morrey et al., 1985; Bandy, Lovelace-Chandler and Holt, 1991). Surgical management is normally favoured because conservative treatment has been said to give a loss of supination power (Morrey et al., 1985; Baker and Bierwagen, 1985). However, the reason for this deficit may be the lack of adequate rehabilitation following conservative management (Bandy, Lovelace-Chandler and Holt, 1991).

Conservative management consists of the RICE protocol to minimize inflammation, with gentle mobility exercises to the elbow within the pain-free range. Exercise therapy is used to maintain shoulder function. Multi-angle isometric training begins as soon as possible to reduce muscle atrophy, the deciding factor for starting this is pain. As pain to resisted movement reduces, dynamic exercise is begun against manual, and later isokinetic, resistance. PNF techniques, combining shoulder flexion/adduction/medial rotation with elbow flexion/supination, are used. Static stretching to elbow and shoulder extension is used. The resistance training programme is progressed with power actions, and functional sporting activities are introduced. The long-term prognosis is good in terms of restoration of function, but a palpable defect will usually remain in the muscle.

Surgery for distal tendon injuries includes reinserting the tendon into the radial tuberosity, or the use of a fascia lata graft if surgery has been delayed and the tendon has retracted. The long head may be reinserted into the supraglenoid tubercle in the case of an avulsion, or in some instances to the wall of the intertubercular groove.

## Triceps

Rupture of the triceps tendon, either partial or complete, is unusual, and the muscle belly itself is even less frequently injured. There is usually a palpable defect in the musculotendinous junction of the muscle, with scarring in the chronic injury. Active extension is lost, and a large haematoma, which later develops into a bruise, is noted locally. The majority of patients are in their 30s or 40s, and the injury almost always occurs either following a fall onto the outstretched hand or a 'chopping' action. In either case, the stress is one of deceleration imposed on an already contracting muscle.

A small fragment of the olecranon may be avulsed and show up on a lateral radiograph of the elbow, and occasionally radial head fractures are associated with the condition. Conservative management is reserved for partial ruptures (Bach, Warren and Wickiewicz, 1987) distinguished by an ability partially to extend the arm against gravity. Surgical management for avulsion injuries involves drilling the olecranon and suturing the muscle. Postoperatively, the patient is immobilized for 3–4 weeks in a cast or splint at 30–45° elbow flexion.

The triceps tendon may occasionally avulse from its glenoid attachment (O'Donoghue, 1976), especially in throwing athletes. Pain occurs to triceps stretching, often palpable at the inferior rim of the glenoid. With rest, a fibrous union will normally fix the fragment back in place, but surgery to remove the avulsed fragment and re-suture the tendon may be required if the injury reoccurs. When the muscle belly itself is injured, it is usually the medial head which is involved and the treatment of choice is conservative (Kunichi and Torisu, 1984).

It is important to note that the normal triceps tendon is capable of sustaining considerable force before it will rupture, making avulsion fracture the more usual injury. Where tendon rupture occurs, an underlying pathology may be present. High-dosage oral steroids may weaken the tendons (Hunter et al., 1986), a situation which is especially important with athletes using heavy resistance exercise, or power movements. Conditions such as rheumatoid arthritis, systemic lupus erythematosus and hormone disorders may also predispose to tendon rupture (Reid and Kushner, 1989).

## Bursitis

*Gray's Anatomy* (Warwick and Williams, 1973) lists some eight bursae around the shoulder joint, but the one most commonly affected in sport is the subacromial (subdeltoid) bursa. This lies between the deltoid and the joint capsule and extends beneath the acromion process and coracoacromial ligament. The bursa extends over the supraspinatus tendon, and does not usually communicate with the joint capsule except in the case of a supraspinatus tear where the bursa may be damaged as well.

Acute subacromial bursitis is unusual and occurs with sudden onset. The whole bursa is inflamed, and this severely limits abduction, but not in the capsular pattern. Pain is acute and is often referred as far down as the wrist in extreme cases. Resisted movements are largely painless, and a painful arc only appears in a sub-acute case, as initially no abduction at all is possible. Treatment in this acute stage aims to reduce the intense pain. The arm is supported in a sling to limit all glenohumeral movement, and anti-inflammatory modalities are used.

Chronic subacromial bursitis occurs when the bursal sac becomes thickened and adherent, but in one part only. The condition is not a progression of acute bursitis, but a separate clinical entity (Cyriax, 1982). The onset is gradual, a painful arc is present, but movements are largely of full range. Injecting the bursa with a local anaesthetic to inflate it is surprisingly effective, and may act mechanically by simply pushing the walls of the bursal sac apart.

## Shoulder instability

Shoulder instability may be caused by either static or dynamic factors. Static factors include damage to the glenoid labrum, anterior capsule and glenohumeral ligaments, while dynamic factors occur as a result of rotator cuff weakness. The strength of the rotator cuff muscles in proportion to that of the deltoid muscle is probably the single most important consideration. As the deltoid contracts, it pulls the humerus up into the glenoid, reducing the subacromial space. One of the functions of the rotator cuff is to depress the humeral head, therefore allowing greater clearance between the tuberosity and the coracoacromial arch. Minimal damage to the rotator cuff muscles may result in reflex weakening of the muscles, disrupting the synchronicity of the shoulder abductors. With further training, the action of the unopposed deltoid muscle leads to an impingement problem.

Static instability may be assessed clinically by the anterior and posterior drawer tests (Gerber and Ganz, 1984). Anterior and posterior instability is initially tested with the athlete in a sitting position. The therapist grasps the athlete's upper arm and applies forward and backward pressure while stabilizing the scapula, comparing the injured and uninjured sides. A more rigorous procedure is to position the athlete in a supine lying position, with the injured shoulder over the table edge. The arm is abducted to 90° and externally rotated, and from this position the examiner applies an anterior or posterior force (Jobe and Bradley, 1988).

Therapeutic exercise after shoulder injury should initially be directed at strengthening the rotator cuff before exercise is attempted for the deltoid. Rotator cuff strength may be regained by performing resisted shoulder rotation with the arm flexed and elbow held into the side of the body. This may be achieved isotonically with a pulley system or powerband (standing) or dumb-bell (sidelying) or isokinetically (Fig. 20.6). The deltoid is then exercised initially from a side lying position moving only to the vertical. This reduces the lever arm as the muscle shortens, and reduces the force

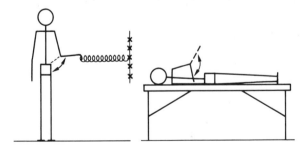

**Figure 20.6** Rotator cuff exercises.

exerted by the middle fibres as the tuberosity approaches the acromion in mid abduction.

In addition to glenohumeral power, the scapulothoracic joint is strengthened by exercising those muscles which control scapular rotation; the serratus anterior (press-ups), latissimus dorsi (pull downs), trapezius (shrugging), levator scapulae and the rhomboids (rowing).

## Glenohumeral dislocation

Dislocation is a commonly seen shoulder injury, with anterior displacement being encountered more often than posterior. Forced movements involving rotation and abduction are common mechanisms, and a fall onto the outstretched arm is also a frequent aetiology. Acute anterior dislocation gives considerable pain. The arm is usually held slightly abducted and externally rotated, and the normal rounded contour of the shoulder is lost. Close inspection shows the acromion process to be more prominent than usual, and a hollow is visible below it. The displaced humeral head can usually be felt on the anterior aspect of the shoulder. The question of whether to reduce an acute injury is one of debate. On the positive side, early reduction of an uncomplicated injury may be achieved without anaesthetic and with little discomfort. If left, muscle spasm sets in, making reduction under anaesthetic necessary. The main problem is the likelihood of further injury by reduction without X-ray by inexperienced staff. Fracture of the head or neck of the humerus may have occurred at the time of injury and epiphyseal displacement is seen in adolescents. Displaced bone fragments may easily be pulled onto the circumflex or radial nerves causing injury, and vascular damage may also occur. For these reasons, an acute injury occurring for the first time should be referred to an orthopaedic consultant.

Recurrent anterior dislocation may be reduced more easily. The forces required to dislocate the shoulder in the first place are considerably less than with the acute injury, and so the chance of associated fracture is minimal. Frequently, the athlete has learnt to reduce the dislocation him or herself, and the joint is fairly lax. The patient is placed in a supine position, on the ground, with the therapist sitting on the patient's injured side. The therapist places his or her stockinged foot just below the ipsilateral axilla, while holding the patient's arm. He or she then simply leans back to provide traction, and may gently rotate the arm to facilitate reduction. The simplest self-reduction procedure is for the athlete to bend his or her ipsilateral leg and grasp the knee with both hands, keeping the arms locked straight. Slowly leaning back produces in-line traction which usually allows the shoulder to reduce. It must be emphasized that these procedures should only be performed in the absence of and spasm. The traction is applied gently, brute force or 'yanking' the arm by another athlete being an obvious contraindication. If the recurrently dislocated shoulder does not reduce readily referral is still necessary.

Acute posterior dislocation is not so obvious as anterior. Pain is still intense, with the arm held adducted and internally rotated. Any attempt to move the arm is resisted by intense muscle spasm. In thin individuals the coracoid process is more visible than usual, and fullness is often apparent posteriorly. Heavy musculature in an athlete will however generally obscure these signs. Posterior dislocations require referral and reduction under sedation. Gentle in-line traction is applied to the adducted/internally rotated arm with gentle pressure over the humeral head.

## Rehabilitation following anterior dislocation

Following reduction, rest and ice are used to limit inflammation. The arm is immobilized in a sling, which may be kept on for three weeks or so, being removed only to exercise. As irritability begins to settle, joint mobilization procedures are begun. These initially aim to reduce pain and then to restore range of motion. Distractions and posterior gliding are performed, large range anterior movements being contraindicated. Exercise therapy may be started early, taking care not to disrupt the healing joint capsule and rotator cuff. Limited range movements are started, beginning with pendular swinging actions, in transverse and sagittal planes. External rotation with abduction, and

hyperextension should be avoided (Kisner and Colby, 1990). Self stretches, such as 'finger walking' along a table top or up a wall, and limited joint distractions are useful (Fig. 20.7). Auto-therapy distractions may be performed in prone kneeling, holding the couch end.

Restoration of shoulder strength and stability is essential, as up to 85% of athletes below 20 years of age may have a recurrence of dislocation (Halbach and Tank, 1990). Pain-free isometric contractions to maintain muscle tone are begun on the first or second day after injury. Isotonic exercises, using short arm levers and limb weight alone, are begun one or two weeks after injury and progress to resisted exercise with powerbands and light weights as pain permits. Strengthening concentrates on medial rotation, to strengthen the subscapularis and support the anterior joint, and limited range adduction to work latissimus dorsi, teres major, the pectorals and coracobrachialis to resist abduction forces. Eccentric activity must be used at some stage, as this is the more functional action to resist abduction and lateral rotation forces. By 4–6 weeks after injury the range of movement is increased and lateral rotation may begin. Abduction is still limited to 90° but flexion and extension may be used overhead. Slow velocity (<90°/s) isokinetics may be used and gradually the velocity is increased to functional sporting levels as the athlete is able to control the movement.

Exercises in the swimming pool are used to incorporate faster actions against the resistance of a

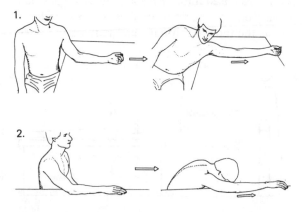

**Figure 20.7**  Self-stretching procedures for the shoulder.

paddle, and range of motion exercise using flotation to take the weight of the arm. PNF techniques involving extension/adduction/medial rotation are used initially against manual resistance, and subsequently with a weight and pulley system. Later, flexion/abduction/lateral rotation is used with caution.

Restoration of kinaesthetic awareness is important after anterior dislocation (Smith and Brunolli, 1989). This may be achieved by using prone kneeling or press-up positions with the arms locked and hands on a balance board, and by performing 'figure drawing' movements in the air with the eyes closed.

## Frozen shoulder

Frozen shoulder or 'adhesive capsulitis' is an increasingly common pathology found in sport. As the number of elderly people involved in sport continues to rise this condition is likely to be seen even more frequently. The problem is more common in females, and presents as a gradual loss of shoulder movement, with or without pain. The initial loss of movement may go unnoticed until function is limited. Patients complain that the activities of everyday living become increasingly difficult. Combing the hair at the back of the head and fastening a bra strap are frequent sources of complaint. Active sportspersons frequently notice the onset of the condition earlier than sedentary individuals. Elderly athletes often complain that their golf swing is affected, or that overhead badminton shots are painful, for example.

The term 'frozen shoulder' is not an accurate diagnosis, but rather a description of the major symptom, which is lack of movement. The condition may be preceded by a number of other pathologies, including rotator cuff injuries, impingement syndrome, traumatic arthritis, osteoarthritis or shoulder joint immobilization (Hertling and Kessler, 1990; Boissonnault and Janos, 1989). The pain from these conditions will reduce the range of movement, and an untreated patient may later develop a frozen shoulder. It is doubtful whether these conditions occur at the same time as a frozen shoulder because the signs in frozen shoulder are

usually of capsular limitation rather than contractile involvement or impingement.

The joint capsule seems to be the major source of limitation. The capsule is thickened and may adhere to the humeral head, with the axillary pouch frequently being obliterated. A reduction in joint volume has been noted on arthrogram (Reeves, 1966). Following immobilization, capsular changes, including abnormal cross bridge formation and orientation, as well as changes in hyaluronic acid and water content have been demonstrated in synovial joints in general (Akeson, Amiel and Woo, 1980) and may be a factor in frozen shoulder.

On examination, movement is usually limited in a capsular pattern (sub-acute) or by muscle guarding (acute), but resisted movements are normally pain free. Accessory movements are limited, particularly inferior and anterior gliding, and the quadrant position is limited and painful when compared with the uninvolved side. Three stages of the condition have been described (Maitland, 1991). In stage one, pain is the dominant feature, which almost completely prevents movement. With stage two conditions, painful limitation is again a feature. This time, however, some movement is present, and when the joint is stretched the pain increases. Stage three lesions have restricted range but very little pain.

The frozen shoulder responds well to joint mobilization techniques. The condition is sometimes self-limiting within a year, but with mobilization it may resolve in a matter of months. Pain may be greatly reduced by postero-anterior (PA) oscillations (Maitland, 1991), and this is the manual treatment of choice for the stage one lesion. The patient lies supine with the arm supported in a pain-free position. The elbow is flexed with a folded towel placed under the arm. The patient's forearm rests on his or her trunk. This position limits adduction, extension and excessive medial rotation. The therapist kneels on the floor and directs his or her thumbs to the posterior aspect of the humeral head. The oscillations are produced by the therapist's arms rather than his or her finger flexors.

With the stage two condition, the pain is limited first, and then stiffness is addressed. As pain is reduced, the starting position is changed to use the patient's upper arm as a lever. The therapist grips the patient's upper arm in his or her cupped hands, high into the axilla. Initially, the arm is by the patient's side. From this position the slack is taken up in the joint by lifting it anteriorly, and then the arm is lifted and lowered to perform the PA glide. As pain lessens and movement returns, the same action is performed with the arm held abducted to 45°, and then in full flexion overhead (Fig. 20.8).

Inferior gliding, if limited, may be regained with the patient's shoulder flexed to 90° and his or her hand on the trapezius (central fibres). The therapist stabilizes the patient's elbow against his or her own shoulder and grips the upper arm in his or her cupped hands. The gliding motion pulls the humeral head inferiorly. As pain reduces, a similar movement may be performed with the patient's arm abducted and supported. The therapist pushes down on the humeral head with the web of his or her free hand (Fig. 20.9).

The final range of movement may be regained using the quadrant position (see above) as a mobilization to stretch the anterior capsule. This is only used when pain is minimal and stiffness is the predominant symptom (late stage two and stage three lesions). The therapist stands at the head of the couch with his or her knee resting on the couch top (Fig. 20.10). The arm is then oscillated through approximately 30° to facilitate a grade II mobilization. A grade IV movement may be used by placing the therapist's nearside arm under the patient's upper rib angles, a small 5° oscillation is all that is required.

Following each treatment, the patient is shown exercise and autotherapy techniques to maintain the new range of motion. Such movements include pendular swinging in the early stages and subsequently overhead reaching into flexion. Cord and pulley exercises are used if abduction is not painful, and rotation movements placing the hand behind the head or the small of the back are begun. Strength development must parallel the restoration of joint mobility.

Although the above discussion has focused on the glenohumeral joint, should the scapulo-thoracic joint have limited movement it too should obviously be mobilized. In addition, re-education of movement must include a restoration of normal scapulo-humeral rhythm and muscular symmetry.

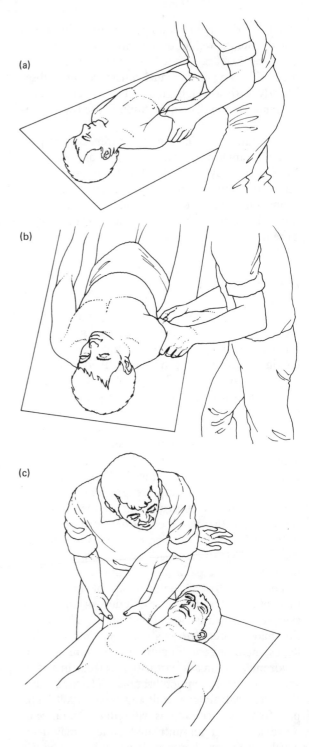

(a)

(b)

(c)

**Figure 20.8** Postero-anterior glenohumeral joint movement. (a) Patient's arm by his or her side. (b) 45° abduction. (c) Maximal flexion-abduction.

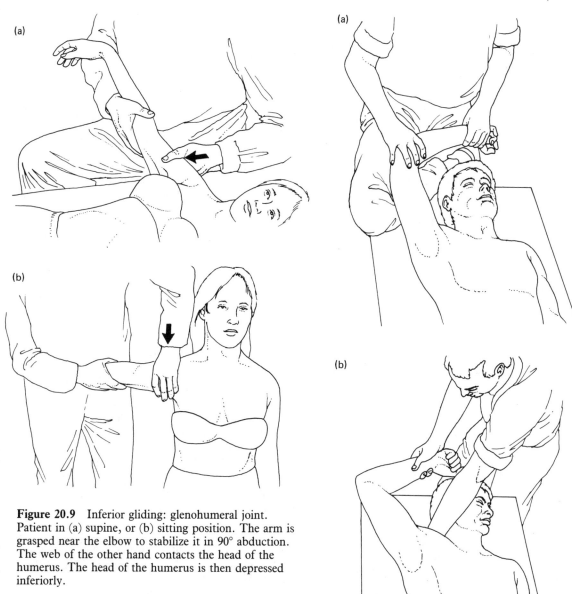

**Figure 20.9** Inferior gliding: glenohumeral joint. Patient in (a) supine, or (b) sitting position. The arm is grasped near the elbow to stabilize it in 90° abduction. The web of the other hand contacts the head of the humerus. The head of the humerus is then depressed inferiorly.

## Snapping scapulae

This unusual condition occurs in particular in adolescent females just after skeletal maturity, and in both sexes following surgery. Patients experience a snapping sensation, which is sometimes audible, near the vertebral border of the scapula. Pain is often localized to the rhomboids and levator scapulae over the medial scapular border or the trapezius over the medial aspect of the scapular spine. It appears to be from tendinitis to these

**Figure 20.10** Glenohumeral mobilizations in the quadrant position to regain final degrees of movement.

muscles. This occurs through microtrauma from excessive shearing forces beneath the scapular due to abnormal scapulo-thoracic rhythm. Management relies on the restoration of a more normal scapulo-thoracic rhythm (Percy, Birbrager and Pitt, 1988).

# References

Akeson, W.H., Amiel, D. and Woo, S. (1980) Immobility effects of synovial joints: the pathomechanics of joint contracture. *Biorheology*, **17**, 95

Bach, B.R., Warren, R.F. and Wickiewicz, T.L. (1987) Triceps rupture. A case report and literature review. *American Journal of Sports Medicine*, **15**, (3) 285–289

Baker, B.E. and Bierwagen, D. (1985) Rupture of the distal tendon of the biceps brachii: operative versus non-operative treatment. *Journal of Bone and Joint Surgery*, **67A**, 414–417

Bandy, W.D., Lovelace-Chandler, V. and Holt, A (1991) Rehabilitation of the ruptured biceps brachii muscle of an athlete. *Journal of Orthopaedic and Sports Physical Therapy*, **13**, (4) 184–190

Boissonnault, W.G. and Janos, S.C. (1989) Dysfunction, evaluation, and treatment of the shoulder. In *Orthopaedic Physical Therapy*, (ed. R. Donatelli and M.J. Wooden), Churchill Livingstone, New York

Crawford-Adams, J. (1976) *Outline of Orthopaedics*, Churchill Livingstone, Edinburgh, pp. 230–231

Cyriax, J. (1982) *Textbook of Orthopaedic Medicine*, Vol. one, 8th edn, Baillière Tindall, London

Cyriax, J.H. and Cyriax, P.J. (1983) *Illustrated Manual of Orthopaedic Medicine*, Butterworth, London

Delport, H.P. and Piper, M.S. (1982) Pectoralis major rupture in athletes. *Archives of Orthopaedic and Traumatic Surgery*, **100**, 135–137

Freidman, E. (1963) Rupture of the distal biceps tendon. Report on 13 cases. *Journal of the American Medical Association*, **184**, 60–63

Gerber, C. and Ganz, R. (1984) Clinical assessment of instability of the shoulder, with special reference to the anterior and posterior drawer tests. *Journal of Bone and Joint Surgery*, **66B**, 551–556

Halbach, J.W. and Tank, R.T. (1990) The shoulder. In *Orthopaedic and Sports Physical Therapy*, (ed. J.A. Gould), 2nd edn, C.V. Mosby, St Louis

Hunter, M.B., Shybut, G.T. and Nuber, G. (1986) The effect of anabolic steroid hormones on the mechanical properties of tendons and ligaments. *Transactions of the Orthopaedics Research Society*, **11**, 240

Jobe, F.W. and Bradley, J.P. (1988) Rotator cuff injuries in baseball: Prevention and rehabilitation. *Sports Medicine*, **6**, 377–386

Kisner, C. and Colby, L.A. (1990) *Therapeutic Exercise. Foundations and Techniques*, F.A. Davis, Philadelphia

Hertling, D. and Kessler, R.M. (1990) *Management of Common Musculoskeletal Disorders*, J.B. Lippincott, Philadelphia

Kretzler, H.H. and Richardson, A.B. (1989) Rupture of the pectoralis major muscle. *American Journal of Sports Medicine*, **17**, 453–458

Kunichi, A. and Torisu, T. (1984) Muscle belly tear of the triceps. *American Journal of Sports Medicine*, **12**, (6) 485

Maitland, G.D. (1991) *Peripheral Manipulation*, 3rd edn, Butterworth–Heinemann, Oxford

Morrey, B.F., Askew, L.J., An, K.N. and Dobyns, J.H (1985). Rupture of the distal tendon of the biceps brachii: a biomechanical study. *Journal of Bone and Joint Surgery*, **67A**, 418–421

Neer, C. (1972) Anterior acromioplasty for the chronic impingement syndrome in the shoulder. *Journal of Bone and Joint Surgery*, **54A**, 41–50

O'Donoghue, D.H. (1976) *Treatment of Injuries to Athletes*, W.B. Saunders, Philadelphia

Percy, E.C., Birbrager, D. and Pitt, M.J. (1988) Snapping scapula: A review of the literature and presentation of 14 patients. *Canadian Journal of Surgery*, **31**, 248–250

Rathbun, J. and Macnab, I. (1970) The microvascular pattern of the rotator cuff. *Journal of Bone and Joint Surgery*, **52B**, 540–553

Reeves, B. (1966) Arthrographic changes in frozen shoulder and post traumatic stiff shoulders. *Proceedings of the Royal Society of Medicine*, **59**, 827

Reid, D.C. and Kushner, S. (1989) The elbow region. In *Orthopaedic Physical Therapy*, (ed. R. Donatelli and M.J. Wooden), Churchill Livingstone, New York

Reut, R.C., Bach, B.R. and Johnson, C. (1991). Pectoralis major rupture: diagnosing and treating a weight-training injury. *Physician and Sportmedicine*, **19**, (3) 89–96

Roi, G.S., Respizzi, S. and Dworzak, F. (1990) Partial rupture of the pectoralis major muscle in athletes. *International Journal of Sports Medicine*, **11**, (1) 85–87

Smith, R.L. and Brunolli, J. (1989) Shoulder kinesthesia after glenohumeral joint dislocation. *Physical Therapy*, **69**, (2) 106–112

Thein, L.A. (1989) Impingement syndrome and its conservative management. *Journal of Orthopaedic and Sports Physical Therapy*, **11**, (5) 183–191

Warwick, R. and Williams, P.L. (1973) *Gray's Anatomy*, 35th edn, Longman, London

# 21 The elbow

The primary purpose of the shoulder was described as positioning the arm to facilitate hand action. The elbow, in turn, functions to shorten or lengthen the arm, largely to allow the hand to be brought to the mouth. The elbow complex consists of the humero-ulnar and humero-radial articulations and the superior radioulnar joint, all of which share the same capsule.

When viewed from the side, the distal end of the humerus is larger anteriorly and inferiorly, and sits at an angle of 45° to the longitudinal axis of the bone. Similarly, the trochlear notch of the ulna bulges, making a comparable angle to its axis (Fig. 21.1). This structure postpones contact between the humerus and ulna on flexion, and allows more space between the bones to accommodate soft

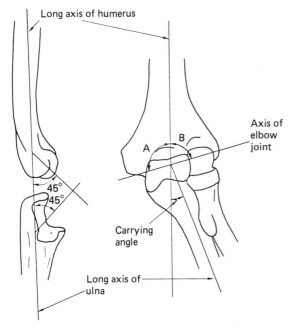

**Figure 21.1** Elbow joint axes. From Palastanga et al. (1989).

tissues. The 'nutcracker effect' is therefore reduced, as the bones come together.

Viewed from the front, the radius and ulna are slanted laterally to the shaft of the humerus, the angulation forming the carrying angle. This is approximately 10–15° for men, increasing to 20–25° for women. This bony alignment means that normally, as the arm is flexed the hand moves towards the shoulder. Variations in carrying angle are seen between individuals, and changes in bony alignment may occur after injury—an important factor in rehabilitation following elbow fractures.

The contact area between the joint surfaces of the elbow complex increases throughout flexion. In full extension the lower medial part of the trochlear notch of the ulna is used, with no contact occurring between the radius and ulna. At 90° the contact area is a diagonal (lower medial to upper lateral) across the trochlear surface, with only slight pressure between the humerus and radial head. In full flexion definite contact occurs between the radius and ulna, and the trochlear contact areas increase (Fig. 21.2). Full flexion is thus required to ensure adequate nutrition of the whole articular cartilage, a situation which is sometimes not possible in obese or heavily muscled individuals due to the approximation of the flexor soft tissues.

As occurs in the knee, the collateral ligaments of the elbow become taut at different degrees of flexion. The anterior fibres of both the medial and lateral collateral ligaments are taut in extension, whereas the posterior fibres are taut in flexion. Protection is provided against valgus and varus strains throughout the whole range of joint movement as a result.

Pronation and supination of the forearm involve not just the superior and inferior radioulnar joints, but also the ulnohumeral, radiohumeral and radiocarpal joints. With pronation, the head of the

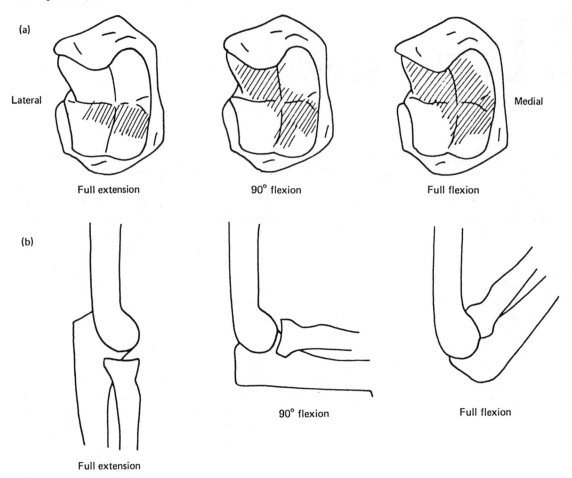

**Figure 21.2**   Contact areas at different elbow positions. (a) The trochlear notch. (b) The head of the radius. From Palastanga et al. (1989).

radius twists on the capitulum and swings on the radial notch of the ulna, tightening the quadrate ligament. The radial head tilts, and is pulled into the capitulotrochlear groove, and the ulna moves into slight extension and abduction at the ulnohumeral joint (Lee, 1986). Consequent to this, at the inferior radioulnar joint the ulnar notch of the radius swings medially over the ulnar head. A traumatic injury to the elbow is therefore likely to affect the wrist, and to be complete a clinical examination should include both joints.

## Screening examination

Following inspection, objective examination begins with flexion and extension, each performed to full range, noting the joint end feel. The normal end feel in extension is hard while that in flexion is soft. Pronation and supination are performed with the elbow held at the side of the body and arm flexed to 90°. The end feel should be springy. Further differentiation may be obtained by combining flexion and extension with abduction and adduction (valgus/varus) stresses, and by assessing gliding motions of the individual component joints of the elbow complex. The capsular pattern is of flexion more limited than extension, and rotations relatively free.

The inferior radio-ulnar joint is stressed by pronation and supination, and may require further examination if pain is produced. Screening examinations of the neck and shoulder are performed if referred pain is suspected, and full neurological examination may be required. The front of the elbow lies within the C5 and C6 dermatomes, while the back of the elbow is in the C7 dermatome. Pain may therefore be referred to the elbow from the cervical nerve roots or the shoulder region.

The contractile structures are examined by resisted movements, performed firstly with the elbow flexed to 90°. One of the therapist's hands supports the elbow to restrict shoulder movement and the other applies resistance to flexion and extension. For pronation and supination, the lower forearm (not the hand) is gripped. The grip must be tight and positioned over the radial styloid to avoid a friction burn to the patient's skin. Resisted wrist flexion and extension are performed with the elbow locked.

## Lateral pain

The term tennis elbow is often used colloquially as a blanket description for any soft tissue pain between the shoulder and wrist, and there has been little agreement in the past as to the exact site of the lesion. The condition was first documented in the late 1800s when it was described as 'lawn tennis arm'. Cyriax (1936) described 26 different lesions to which the condition had been attributed, while Lee (1986) cited 12 more general causes as shown in the list below. The terms lateral and medial tennis elbow have been used (Nirschl, 1986), but in this text the name tennis elbow is used to describe lateral epicondylitis, while 'golfers elbow' refers to medial epicondylitis. The ratio of lateral to medial epicondylitis encountered clinically has been shown to be 7:1 (Leach and Miller, 1987). Some documented causes of lateral elbow pain are:

Radiohumeral bursitis
Periostitis of the common extensor tendon
Tendinitis: extensor carpi radialis brevis, supinator
Microtendonous tears of the common extensor tendon with subtendonous granulation and fibrosis
Myofasciitis
Radial head fibrillation/chondromalacia
Calcification
Radial nerve entrapment and subsequent fibrosis
Stenosis of the orbicular ligament
Hyperaemic synovial fringe
Inflammation of the annular ligament
Cervical radiculopathy

Tennis elbow is a lesion to the common extensor origin (CEO), the primary site being the tendon of extensor carpi radialis brevis. Less frequently, the extensor carpi radialis longus is affected at its attachment to the supracondylar ridge, and in some cases the anterior portion of the extensor digitorum. Most commonly, the injury is at the tenoperiosteal junction but scar tissue may form on the tendon itself, or on the musculotendinous junction. Repeated activity causes microtrauma, with subsequent granulation tissue formation on the underside of the tendon unit and at the tenoperiosteal junction. The granulation tissue formed appears to contain large numbers of free nerve endings, hence the pain of the condition. The major problem is that the granulation tissue does not progress quickly to a mature form, and so healing fails to take place, almost a type of tendinous 'non-union' (Goldie, 1964; Bernhang, 1979).

### Clinical presentation

Tennis elbow usually presents as pain over the region of the lateral epicondyle, extending distally. The pain may build up slowly (due to overuse) or may be the result of a single incident (trauma). Pain is usually increased with resisted wrist extension. Depending on the site of the lesion, pain can be made worse by adding forearm supination (but see radial tunnel syndrome below), and radial deviation of the wrist (Hall, Franklin and Karalfa, 1986). Performing resisted wrist extension with the elbow fully extended will usually elicit pain even in mild cases.

The condition is most common in athletes over 30 years of age, and occurs normally when repeated wrist extension is combined with forearm supination. Racquet sports involve this action, but several occupational stresses can also be causal factors. Hammering, painting and using heavy spanners will all exacerbate the problem, so any training modification which is prescribed must also take into account an athlete's job. Pain usually increases when small objects are gripped, as this hand position places additional stretch on the forearm extensors.

As with most overuse syndromes, the ache initially may subside when the stressful activity is discontinued, but as the condition progresses, pain occurs even at rest. Patients complain of a weak grip, and wasting of the affected muscles may be seen in long-standing cases. Close inspection will often reveal slight swelling over the affected area, but this is rarely obvious to the patient.

### Treatment

Treatment aims initially to reduce pain and swelling. The RICE protocol is used, and several authors have reported good results using ultrasound, either alone or with hydrocortisone gel (Griffin and Touchstone, 1963; Klienkort and Wood, 1975; Halle, Franklin and Karalfa, 1986). It is important to reduce the stress applied to the tendon. Rest from exacerbating activities, and the use of counterforce bracing is effective. The counterforce brace consists of a tight strap which is placed around the upper forearm, to create a lateral pressure when an object is gripped (Fig. 21.5a). The aim is to redirect and disperse overload to healthy tissue or to the band itself, and in so doing reduce painful inhibition and permit a more forceful contraction. Using this technique grip strength has been shown to improve (Burton, 1985; Wadsworth et al., 1989), and a positive effect has been shown using biomechanical analysis and technique correction of tennis serves and backhand strokes (Groppel and Nirschl, 1986).

As the local swelling adheres and shrinks, inelastic scar tissue is formed. Stretching exercises are

therefore of particular value. A useful forearm extensor stretch may be performed with the athlete facing a wall (Fig. 21.3). The dorsum of the hand is placed flat onto the wall, and the elbow remains locked. By leaning forwards the wrist is forced into 90° flexion, stretching the posterior forearm tissues. Wrist flexion may be combined with a pronation stretch. Keeping the elbow locked, the forearm is maximally pronated and the wrist flexed. Overpressure is applied with the other hand and a static stretch performed. The scar tissue is more pliable when warm and so the athlete is advised to practise stretching after a hot bath or shower.

Resistance exercises (weight or powerband) are used to re-strengthen the forearm extensors. Wrist extension may be performed holding a small (2 kg) dumb-bell. The forearm is supported on a block or over the couch side and full range movement is attempted. Powerband extension is performed with the athlete sitting. One end of the band is placed beneath the foot and the other end gripped. The forearm is supported along the athlete's thigh. One word of caution, negative transfer effects (see p. 93), have been described by Nirschl and Sobel (1981) when using high weight low repetition training following tennis elbow. To avoid this they recommended the use of high speed skill training as part of the total rehabilitation programme.

Manual therapy, including local massage to reduce swelling and produce hyperaemia, and transverse frictions to form a mobile scar, are both of use. It is important to locate the exact site of

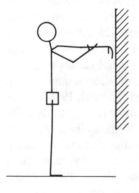

**Figure 21.3** Forearm extensor stretch.

injury for transverse frictions to be effective. The forearm should be pronated and supinated while the area is palpated to find the exact site of the CEO. The lateral epicondyle should be identified, as should the supracondylar ridge, and each considered as a possible source of pain. The teno-osseous junction is best frictioned with the forearm in mid position to let the CEO relax slightly and allow the palpating finger to get right on to the bony surface. The tendon itself is treated on stretch with the elbow and wrist flexed, and forearm pronated.

Mills manipulation (Mills, 1928), although originally designed to stress the annular ligament, can be performed to stretch the CEO. The patient's arm is held in extension at the shoulder, with the elbow comfortably flexed, and wrist and forearm fully flexed and pronated. A high velocity low amplitude thrust is applied to the elbow to fully extend it. Cyriax and Cyriax (1983) claimed this procedure would pull apart the tissue surfaces joined by a painful scar, the fresh tear being replaced by new fibrous tissue under no tension.

Accessory movements of the elbow should be assessed, and mobilization used to reduce pain or resistance. Flexion or extension combined with abduction or adduction may be used together with distraction techniques.

### Sports ergonomics

Ergonomics plays an important part in the management of this condition. Enlarging the grip of any object being held, be it a racquet or a spanner, is important in most cases. The correct grip size can be calculated by measuring from the tip of the ring finger to the bottom lateral crease of the palm, directly below (Fig. 21.4). The figure obtained represents the circumference of the racquet handle. Placing a thick piece of sponge around a handle is also useful to enlarge the grip and reduce shock travelling from the handle to the hand. In some cases, a grip which is too large may also be a problem, so to assess whether grip size is a relevant feature, ask the patient to grip a thin object (a pencil) and a large one (a bottle) and say which gives less pain.

In tennis, higher impact and torsion forces are produced by a wet, heavy ball, or a racquet which

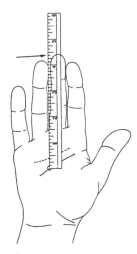

**Figure 21.4** Hand size measurement to determine proper grip handle size. The distance from the proximal palmar crease to the tip of the middle finger determines the proper size. From Nirschl (1988), with permission.

is too tightly strung. The closer the ball is to the centre of percussion (the mathematical point on the racquet face where no torsion will occur on impact) the less strain there is on the elbow tissues.

Oversized racquets, by increasing the likelihood of keeping the ball away from the frame, may reduce torsion and in turn overload stress on the elbow. In addition, leverage forces may be reduced in these racquets by moving the centre of percussion closer to the racquet handle (Nirschl and Sobel, 1981). A heavier racquet will have more momentum, and will place a greater strain on the forearm. Nirschl (1988) recommended a mid-sized (90–100 square inch) graphite composite lightweight racquet to give the best protection, and Bullard (1982) recommended fibreglass or graphite as the best materials to absorb vibration.

### Osteochondrosis

The most common site for osteochondrosis in the elbow is the anterolateral surface of the capitulum (Panner's disease). The aetiology is generally either traumatic or vascular, although some familial tendency may be present. The condition is most commonly related to throwing or racquet sports. In throwing, the angular velocity experienced at the joint may exceed 300°/s (Jobe and Nuber, 1986). This, coupled with a valgus force and an extension stress, causes the radial head to impinge against the capitulum. Ultimately, a breakdown can occur in the capitulum surface and the radial head may hypertrophy.

The vascular supply to the area can be disrupted by this repeated trauma. Up until the age of 5 years the capitulum has a good blood supply, but later the nucleus of the capitulum receives only one or two vessels. These pass into the area posteriorly through soft, compressible cartilage—a possible site of damage.

The typical patient is an athlete in early adolescence (usually male) who shows limitation of elbow extension with local swelling. Onset is often insidious and the patient may report that he or she has been experiencing difficulties over a protracted period. If the osteochondrotic fragment is free within the joint, locking or catching may be experienced with certain movements. Radiographs may show blunting of the capitulum with enlargement of the radial head. Often an island of bone is seen surrounded by an area of rarefaction. Premature epiphyseal closure may also be noted to either the humerus or proximal radius.

In the initial stages of the condition with a young athlete, rest is all that is required, splinting being indicated if the patient fails to heed this advice. If stress has been allowed to continue and bony degeneration has occurred, drilling or grafting of the attached fragment may be required. In late stage conditions loose bodies may need to be removed, and unfortunately the prognosis is sometimes poor.

## Medial pain

Lesions to the medial side of the joint occur most often with throwing actions. Although different sports demand different throwing techniques, similarities still exist. Initially, the shoulder is abducted and taken into extreme external rotation and extension, while the elbow remains flexed. Then, the shoulder and trunk rapidly move forward, leaving the arm behind. This action imposes a valgus stress on the joint and stretches the ulnar collateral ligament in particular. The shoulder flexors and internal rotators contract powerfully, flinging the arm forward and resulting in stress to the olecranon as the arm extends rapidly to full range.

The throwing action imposes a number of stresses on the elbow. The lateral joint line is subjected to compression forces, in the olecranon fossa on the posterior aspect of the joint there are shearing forces, while the medial joint line experiences tensile forces (Jobe and Nuber, 1986). These forces, if repeated, can give rise to specific injuries and general degeneration reflecting the stress imposed on the elbow structures (Table 21.1).

## Medial epicondylitis

This is a lesion of the common flexor origin (CFO) on the medial epicondyle, and is commonly called golfer's elbow. The primary site is the origin of pronator teres and flexor carpi radialis on the medial epicondyle. The flexor carpi ulnaris may occasionally be affected. Golfer's elbow is less common than tennis elbow, occurring at a ratio of about 1:15 (Coorad and Hooper, 1973). The injury can be complicated by ulnar nerve involvement, the nerve being compressed at a point distal to the medial epicondyle. Sensory symptoms are often present and Tinels sign is positive (Nirschl, 1986).

**Table 21.1 Throwing injuries to the elbow**

| Force | Injury |
|-------|--------|
| Medial tension | Muscular overuse<br>Ligamentous injury<br>Capsular injury<br>Ulnar traction spur<br>Medial epicondylitis |
| Lateral compression | Osteochondrosis<br>Fractured capitulum<br>Lateral epicondylitis |
| Posterior shear | Muscular strain<br>Impingement<br>Olecranon fracture<br>Bony hypertrophy<br>Loose bodies |

In chronic conditions calcium deposits may develop within the tendon itself (Leach and Miller, 1987).

Pain is felt more locally than with tennis elbow, and is increased on resisted wrist flexion and sometimes forearm pronation. The condition may be differentiated from chronic medial ligament sprain by applying the valgus stress test, which should not give pain or laxity in epicondylitis.

The treatment is for the most part like that for tennis elbow, including soft tissue techniques and ergonomics. Transverse frictions are performed with the elbow and wrist in extension, with the forearm supinated. Counterforce bracing is again used, but this time the brace is of a different design, to bring it up to the medial epicondyle without interfering with elbow flexion (Fig. 21.5).

## Medial collateral ligament

Repetitive stresses to this ligament are common in throwing athletes, particularly in events such as the javelin. Pain is generally quite localized over the

(a)

(b)

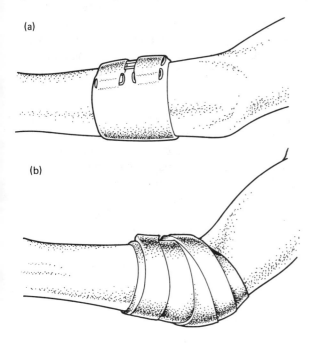

**Figure 21.5** (a) Lateral counterforce elbow brace. (b) Medial counterforce elbow brace. From Nirschl (1988), with permission.

medial joint line, and is exacerbated by applying an elbow abduction stress test, forcing a valgus strain on the joint in 20° flexion. In severe injuries, gapping of the joint may be apparent.

Initial treatment is to remove the causal stress and rest from throwing. Operative repair of a ruptured medial collateral ligament is often recommended for athletes and those involved in heavy manual labour. The theory is that instability may produce problems later in life. However, Kuroda and Sakamaki (1986) reported surgical repair in ten patients and conservative management in three others. Before surgery valgus instability averaged l4.9°. Those treated surgically later showed average laxity of 5.1° while those managed conservatively had average values of 8.0°. With figures for instability which are so similar, it is questionable whether surgery offers any substantial advantage over conservative management in most cases.

## Posterior elbow pain

Pain at the back of the elbow is common in sports which rapidly extend or hyperextend the joint. These include the throwing sports, punching in martial arts, and pressing actions in weight training. Structures involved, either individually or in combination, include the insertion of the triceps, the olecranon bursa, and the olecranon itself.

### Olecranon burstitis

The olecranon bursa is placed at the bony point of the elbow, over the olecranon process subcutaneously. A deeper bursa is sometimes present between the capsule and triceps. When the elbow is extended, the margins of the olecranon bursa cause a circular ridge of skin about 1.5–2 cm in diameter to be pulled up on the posterior aspect of the elbow.

The bursa can become inflamed by leaning on the elbow for a prolonged period (student's elbow), or due to a direct fall onto the point of the elbow. This latter case may induce haemorrhage into the bursal sac itself. Examination of the joint reveals no abnormality, but pain and thickening occur to direct palpation over the bursa. Treatment is to remove the cause, pad the point of the elbow, and aspirate the fluid.

### Triceps insertion

Repeated strain on the triceps, particularly through excessive weight-training activities by young males, may cause inflammation of the triceps tendon, with damage to the musculotendinous or teno-osseous junctions. Cessation of activity and correction of technique, coupled with modalities to reduce local inflammation and pain are usually curative.

## Posterior impingement

Posterior impingement of the olecranon into its fossa is common in sports where the elbow is 'snapped back'. This is especially the case with rapid weight (circuit) training, and martial arts where athletes 'punch the air' while performing forms. Throwing events will tend to cause impingement of the medial aspect of the olecranon on the follow-through movement.

Examination usually reveals point tenderness over the posterior or posteromedial aspect of the olecranon. This is made worse by forced extension, and extension/abduction. Chronic injuries may show osteophyte formation posteromedially. Cortical thickening is also usually seen on radiograph, but this is thought to represent adaptation of the bone to repetitive stress (Garrick and Webb, 1990).

Treatment is initially to limit extension and valgus stress by strapping, or if this fails, to rest the elbow completely. The elbow flexors are strengthened (especially eccentrically) to enhance their action as decelerators of elbow extension, and to shorten them and therefore limit hyperextension.

## Muscular injury

The biceps, triceps and brachialis may all be injured in sport. The most common injury for the biceps is to its long head (see p. 283), but its lower insertion may also be injured occasionally. Pain is reproduced to resisted elbow flexion and supination, and passive pronation, resisted shoulder flexion may also be added. If resisted flexion is painful but supination is not, the brachialis is indicated. The site of pain is the centre of the front of the arm, often radiating as far as the wrist in severe cases.

The usual site for injury to the triceps is the musculotendinous junction, but the muscle belly may be injured. Pain on resisted elbow (and shoulder) extension is the clinical sign, but when this test gives pain in the upper arm felt nearer to the shoulder, referred pain from impingement of a shoulder structure should be considered. In this case the triceps contraction pulls the humerus up into the acromion approximating the joint.

## Myositis ossificans traumatica

Injury to the brachialis should always be treated with caution, because this muscle shares with the quadriceps the potential for myositis development (see pp. 43, 160).

The history is usually that of a direct blow, for example from a knee or head in rugby or a foot in martial arts. Most commonly, a second blow has been experienced to the same area. The typical findings are tenderness persisting for two to three weeks after injury, and difficulty in regaining full range motion. On examination, a fibrous mass is often palpable within the muscle over the anterior aspect of the arm. Where these findings are present, X-ray examination is required. Often heterotrophic bone formation is seen, showing a diffuse fluffy callous. As the callus matures it will shrink and its margins become better defined. A bone scan will reveal whether the condition is still active.

Management aims initially to minimize the damage. Local swelling is reduced where possible, and activity limited. Mobility exercise is begun with caution when radiographic evidence shows that the condition is no longer active. Resisted work is the last exercise to be started, and when sport is resumed, the area is protected with padding.

## Elbow dislocations

Posterior or posterolateral dislocation of the elbow is seen following a fall onto the outstretched arm, sometimes associated with a fracture to the olecranon or coronoid process. This is common when falling from a horse or bicycle, and from gymnastic accidents. Rollerskating, and skateboarding are also prime causes, as the athlete usually falls backwards onto an abducted straight arm. There is often a snap or crack at the time of injury with immediate swelling. On examination, the arm is held flexed, and a gross deformity is apparent on the posterior aspect of the elbow. The normal triangular alignment of the olecranon and two epicondyles is lost. Radiographic examination is required to assess bony damage, and on no account should reduction on the field be attempted because of the risk of neural complications. Reduction is achieved by downward pressure on the forearm, initially to disengage the coronoid from the olecranon fossa and then the forearm is brought forwards. As with the shoulder, reduction, unless immediate, will usually require analgesia. Operative intervention has often been recommended if reduction is unstable due to ligament avulsion. However, Josefsson et al. (1987) compared the results of patients treated by primary surgical repair with those treated by closed reduction. Although the surgery group included those with complete collateral ligament ruptures or avulsions (all patients) and muscle origin tears from the humeral epicondyles (half the patients) the results from the two groups were the same.

If the arm is immobilized for more than a week, the resting position should be in as much extension as possible (Garrick and Webb, 1990). This is important because reduced flexion is far easier to regain during rehabilitation than is extension. With an uncomplicated injury, gentle isometric exercise is begun as pain and swelling settles. After 2–3 days, active mobility exercise is started with caution in the pain-free range, the athlete wearing a sling between exercise periods for protection.

Early mobilization of this injury is essential. Mehlhoff et al. (1988) described 52 adults with elbow dislocation. Those immobilized for less than 18 days showed significantly better results than those inactive for longer periods, and patients immobilized for more than 4 weeks all showed only fair or poor results. None of the patients redislocated.

Following this injury, there is normally a slight loss of extension. If the elbow had previously hyperextended, this is not usually a problem.

However, if the arm remains slightly flexed, weight-bearing activities, such as handstands and cartwheels, will tend to push the arm into flexion. To stabilize the arm and obtain some degree of functional locking, the triceps must be built up extensively.

## Radial head

Compression fracture of the radial head may occur with a vertical fall onto the outstretched arm, but more commonly the injury which affects the radial head is a dislocation. This is usually seen in children, where the radial head is pulled through the annular ligament, limiting extension. Reduction, if performed before muscle spasm sets in, may be accomplished by holding the elbow flexed to 90° and lightly rotating the forearm. At the same time, the radius and humerus are gently pulled together and the radial head is felt to click back beneath the annular ligament on full supination. This condition often reduces spontaneously.

## Nerve involvement

### Ulnar nerve

The ulnar nerve may be involved with medial collateral ligament injuries of the elbow, as stated above. Friction against this nerve or its sheath may give rise to symptoms, described by Wadsworth and Williams (1973) as the cubital tunnel syndrome.

Since the sensory fibres of the ulnar nerve are more superficial than the motor fibres, sensory symptoms are more prevalent, with paraesthesia occurring in the fourth and fifth fingers.

The nerve passes through the groove behind the medial epicondyle and is covered by a fibrous sheath, forming the cubital tunnel. The roof of the tunnel is the aponeurosis of the two heads of flexor carpi ulnaris. This is taut at 90° flexion, constricting the tunnel, and slack on extension. The floor of the cubital tunnel is formed from the tip of the trochlea and the medial collateral ligament. The ligament bulges with elbow flexion, an additional factor leading to nerve compression, especially with prolonged periods of end range flexion.

Dislocation of the nerve from the ulnar groove can also occur following fracture and is accompanied by a persistent tingling sensation with certain elbow actions.

## Radial nerve

The radial nerve can be injured in the elbow region. The nerve travels in front of the lateral condyle of the humerus to divide into deep (posterior interosseous) and superficial branches. The superficial branch may be exposed to direct trauma, sometimes being damaged as a complication of fractures to the radial head or neck.

Radial tunnel syndrome (Roles and Maudsley, 1972) occurs when the deep branch of the radial nerve is compressed as it passes along the fibrous edge of the supinator muscle (arcade of Frohse). Pain is produced when the arm is fully pronated with the wrist flexed.

Differential diagnosis of radial tunnel syndrome is made by eliciting pain by palpation of the radial head, and pain on resisted supination. True tennis elbow will give pain over the lateral epicondyle (not the radial head), with pain on resisted wrist extension but not supination alone (Lee, 1986). The condition is seen following repeated contraction of the wrist extensors and forearm supinators against resistance, as in racquet sports in a novice sportsperson (Cailliet, 1983).

## Testing the elbow following injury

A sportsperson must be able to perform actions relevant to his or her sport and to his or her competitive role within that sport (Wright, 1981). Maximal functional work of the biceps may be performed by the subject chinning a bar, and for the triceps, dipping between two chairs, or performing a push-up with the feet on a chair, both of these actions should be slow and controlled until confidence is built. Faster, more demanding actions include press-ups with a clap in between each repetition, and walking hand to hand while hanging at arm's length from a horizontal ladder.

Racquet sportspeople should mimic their stroke action with a weighted racquet or heavy club, and can assess their resilience to jarring strains by hitting a club or bat against a firm surface (a medicine ball is ideal). The elbow must be able to take repeated traction and approximation strains, and be pain-free when the arm is locked while holding a weight at arm's length.

## References

Bernhang, A.M., Dehner, W. and Fogerty, C. (1974) Tennis elbow. A biomedical approach. *American Journal of Sports Medicine*, 2, 235–258

Bernhang, A.M. (1979) The many causes of tennis elbow. *New York State Journal of Medicine*, 1363–1366

Bullard, J.A.A (1982) Tennis elbow. *Canadian Family Physician*, 28, 961–963

Burton, A.K. (1985) Grip strength and forearm straps in tennis elbow. *British Journal of Sports Medicine*, 19, 37–38

Cailliet, R. (1983) *Soft Tissue Pain and Disability*, F.A. Davis, Philadelphia

Coorad, R.W. and Hooper, W.R. (1973) Tennis elbow: course, natural history, conservative and surgical management. *Journal of Bone and Joint Surgery*, 55A, 1177

Cyriax, J.H. and Cyriax, P.J. (1983) *Illustrated Manual of Orthopaedic Medicine*, Butterworth, London

Cyriax J. (1936) Pathology and treatment of tennis elbow. *Journal of Bone and Joint Surgery*, 18, 921

Garrick, J.G. and Webb, D.R. (1990) *Sports Injuries: Diagnosis and Management*, W.B. Saunders, London

Goldie, I. (1964) Epicondylitis lateralis humeri: a pathological study. *Acta Chirurgica Scandinavica* (suppl.), 34, 339

Griffen, J.E. and Touchstone J.C. (1963) Ultrasonic movement of cortisol into pig tissues. (I). Movement into skeletal muscle. *American Journal of Physical Medicine*, 43, 77

Groppel, J.L. and Nirschl, R.P. (1986) A mechanical and electromyographical analysis of the effects of various joint counterforce braces on the tennis player. *American Journal of Sports Medicine*, 14, 195–200

Halle, J.S., Franklin, R.J. and Karalfa, B.L. (1986) Comparison of four treatment approaches for lateral epicondylitis of the elbow. *Journal of Orthopaedic and Sports Physical Therapy*, 8, (2) 62–69

Jobe, F.W. and Nuber, G. (1986) Throwing injuries of the elbow. *Sports Medicine*, 5, (4) 621–635

Josefsson, P.O., Gentz, C., Johnell, O. and Wendeberg, B. (1987) Surgical versus non-surgical treatment of ligamentous injuries following dislocation of the elbow joint: a prospective randomized study. *Journal of Bone and Joint Surgery*, 69A, 605–608

Kleinkort, J.B. and Wood, F. (1975) Phonophoresis with 1% versus 10% hydrocortisone. *Physical Therapy*, 55, 1320

Kuroda, S. and Sakamaki, K. (1986) Ulnar collateral ligament tears of the elbow joint. *Clinical Orthopaedics*, **208**, 266–271

Leach, R.E. and Miller, J.K. (1987) Lateral and medial epicondylitis of the elbow. *Clinics in Sports Medicine*, **6**, (2) 259–272

Lee, D.G. (1986) Tennis elbow: a manual therapists perspective. *Journal of Orthopaedic and Sports Physical Therapy*

Mehlhoff, T.L., Noble, P.C., Bennett, J.B. and Tullos, H.S. (1988) Simple dislocation of the elbow in the adult: Results after closed treatment. *Journal of Bone and Joint Surgery*, **70A**, 244–249

Mills, G.P. (1928) Treatment of tennis elbow. *British Medical Journal*, **1**, (12)

Nirschl R.P. (1975) The etiology and treatment of tennis elbow. *Journal of Sports Medicine*, **2**, 308–319

Nirschl, R.P. (1986) Soft tissue injuries about the elbow. *Clinics in Sports Medicine*, **5**, (4) 637–652

Nirschl, R.P. (1988). Prevention and treatment of elbow and shoulder injuries in the tennis player. *Clinics in Sports Medicine*, **7**, (2) 289–309

Palastanga, N., Field, D. and Soames, R. (1989) *Anatomy and Human Movement: Structure and Function*, Butterworth–Heinemann, Oxford

Roles, N.C. and Maudsley, R.H. (1972) Radial tunnel syndrome. Resistant tennis elbow as a nerve entrapment. *Journal of Bone and Joint Surgery*, **54**, 499–508

Wadsworth, C.T., Nielsen, D.H., Burns, L.T., Krull, J.D. and Thompson, C.G. (1989) Effect of the counterforce armband on wrist extension and grip strength and pain in subjects with tennis elbow. *Journal of Orthopaedic and Sports Physical Therapy*, **11**, 192–197

Wadsworth, T.G. and Williams, J.R. (1973) Cubital tunnel external compression syndrome. *British Medical Journal*, **1**, 662

Wright, D. (1981) Fitness testing after injury. In *Sports Fitness and Sports Injuries*, (ed. T. Reilly), Faber and Faber, London

# 22 The wrist and hand

The wrist area has a series of articulations between the distal end of the radius and the carpal bones (radiocarpal joint), and between the individual carpals themselves (intercarpal joints). The radiocarpal joint is formed between the distal end of the radius and the scaphoid, lunate and triquetral. The end of the radius is covered by a concave disc. The eight carpal bones are arranged in two rows, the junction between the rows forms the mid-carpal joint. This joint is convex laterally and concave medially, giving it an 'S' shape.

The wrist is strengthened by collateral, palmar and dorsal ligaments. The ulnar collateral ligament is a rounded cord stretching from the ulnar styloid to the triquetral and pisiform. The radial collateral ligament passes from the radial styloid to the scaphoid and then to the trapezium. The dorsal radiocarpal ligament runs from the lower aspect of the radius to the scaphoid, lunate and triquetral. On the palmar surface, the radiocarpal and ulnocarpal ligaments attach from the lower ends of the radius and ulna to the proximal carpal bones.

The available range of movement at the wrist is a combination of radiocarpal and midcarpal movement. Flexion occurs more at the midcarpal joint, while extension is greater at the radiocarpal joint, but the combined movement is about 85° in each direction. Abduction occurs mostly at the midcarpal joint and has a range of about 15° whereas adduction involves most movement at the radiocarpal joint and has a range of motion of 45° (Palastanga, Field and Soames, 1989). The difference in range is because the radial styloid comes down further than the ulnar styloid, and so is more limiting to abduction.

The carpal bones form a transverse arch, concave on their palmar aspect. This arch is maintained by the flexor retinaculum, which attaches medially to the pisiform and the hook of hamate. Laterally, the retinaculum binds to the scaphoid tubercle and to the groove of trapezium, through which runs the tendon of flexor carpi radialis. The space formed beneath the retinaculum is called the 'carpal tunnel', and the tendons of flexor pollicis longus, flexor digitorum profundus, flexor digitorum superficialis and the median nerve pass through it. On the posterior aspect of the wrist the extensor retinaculum stretches from the radius to the hamate and pisiform bones and extends inferiorly to form six longitudinal compartments for the passage of the extensor tendons (Fig. 22.1).

## Grip

Prehension is an advanced skill in humans, resulting largely from the ability of the thumb to oppose the fingers. Two types of grip may be described, 'precision' involving the thumb and fingers and 'power', involving the whole hand.

With precision grip, the object is usually small and light. The grip is applied with the nails or fingertips (terminal opposition), pads of the fingers (subterminal opposition), or the pad and side of another finger (subterminal-lateral opposition). This action involves rotation of both the carpometacarpal joints of the thumb and fingers involved in the gripping action. The small finger muscles work in combination with the flexor digitorum profundus and superficialis as well as the flexor pollicis longus.

In power grips the long flexors and extensors work to lock the wrist and grip the object. In the palmar grip, the whole hand surrounds the object, and the thumb works against the fingers. The shape taken up by the hand is largely determined by the size of the object, but the grip is strongest when the thumb can still touch the index finger.

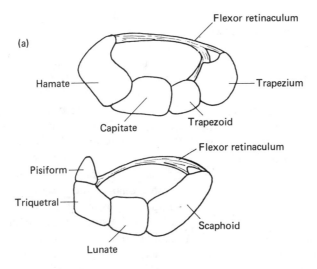

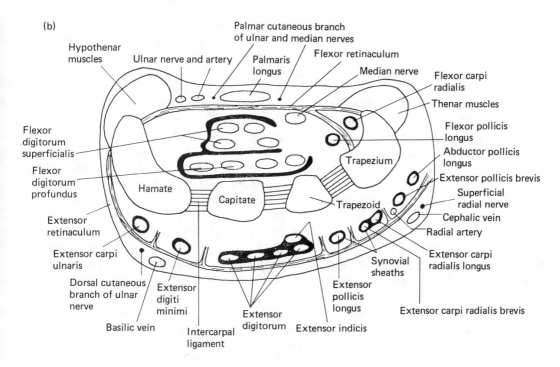

**Figure 22.1** (a) Arrangement of the carpal bones and attachment of the flexor retinaculum. (b) Transverse section through the wrist region showing the relationships of the various structures which pass into the hand. From Palastanga, Field and Soames (1989), with permission.

This is the type of grip used when holding a racquet or javelin. When the fingers are closed firmly, the fourth and fifth metacarpals move over the hamate bone to further tighten the grip and prevent a smooth object from slipping out of the hand. The hook grip is used when lifting something with a handle, such as a suitcase. Now, the object is held between the flexed fingers and palm, the thumb not being used. Although the grip is quite powerful, the power is in one direction only.

## Screening examination

Initial examination of the wrist utilizes a number of movements to cover all the joints involved in wrist articulation. The superior and inferior radioulnar joints are stressed by passive pronation and supination. The wrist itself is assessed by flexion, extension, abduction and adduction, performed both passively and against resistance. At the same time as the wrist is examined, the fingers are also assessed as the two areas are intimately linked. Passive and resisted movements are performed at the thumb and finger joints. Again, flexion, extension, abduction and adduction are used. The capsular pattern for the wrist joint is an equal limitation to passive flexion and extension. Painful resisted movement at the wrist indicates that the lesion is not local, but higher up in the muscle bellies, whereas pain to resisted finger movements may give local pain. In addition to pain, crepitus to active movements is an important sign for the long finger tendons.

This examination, described by Cyriax (1982) provides the examiner with enough information to establish whether a lesion is intracapsular or not, and whether contractile tissue is affected. For the physiotherapist, further assessment is usually required to assess and record range of motion and accessory movements. In addition, specific tests are used once the screening examination has focused the therapist's attention onto a specific area or series of tissues.

## Scaphoid fracture

The important feature of this fracture is not the frequency with which it occurs, but the number of times it is missed, with pain so often being attributed to 'just a sprain'. The usual history is of a fall onto the outstretched arm with the wrist fully extended. When the hand is locked into extension, the athlete is more likely to sustain a scaphoid fracture, this can occur with a vertical fall from gymnastic apparatus for example. When the hand is more relaxed and the force has some horizontal component, as with a fall when running, the distal radius will usually break (Colles' fracture). The scaphoid fracture is common in the young athlete, while the Colles' fracture is seen more frequently in the elderly. This is partially due to the weakness of the radius with the onset of osteoporosis in the aged. A further cause of injury to the scaphoid is striking an object with the heel of the hand, a mechanism seen in contact sports, such as the martial arts, or in a collision with another player.

The major symptom is one of well-localized pain to the base of the thumb, within the 'anatomical snuffbox'. In addition, pain is exacerbated by longitudinal compression of the first metacarpal against the scaphoid by pressing the thumb proximally. Radiographic examination is helpful, but a negative X-ray does not eliminate the possibility of a fracture (Garrick and Webb, 1990). Non-displaced fractures are often normal to begin with and only become positive when some bone reabsorption has occurred, the fracture line beginning to show up 2–4 weeks after injury.

The blood supply to the scaphoid is confined to its distal pole in some subjects. The fracture, which usually travels transversely through the neck of the bone, can cut off the blood supply to the proximal fragment, making non-union or mal-union more likely. Scaphoid fracture requires prolonged immobilization of the wrist and thumb. The cast usually extends to the interphalangeal (IP) joint of the thumb to just below the elbow. In some cases an above-elbow splint is used to limit pronation and supination. Uncomplicated fractures of the scaphoid tubercle may heal in as little as 4 weeks, but fracture to the proximal part of the bone may take as much as 20 weeks to heal.

Complications to scaphoid fracture have a poor prognosis. Avascular necrosis may require excision of the avascular fragment, or prosthetic replacement of the whole bone. Non-union usually demands bone graft or screw fixation, but the failure rate can be high. A relatively new development in the management of scaphoid non-union is the use of the Herbert differential pitch screw, which is completely buried in the bone. Bunker, McNamee and Scott (1987) described successful union in 90% of patients treated using this procedure combined with bone grafting.

## Wrist pain

### Sprains

A 'sprained wrist' is a common 'diagnosis', but this really only indicates the area of pain, and the fact that soft tissue is the likely structure affected. The most common tissues injured are the intercarpal ligaments, with or without subluxation of a carpal bone. Pain is reproduced to passive wrist flexion and is generally well-localized to the particular tissue affected. Common ligaments involved include the lunate-capitate (Cyriax, 1982) and scapho-lunate (Wilkes, 1989). Transverse frictions to the ligament with the wrist flexed is effective, but manipulation to rupture adhesive scarring is not (Cyriax, 1982).

Sprain to the ulnar or radial collateral ligaments is rare, but if present gives pain to end range passive abduction and adduction.

### Carpal dislocation

Subluxation or dislocation of a carpal bone, rather than a scaphoid fracture, may occur from a fall on to the outstretched hand. The bone most commonly affected is the lunate, although the capitate may also sublux (Cyriax and Cyriax, 1983). Movement is generally limited in one direction only (contrast the capsular pattern). Pain is localized by palpating in a line along the third finger to reach the third metacarpal. In the normal hand the capitate lies in a hollow just proximal to the base of

the third metacarpal and the lunate is felt proximal to this, and slightly towards the ulna.

When the capitate subluxes, the wrist is held in flexion, and a prominent bump is seen over the dorsum of the wrist as the capitate stands proud of its neighbours. Reduction of a minor subluxation is often spontaneous, but if not, may be achieved during traction by a repeated anterior and posterior glide, with the wrist positioned over the edge of the treatment couch. The wrist is immobilized in a splint until the acute pain subsides, when rehabilitation is begun.

Full dislocation of the lunate may occur with a fall on to the extended wrist. The shape and position of the lunate lying between the lower radius and capitate make it prone to dislocation. On forced wrist extension, the wedge-shaped lunate is squeezed out from between the two bones to lie on the palmar surface of the carpal region (Fig. 22.2) as an apparent 'swelling'. The scaphoid-lunate ligament usually ruptures and the lunate rotates. Radiographs taken with the forearm fully supinated show a separation of the scaphoid-lunate joint of more than 2 mm (Corrigan and Maitland, 1983). The dislocated lunate may impinge on the

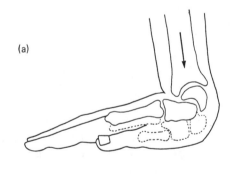

(a)

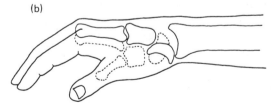

(b)

**Figure 22.2** Lunate dislocation. (a) The injury occurs when the radius forces the lunate in a palmar direction, resulting in dislocation. (b) From Hertling and Kessler (1990), with permission.

median nerve, and the flexor tendons may be compressed within the carpal tunnel.

Reduction under anaesthesia is possible if the condition is diagnosed early, with the wrist initially immobilized in some degree of flexion, and then protected from forced extension when sport is resumed. If left, damage to the median nerve is more likely and open reduction is usually required.

Occasionally, the lunate may stay in place against the radius, and the carpal bones surrounding it dislocate posteriorly to give a perilunar dislocation. This normally occurs in association with a scaphoid fracture, part of the fractured bone remaining with the radius and lunate (Williams and Sperryn, 1976 O'Donoghue, 1976).

## Wrist pain in gymnasts

Repetitive forced extension causes compression and impaction forces on the wrist. This type of movement is common in gymnastics, and in exercises such as the 'press-up with clap', in addition, heavy bench press exercises used in training or powerlifting forces extension. When this occurs, the athlete may experience pain over the dorsum of the wrist, and end range flexion and extension are painfully limited. The main fault initially may be an impingement of the dorsal wrist structures, resulting in capsular inflammation (Aronen, 1985). If impact forces continue, however, carpal subluxation or fracture may occur in the adult, and epiphyseal damage in the adolescent.

The distal end of the ulna has a fibrocartilage disc which separates it from the lunate. The disc prevents ulnocarpal abutment by cushioning forces between the ulna and lunate. Trauma may cause thinning of the articular disc, and a reduction in shock-absorbing capacity. Studies of cadavers have shown that the radius takes 60% of axial loading to the wrist when the articular disc is intact, but that this is increased to 95% when the disc is excised (Palmer and Werner, 1981).

Forced extension is of particular concern in the child. Normally, closure of the distal ulnar growth plate should precede that of the radius. However, the structure and function of the distal radial growth plate can be altered by repetitive loading in gymnastics or other sports, and may fuse prematurely, giving radial shortening with respect to the normal ulna (Albanese et al., 1989). On posterior-anterior radiographs, the position of the ulna may be compared with that of the radius. If the ulna is longer, positive ulnar variance exists, if shorter, negative variance is present. As the radial growth plate closes after that of the ulna, negative ulnar variance is the norm. However, gymnasts have been shown to have significant positive ulnar variance when compared with controls (Mandelbaum et al., 1989).

With positive variance, in addition to bone changes, the disc between the ulna and lunate may be thinner, and less stable. The combination of reduced shock absorption and stability may lead to a chronic degenerative condition.

In the adolescent, rest from activities involving extension and loading of the wrist is essential. Carter et al (1988) have demonstrated significant healing of this condition within three months following cessation of gymnastics.

## Kienbock's disease

This is an aseptic necrosis (osteochondritis) of the lunate. The condition may result from direct trauma, such as a compression fracture (Cetti, Christensen and Reuther, 1982), or following repeated micro-trauma from impact stresses. Industrial stresses, such as hammering, and impact forces in sports, such as tennis, karate, volleyball and golf, have been identified as factors (Nakamura et al., 1991). Although the progress of the condition is similar in both sporting and non-sporting populations, athletes develop symptoms more quickly.

The condition is seen from adolescence up to the mid-30s. The lunate atrophies, becomes sclerosed, and later decalcifies, showing flattening and fragmentation on X-ray. The main symptom is wrist pain, with range of motion and grip strength reducing.

Marked deformity of the bone occurs, unless the condition is identified early enough, when pressure on the wrist during sport should be eliminated. If the condition is too advanced to respond to conservative management, surgery is required. As the patients are young, and remodelling of the lunate can be expected, osteotomy is frequently performed rather than carpectomy (Nakamura et al., 1991).

## Compression neuropathies

### Carpal tunnel syndrome

Carpal tunnel syndrome is a compression neuropathy of the median nerve as it passes beneath the transverse carpal ligament. It is more common in women than men, and occurs typically later in life (40–60 years), although it is seen in younger individuals secondary to trauma. Paraesthesia (numbness, burning and tingling) is felt over the first three fingers and the radial half of the fourth. Pain is made worse with repeated movements, and prolonged wrist flexion can reproduce the symptoms (Phalen's test). Percussion of the medial nerve (Tinel's sign) within the carpal tunnel with the wrist extended may also be positive.

A number of factors may contribute to the condition, and these generally fall into one of two categories. First, factors which increase the size of the structures within the carpal tunnel. This could be through swelling of the flexor tendon sheaths (tenosynovitis) as a result of repeated or sustained flexor activity (for example, in gymnasts, cyclists and weightlifters). Secondly, factors which reduce the size of the carpal tunnel itself, such as arthritic changes secondary to a Colles' fracture, fluid retention during pregnancy, and obesity. The condition must be differentiated from vascular insufficiency, which usually gives a glove-like distribution of symptoms, and entrapment of the C6/C7 nerve root, which does not give increased pain to repeated wrist movements.

Management of the condition is initially to rest the wrist in a splint (day and night), as in the neutral position there is less pressure within the carpal tunnel (Hertling and Kessler, 1990). In addition, the flexor retinaculum may be stretched by separating the pisiform and hamate from the trapezium and scaphoid (Maitland, 1991). It is interesting to note that vitamin B6 may facilitate healing in this condition (Diamond, 1989).

### Ulnar nerve compression

Ulnar nerve compression (cyclist's palsy) is an unusual condition. The nerve passes into the hand through a shallow trough (canal of Guyan) between the pisiform and the hook of hamate, to emerge and divide into two. During cycling, the nerve is stretched by hyperextension and ulnar deviation of the wrist. The stresses taken by the hand in cycling can be greater than the athlete's bodyweight (Haloua, Collin and Coudeyre, 1987), and altered conduction velocity of the distal ulnar nerve has been shown in long-distance cyclists (Wilmarth and Nelson, 1988).

Motor and sensory symptoms may be caused, affecting the fourth and fifth fingers. Weakness and clumsiness of fine finger movements may be seen with a reduction in pinch grip strength. Initial management is by ensuring a correct cycle frame size to prevent the athlete overstretching. Extra padding on the handlebars or in cycling gloves will reduce compression stress, but if symptoms persist, the athlete should refrain from cycling for as long as 4 months to allow recovery of motor function.

## Thumb

### Ulnar collateral ligament rupture

Injury to the ulnar collateral ligament (UCL) of the metacarpophalangeal (MCP) joint of the thumb is common in any sport in which the thumb is forced into excessive abduction. This may occur in alpine skiing, in which the strap of the ski pole pulls the thumb. It has been estimated that around 10% of all alpine skiing injuries involve this ligament, giving a total of 50 000–200 000 injuries per year (Peterson and Renstrom, 1986). The injury also occurs less commonly in contact sports when the thumb becomes trapped as a player falls.

Chronic insufficiency of the ligament (Gamekeeper's thumb) is distinct from complete rupture (skier's thumb). Complete rupture usually occurs from the distal attachment at the base of the proximal phalanx and in about 30% of cases an avulsion fracture occurs. The UCL lies beneath the adductor pollicis, and with complete rupture the aponeurosis of this muscle may be trapped between the pieces of torn ligament—a so called 'Stener lesion' (Stener, 1962). When the ligament is completely ruptured, contraction of the adductor pollicis will tend to sublux the joint rather than give true adduction, and so grip is weakened.

Symptoms are reproduced by passive extension and abduction of the thumb, and the pain is usually well localized to the ulnar side of the joint. A valgus strain to the MCP joint will stretch the ligament and again gives pain. In complete rupture, the end feel of the joint is limp, and a dorsal haematoma may be visible over the thumb interphalangeal joint, indicating that blood has diffused along the extensor pollicis longus (Moutet et al., 1989). Treatment of a grade I injury is initially by rest and ice in the acute phase and then the joint is actively mobilized as pain and swelling settle. Grade II injuries require immobilization in a strapping or splint for as much as 4 weeks to limit abduction, and in severe cases a cast may be required. Complete ligamentous ruptures generally require surgery, and about a quarter may be expected to have displaced bone fragments (Moutet et al., 1989) which will require fixation by Kirschner wires. Following surgical repair, the thumb is immobilized in a cast for 4–6 weeks, and later a full rehabilitation programme is begun.

## De Quervain's tenovaginitis

This is an inflammation and thickening of the synovial lining of the common sheath of the abductor pollicis longus and extensor pollicis brevis tendons. The thickening occurs particularly at the point where the tendons pass over the distal aspect of the radius. The history is usually of overuse, and the condition represents a common occupational injury, but is also seen in rock climbers. There is pain to resisted thumb extension and abduction. In addition, pain is caused by passively ulnar deviating the wrist, while keeping the thumb fully flexed, a movement which stretches the tendon and sheath. Local tenderness is found to palpation,

again with the tendon on stretch. Crepitus is often present to repeated movements. The condition must be differentiated from arthritis of the carpometacarpal joint of the thumb which will not give pain on resisted movements, and tendon stretch which will give pain in roughly the same area.

De Quervain's tenovaginitis responds well to frictional massage with the tendon on stretch, and immobilization of the thumb in a splint. Treatment by corticosteroid injection into the tendon sheath is reserved for persistent cases.

## Arthrosis

The capsular pattern at the carpo-metacarpal joint is a limitation of abduction only. By far the most common intra-articular lesion is osteoarthrosis. The condition is more usual in women and is frequently bilateral, but can also occur secondary to Bennett's fracture. The typical patient seen by the sports physiotherapist is a mature female who plays casual racquet sports. The pain is made worse with increasing frequency of play, particularly with a sustained grip. Pain is well localized to the base of the thumb and must be distinguished from tenovaginitis (see above). Sudden shooting pains may often cause the patient to drop an object in extreme cases, and accessory movements are limited and painful, particularly axial rotations. Pinch grip power is reduced.

Splinting the joint may allow the acute inflammation to subside. Joint mobilization, including longitudinal oscillations, and abduction/adduction while stabilizing the trapezium are effective for pain relief or increasing motion.

## Fracture

The base of the first metacarpal is often fractured from a longitudinally applied force, as occurs from a punch in sports such as boxing and karate. Transverse or oblique fracture lines may occur, and if the fracture line affects the joint surface (Bennett's fracture), secondary osteoarthritis may occur in later years. Oblique fractures are often displaced and will require manipulation under anaesthetic. Maintenance of reduction is by casting the thumb, wrist and forearm, keeping the first metacarpal in extension. Fixation may be required if the joint surface is involved, to improve the alignment of the bone fragments.

Immobilization is usually for a period of about 3 weeks. Active mobility exercises are begun immediately the cast is removed, as stiffness is a severe impairment to normal hand function.

## The fingers

The fingers are commonly injured in sport by being 'pulled back' when hit by a ball or an opponent. In addition, sports which place great strain on the fingers, such as rock climbing and certain martial arts, may also cause problems.

### Dislocation

Dislocations of the proximal interphalangeal (PIP) joints, especially that of the fifth finger, are the most commonly seen types. These result from a hyperextension force, with posterior dislocation being most common. The radiographic appearance is of the middle phalanx overriding the proximal, a condition which is often associated with detachment of the palmar ligament (volar plate) from the base of the middle phalanx. Once reduced, these injuries should be protected in a splint which prevents hyperextension, but allows early flexion. If the force is less severe, dislocation may not occur, but the palmar ligament may still be disrupted. The anterior aspect of the joint is tender to palpation, and the joint is splinted as for a dislocation.

Fracture dislocation can result when an axially directed force is imposed on a semi-flexed finger. The middle phalanx shears and hits onto the condyle of the proximal phalanx dislodging a bony fragment. When the fragment involves less than one third of the articular line (Fig. 22.3) the collateral ligament usually remains intact and ensures joint stability. Closed reduction is used, with splinting to prevent the last 15% of extension. Where the joint surface is fragmented the collateral ligament will usually be disrupted, and repeated subluxation is likely to occur. Open reduction with internal fixation is therefore required (Isani, 1990).

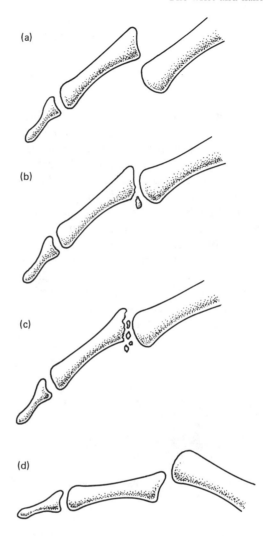

**Figure 22.3** Dislocations of the proximal interphalangeal joint. (a) Reducible dislocation. (b) Fracture-dislocation involving less than one third of the articular base. (c) Articular fragmentation involving more than one third of the articular base. (d) Anterior (volar) dislocation.

It is often tempting to reduce finger dislocations immediately, and this is certainly easier than when muscle spasm has set in. As the joint capsule is intact the procedure is usually quite successful. However, the danger of fracture dislocation or the imposition of soft tissue between the bone ends makes it necessary to err on the side of caution. Close examination is needed, and longitudinal traction should be applied gently. The joint may reduce easily, but this should be checked by X-ray (Rimmer, 1981).

## Collateral ligament injuries

The MCP and IP joints have loose capsules which are lax in extension. Each joint has obliquely placed collateral ligaments which become increasingly tight with flexion. In addition, the palmar ligaments are fibrocartilage structures attached loosely to the metacarpals but firmly to the bases of the proximal phalanges. Proximally, the palmar ligament thins out to become membranous. During flexion, this thin portion folds like a bellows, but with hyperextension it is stretched and provides the support lacking from the joint capsule (Fig. 22.4). The fibrous flexor sheaths (containing the tendons of flexor digitorum superficialis and flexor digitorum profundus) in turn attach to the palmar ligaments.

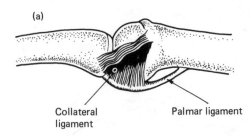

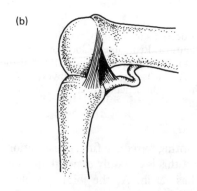

**Figure 22.4** Interphalangeal joint of the finger. (a) Extension — collateral ligaments lax, palmar ligament tight. (b) Flexion — collateral ligament tight, palmar ligament lax. From Hertling and Kessler (1990), with permission.

Valgus and varus forces directed against the PIP joints will usually result in partial tearing of the collateral ligaments but leave the joint stable. The injuries respond to strapping to the adjacent finger (buddy splinting) to protect the joint and at the same time facilitate early mobility.

Complete ligamentous disruption may warrant surgical intervention, especially where the radial collateral ligament of the index or little finger is affected, as these are subjected to greater stress in normal gripping activities (Isani, 1990). The ligament normally ruptures at the level of the joint line, possibly with avulsion. After suture repair, the finger is maintained in 60° flexion for 3 weeks (Rimmer, 1981).

## Muscles

The muscles most commonly injured in the hand are the interossei, usually by overstretching the fingers. Pain is highly localized, and increased to abduction (dorsal interossei) or adduction (plantar interossei). As the muscle fibres travel parallel to the finger, transverse friction massage is given by the therapist placing his or her finger between those of the athlete and using a rotation action by pronating and supinating his or her own forearm.

## Tendon injury

Prolonged gripping with the tips of the fingers, such as may occur in rock climbing, can cause injury to the flexor tendons. The distal IP joint is extended, while the proximal IP is flexed, stressing the flexor digitorum profundus. Long term exposure to this type of stress may also damage the flexor sheath, increasing the bowstringing effect to resisted finger flexion (Bollen, 1988).

Hyperflexion may disrupt the extensor tendon, and avulse it from the base of the distal phalanx (Mallet finger) or cause the middle section of the tendon to rupture (Boutonniere or 'button hole' deformity) (Fig. 22.5). This can occur when the end of the terminal phalanx is struck by a ball for example. When the extensor mechanism is disrupted in this way, the athlete can flex the finger, and while elastic recoil enables the joint to extend slightly, normal extension is impossible. With mal-

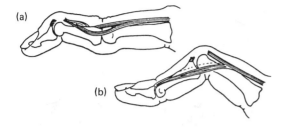

**Figure 22.5** Results of injury to the extensor tendon mechanism. (a) Mallet deformity. (b) Buttonhole deformity. From Reilly (1981), with permission.

let finger, tenderness occurs at a point between the nail and the distal IP joint, and the fingertip is held slightly flexed when resting. In a buttonhole deformity, tenderness is more proximal, and the finger is hyperextended at the distal interphalangeal joint. Radiographs reveal the avulsed fragment. Treatment is by immobilization in a splint which maintains hyperextension of the distal IP joint, or occasionally by surgical intervention.

Inflammation of the extensor tendons (tendonitis), or tendon sheaths (tenosynovitis) may occur with repetitive finger movements. Although more common as an occupational injury (for example, in keyboard operators), the condition can occur through excessive training activities. Pain and crepitus occur to repeated movements, with pain localized to the extensor tendon sheaths. Treatment is to remove the stressor and reduce the inflammation with ice and modalities.

## Rehabilitation of wrist and hand injuries

There is often a tendency for athletes to play down wrist and finger injuries. Because they can run, and because they largely look normal, athletes may often be found some years later to still have a lack of movement or strength in an injured hand when compared with the uninjured side. This, of course, leads to faults in sports technique in those areas in which the hand is used extensively, and lays the foundation for arthritis in later years. Hand rehabilitation is no less important than that of, for example, a hamstring or injured collateral ligament of the knee, and this must be stressed strongly.

For soft tissue injuries, especially those affecting the fingers, mobility following injury is the all-important factor. Where splinting is required, this should be in the 'protective position', which prevents capsular and ligamentous contracture while protecting the joint from further injury. The IP joints are immobilized in extension, the MCP joints in flexion, and the thumb in abduction (Isani, 1990). Movement must be begun as soon as possible after injury. Gentle isometric exercises and mobility exercise within the pain-free range can usually be begun one or two days after injury. Following this, exercise progresses as hand function returns. For convenience, wrist and finger exercises will be dealt with separately, although many of the exercises will be used together.

### Wrist exercise

Three exercises can be used to form a basis for regaining wrist mobility. The first two are performed with the hand flat on a table top. Initially, the hand is placed palm down on the table surface, with the wrist crease at the table edge. The contralateral hand is placed on top of the injured one, and the elbow is moved up and down to produce flexion and extension of the wrist. The leverage of the forearm and bodyweight may be used to actively assist movement at end range (Fig. 22.6a). The hand is then moved into the centre of the table, so that the whole forearm is supported, again the contralateral hand holds the injured one flat against the table surface, stopping it moving. The elbow on the injured side is moved from side to side, sliding over the table surface to perform abduction and adduction of the injured wrist (Fig. 22.6b). Finally, the arm is held at 90° flexion with the elbow held close into the side of the body, the injured forearm supported by the cupped contralateral hand. A stick is held in the hand, and pronation and supination performed, aiming to move the stick into a horizontal position (Fig. 22.6c). The range of motion is measured regularly and realistic targets are set for the athlete to achieve.

Strength of the wrist is regained by performing movements against the resistance of a powerband or small weight. Flexion/extension may be per-

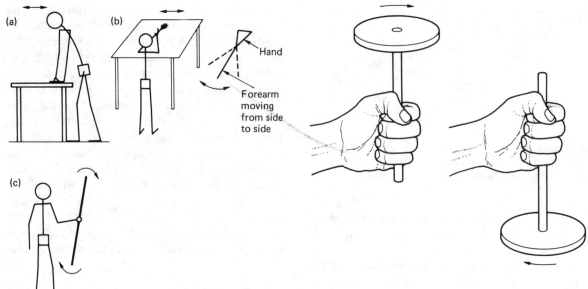

**Figure 22.6** Autotherapy wrist mobilizations. (a) Flexion/extension of the wrist. (b) Abduction/adduction. (c) Pronation/supination with broom handle.

**Figure 22.7** Wrist abduction/adduction using a modified dumb-bell.

formed holding a light dumb-bell, with the forearm supported. The other movements are performed with one weight of the dumb-bell removed (hammerbell), or using a hammer. The forearm is positioned with the side supported, and the hand holds the free end of the dumb-bell. Abduction is performed with the dumb-bell weight above the hand, and adduction with it below, in each case a 'chopping' action is used (Fig. 22.7). Pronation and supination are again executed using the hammerbell. The forearm is supported, and pronated and supinated to perform an arc with the hammerbell weight.

In addition to mobility and strength, compression, distraction and combined movements using functional activities are important. The ability of the wrist to take weight (press-up, bench press), to lock (straight arm actions holding a dumb-bell), and to take tension (chinning a bar) must be redeveloped. Rapid actions such as punching, catching, and throwing all form part of the late stage rehabilitation programme.

### Finger exercise

Many finger exercises may be begun using simple pinch grip and power grip actions. Grip and release movements, holding, and lifting may be performed using small objects with two fingers (pinch) or larger objects and all the fingers (power). Mobility may be performed by isolating the movement to the affected joint and simply teaching the athlete to perform autotherapy activities with the other hand. These are easier when the joint is warm and any tight skin is made more flexible, so hot soaking and the use of oil or cream is encouraged.

Isolation exercises for strength may be accomplished using therapeutic putty, rubber bands of varying sizes, and small weights. Again functional activities, the ability to push, pull, and lock, and rapid grip and release actions are important. Simple actions, such as screwing and unscrewing varying sized nuts and bolts, improve dexterity. Pushing with the finger straight into a thick piece of foam rubber, and pulling using pinch, ring, power and key grips help to restore tension and compression ability. Rapid throwing and catching actions with objects of varying sizes and weight rehabilitate grip and release.

# References

Albanese, S.A., Palmer, A.K., Kerr, D.R., Carpenter, C.W., Lisi, D. and Levinsohn, E.M. (1989) Wrist pain and distal growth plate closure of the radius in gymnasts. *Journal of Pediatric Orthopaedics*, **9**, 23–28

Aronen, J.G. (1985) Problems of the upper extremity in gymnasts. *Clinics in Sports Medicine*, **4**, (1) 61–71

Bollen, S.R. (1988) Soft tissue injury in extreme rock climbers. *British Journal of Sports Medicine*, **22**, (4) 145–147

Bunker, T.D., McNamee, P.B. and Scott, T.D. (1987) The Herbert screw for scaphoid fractures: a multicentre study. *Journal of Bone and Joint Surgery*, **69B**, 631–634

Carter, S.R., Aldridge, M.J., Fitzgerald, R. and Davies, A.M. (1988) Stress changes of the wrist in adolescent gymnasts. *British Journal of Radiology*, **61**, l09–112

Cetti, R., Christensen, S.E. and Reuther, K. (1982) Fracture of the lunate bone. *Hand*, **14**, 80–84

Corrigan, B. and Maitland, G.D (1983) *Practical Orthopaedic Medicine*, Butterworth, London

Cyriax, J. (1982) *Textbook of Orthopaedic Medicine*, Vol. one, 8th edn, Baillière Tindall, London

Cyriax, J.H. and Cyriax, P.J. (1983) *Illustrated Manual of Orthopaedic Medicine*, Butterworth, London

Diamond, M.R. (1989) Carpal tunnel syndrome: a review. *Chiropractic Sports Medicine*, **3**, (2) 46–53

Garrick, J.G. and Webb, D.R. (1990). *Sports Injuries: Diagnosis and Management*, W.B. Saunders, London

Haloua, J.P., Collin, J.P. and Coudeyre, L. (1987) Paralysis of the ulnar nerve in cyclists. *Annales de Chirugie de la Main*, **6**, 282–287

Hertling, D. and Kessler, R.M. (1990) *Management of Common Musculoskeletal Disorders*, J.B. Lippincott, Philadelphia

Isani, A. (1990) Prevention and treatment of ligamentous sports injuries to the hand. *Sports Medicine*, **9**, (1) 48–61

Maitland, G.D. (1991) *Peripheral Manipulation*, 3rd edn, Butterworth–Heinemann, London

Mandelbaum B.R., Bartolozzi, A.R., Davis, C.A., Teurlings, L. and Bragonier, B. (1989) Wrist pain syndrome in the gymnast: Pathogenetic, diagnostic and therapeutic considerations. *American Journal of Sports Medicine*, **17**, (3) 305–317

Moutet, F., Guinard, D., Lebrun, C., Bello-Champel, P. and Massart, P. (1989) Metacarpo-phalangeal thumb sprains: based on experience with more than 1000 cases. *Annales de Chirurgie de la Main*, **8**, 99–109

Nakamura, R., Imaeda, T., Suzuki, K. and Miura T. (1991) Sports-related Kienbock's disease. *American Journal of Sports Medicine*, **19**, (1) 88–91

O'Donoghue, D.H. (1976) *Treatment of Injuries to Athletes*, W.B. Saunders, Philadelphia

Palastanga, N., Field, D. and Soames, R. (1989) *Anatomy and Human Movement*, Heinemann Medical, Oxford

Palmer, A.K. and Werner, F.W. (1981) The triangular fibrocartilage complex of the wrist—anatomy and function. *Journal of Hand Surgery*, **6**, 153–162

Peterson, L. and Renstrom, P. (1986). *Sports Injuries*, Martin Dunitz, London

Reilly, T. (1981) *Sports Fitness and Sports Injuries*, Faber and Faber, London, p. 227

Rimmer, J.N. (1981) Injuries to the hand in sport. In *Sports Fitness and Sports Injuries*, (ed. T. Reilly), Faber and Faber, London

Stener, B. (1962) Displacement of the ruptured ulnar collateral ligament of the metacarpophalangeal joint of the thumb: a clinical and anatomical study. *Journal of Bone and Joint Surgery*, **44B**, 869

Wilkes, J.S. (1989) Reconstructive surgery of the wrist and hand. In *Orthopaedic Physical Therapy*, (ed. R. Donatelli and M.J. Wooden), Churchill Livingstone, London

Williams, J.G.P. and Sperryn, P.N. (1976) *Sports Medicine*, Edward Arnold, London

Wilmarth, M.A. and Nelson, S.G. (1988) Distal sensory latencies of the ulnar nerve in long distance bicyclists: pilot study. *Journal of Orthopaedic and Sports Physical Therapy*, **9**, 370–374

# Index